Health and Fitness Through Physical Education

Russell R. Pate, PhD
Richard C. Hohn, EdD
University of South Carolina

Editors

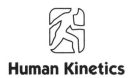

Human Kinetics

Library of Congress Cataloging-in-Publication Data

Health and fitness through physical education / Russell R. Pate,
    Richard C. Hohn, editors.
        p. cm.
    Includes index.
    ISBN 0-87322-490-6
    1. Physical fitness.   2. Physical education and training.
    I. Pate, Russell R., 1946-   II. Hohn, Richard C., 1941-
    GV481.H33   1994
    613.7--dc20   93-39707
                                                              CIP

ISBN: 0-87322-490-6

Developmental Editor: Rodd Whelpley
Assistant Editors: Sally Bayless, Jacqueline Blakley, Dawn Roselund, Lisa Sotirelis, John Wentworth
Copyeditor: Peggy Darragh
Proofreader: Dianna Matlosz
Indexer: Theresa Schaefer
Production Director: Ernie Noa
Production Manager: Kris Slamans
Typesetter: Sandra Meier
Text Designer: Keith Blomberg
Layout Artist: Denise Lowry
Cover Designer: Jack Davis
Illustrator: Thomas E. Janowski
Printer: United Graphics

Printed in the United States of America

10 9 8 7 6 5 4 3 2 1

Human Kinetics
P.O. Box 5076, Champaign, IL 61825-5076
1-800-747-4457

Canada: Human Kinetics, Box 24040, Windsor, ON N8Y 4Y9
1-800-465-7301 (in Canada only)

Europe: Human Kinetics, P.O. Box IW14, Leeds, LS16 6TR, England
0532-781708

Australia: Human Kinetics, P.O. Box 80, Kingswood 5062, South Australia
618-374-0433

New Zealand: Human Kinetics, P.O. Box 105-231, Auckland 1
(09) 309-2259

Contents

Preface

In September 1990, the South Carolina Association for Health, Physical Education, Recreation and Dance (SCAHPERD) hosted a conference it called Fitness Through Physical Education. Many contributors to this book participated in that conference whose fundamental purpose was to call for a basic change in the way school-based physical education is conceptualized, designed, and delivered to American youngsters. As an outgrowth of that conference, *Health and Fitness Through Physical Education* reiterates its call for change.

In our view, powerful societal trends now make it mandatory that physical education adapt if it is to halt the slow deterioration evident during the past decade or longer. Key elements of today's environment include both an increased recognition of the health benefits accruing from lifelong physical activity and a decreased financial support for the public schools. Between these two elements the accountability gap is widening in physical education. We believe that parents, school boards, and school administrators believe intuitively that physical education carries important potential benefits. We also believe these groups doubt that physical education in its present form effectively promotes lifelong health. Amid great financial stress, this lack of effectiveness constitutes a major threat to the future of the physical education profession.

Although there is cause for alarm about the current state of the profession, there is also reason for optimism: signs that physical education is poised for change. One overt sign is that many leaders and practitioners have begun the difficult process of self-examination that must precede meaningful change. This book provides examples of that self-examination in the thoughts and recommendations of key theoreticians and practitioners from all levels of the educational world.

We hope this book will attract a diverse readership. It was designed for a broad range of professionals who want to see school-based physical education realize its potential for promoting health. Accordingly, the material in this book should interest in-service physical educators and health educators, undergraduate and graduate students in physical education, professional preparation specialists, physical education and exercise science researchers, and other professionals who believe the schools have a central role in promoting physical activity in the American population.

This book has three major sections. The first series of chapters summarize the rationale for and scientific basis of health-related physical education. The second section, the longest, presents various curricular and methodological elements of health-related physical education. The final section gives examples of health-related physical education. Hence, this volume spans a full range, from theoretical to practical.

As an edited volume, *Health and Fitness Through Physical Education* provides a considerable diversity of perspectives on a wide range of related issues. A clear common theme threads its way through the book: School-based physical education has an enormous potential for promoting the public health, but to realize this goal it will have to realize profound change. We are optimistic that physical education can, and will, change profoundly enough to become a central element in America's public health.

Acknowledgments

The funding to support the production of this volume came from the South Carolina Association for Health, Physical Education, Recreation and Dance (SCAHPERD) and from corporate sponsors that SCAHPERD solicited: the South Carolina Electric and Gas Company, Stanley Smith and Son, and NationsBank. The editors of this book are deeply indebted to SCAHPERD and the corporate sponsors for this essential financial backing.

Many individuals made enormous personal contributions to this project, but I shall name only three of them. Trudy Leas, administrative assistant to the Department of Exercise Science at the University of South Carolina, assumed much of the burden of communicating among the many participants in this project. She singlehandedly executed the enormous volume of clerical work for producing the manuscript, always performing these duties in a conscientious, competent, and cheerful manner. Robert Hampton, executive director of SCAHPERD, in many ways was the driving force behind this undertaking. His persistence, patience, and farsightedness ensured this project's successful conclusion. Hampton is an administrator of the first order, and I consider it my good fortune to have been associated with him throughout my career. Richard Hohn, my co-editor, was there for every step of a very long process. He generated the proposal for the 1990 conference and became directly involved in every stage of the arduous editorial process that produced this book. Dick has been a good friend and a valued professional colleague for nearly two decades. I am sure that my fondest memory of this project will be the opportunity it provided to work closely with a gentleman whom I respect so greatly.

I wish to express my sincerest thanks to the authors who contributed chapters to this book. They are a diverse group—teachers and researchers, physical educators and exercise scientists, physiologists and psychologists—who share at least two characteristics. First, they all are innovative. Second, they all believe that physical education has the potential to be among the most powerful, effective health modalities in American society. This group of very creative people present a vision of what physical education can be. I know they share with me the hope that health-related physical education will become the norm in the 21st century.

Finally, I must recognize the people who, in the most fundamental sense, are responsible for the great personal satisfaction that I derive from professional projects, such as this book. My parents Robert and Doris Pate are the models of social conscience and dedication to education whom I have proudly endeavored to emulate. My dad's lifelong commitment to the physical education profession is clearly evident in the pages of this book. My wife Angie and my children Kim, Colin, and Amy provide the inspiration that gives meaning to professional accomplishments. Without their support this project could not have been successfully completed.

—Russell R. Pate

Introduction

A Contemporary Mission for Physical Education

Russell R. Pate
Richard C. Hohn
University of South Carolina, Columbia

With origins reaching back to the early 19th century, the physical education profession has a long and proud history in the United States. Physical education is an established component of schooling and is required today in 45 states (20). Most students receive instruction from a state-certified specialist (14), and most schools have athletic facilities. Over 700 colleges and universities offer specialized curricula for preparation of teachers of physical education (3). In 1991 more than 100,000 teachers were engaged in teaching physical education in U.S. schools (14), and the membership of the American Alliance of Health, Physical Education, Recreation and Dance exceeded 35,000. As we approach the year 2000, it seems certain that American society has made a major commitment to the delivery of school-based physical education programs. Clearly, when viewed comprehensively and from a national perspective, physical education in the United States represents an enormous societal investment of school time, space, and personnel.

However, there are indications that society questions whether its considerable investment in physical education is yielding a reasonable return. Professional physical education groups complain chronically, we think with justification, that insufficient time and space are allocated for physical education (22). In many school districts administrators have assigned ill-prepared and disinterested classroom teachers to physical education instruction (20,21). State requirements for PE have been gradually eroded and, in at least one case, serious consideration has been given to total elimination of state support for physical education (20). Such trends indicate that, when confronted with financial restrictions and public concerns about academic achievement, school administrators often respond by transferring resources away from physical education to other school programs. This tendency, we feel, indicates that interest groups (e.g., parents, school boards, and business leaders) tend to see physical education (distinct from school athletic programs) as a low-priority, potentially expendable program.

So, at present we have a situation that manifests both positive and negative elements. On the positive side, society has made a sizable commitment to school physical education, and physical education has become an institutionalized component of the American educational system. Yet on the negative side, society's support for school-based physical education appears to be declining, and the field seems to be facing a very uncertain future.

A major purpose of this introductory chapter is to briefly analyze society's apparent ambivalent attitude toward physical education. The second purpose is to lay out our thoughts concerning a contemporary mission for physical education—one that we feel will both engender societal support and be professionally appropriate in the 21st century. The overall goal of this chapter is to provoke the reader, to challenge him or her to think open-mindedly about the purposes of physical education. We believe that the future of physical education is on the line and that long-term survival and advancement will require fundamental change.

An Analysis of the Problem

Consideration of recent exercise and fitness trends in American society reveals a striking and troubling paradox. During the 1970s and 1980s adult Americans experienced a "fitness revolution." The evidence to support this conclusion is voluminous and compelling. Although there are still a great many sedentary adults, regular exercise is now seen as an appropriate and important component of a healthy adult lifestyle. For example, Gallup Poll results indicate that between 1961 and 1984 the percentage of adults reporting regular involvement in physical activity for fitness increased from 25% to 59% (24). So it is particularly remarkable that during these same decades school physical education programs failed to grow and probably shrank.

So what is the message? In our view, the proper interpretation of these contradictory trends is not that society has come to care less about youth activity and at the same time more about adult fitness. To the contrary, we suspect that overall concern and probably financial investment in physical activity programs for youth have grown along with the expansion of adult fitness programs. However, this growth has taken place outside the school setting. The past two decades have witnessed remarkable development of youth sport programs, fitness-oriented recreational programs for youth (e.g., private swim clubs and gymnastics centers), and agency-based fitness activities for kids (e.g., YMCA programs and daycare center activity programs).

What does all this mean? We readily acknowledge that we can only advance an hypothesis because of insufficient supporting data for a firm conclusion. Nonetheless, we propose that societal support for school physical education has decreased, despite an overall increase in support for activity and fitness programs, because it is society's perception that physical education has not "delivered the goods." We suspect that society's collective attitude toward physical education is fundamentally ambivalent.

In our view, tax-paying adults are convinced, on the one hand, that children need exercise, that they should develop reasonable levels of fitness, and that they should master fundamental motor skills. Yet, on the other hand, these same taxpayers appear skeptical that school physical education is contributing much to these goals. We suspect that this skepticism is fueled by the largely negative recollections that many adults have of their own experiences in PE. We fear that many adults associate physical education with embarrassment, pain, boredom, triviality, and irrelevance. The net effect is that physical education survives in most school districts, but it rarely receives the type of support that would allow it to rise above mediocrity. Society seems unable to eliminate physical education, yet it is also unwilling to support PE at a level that will allow it to function satisfactorily.

The Muddled Mission of Physical Education

We do not claim to fully understand why the field of physical education resides in the doldrums of the American educational establishment. However, one major reason may be absence of a clear, focused, and realistic sense of purpose. There seems to be a lack of consensus among individual professionals and among the divergent groups making up the profession. Some appear to value only motor skill enhancement, others focus largely on short-term fitness gains, still others give priority to social outcomes, and some behave as if their only serious interest is athletic coaching. Clearly, there is considerable diversity among physical educators in both philosophical bent and curricular emphasis. It is our view that this diversity hurts the profession because it limits our ability to communicate our purpose to the various constituencies that we serve.

A closely related problem concerns the profession's tendency to take on, at least philosophically, far too many objectives. Perhaps in an effort to legitimize ourselves, our profession has generated rather lengthy lists of goals and objectives. Table 1 lists objectives that have been espoused by some leaders of the physical education profession. Regrettably there is scant evidence to indicate that many of these objectives are realistic (26).

Table 1 Objectives of Physical Education

A. To promote motor skill acquisition
   - Fundamental movement patterns
   - Sports skills

B. To promote short-term improvements in physical fitness
   - Motor fitness
   - Health-related physical fitness

C. To promote cognitive learning
   - History of sport
   - Game and sport rules
   - Scientific basis of movement
   - Physical fitness concepts and procedures

D. To promote social development
   - Self-concept
   - Interpersonal skills

E. To promote cultural awareness
   - Role of sport in society

F. To promote academic performance
   - Classroom behavior
   - Academic learning

G. To promote lifelong physical activity and fitness
   - Skill in lifetime recreational activities
   - Skill in lifetime fitness activities
   - Adoption and maintenance of an active lifestyle

Note. As identified by selected professional leaders (references 4, 5, 9, 15, 16, 21, 22, 27).

Also, in some areas the educators' ideology gives little evidence that physical education has a unique contribution to make. For example, social skills development is an objective that is shared by all components of the educational system and certainly is not restricted to physical education.

It would be desirable if enhancement of academic performance could be promoted by physical education, but in our view the evidence to support such an effect is quite limited. Therefore, presenting enhanced academic performance as an objective of physical education is at best risky and at worst corrupt.

We believe that elevating the status of these peripheral objectives to *purposes* of the profession raises unrealistic expectations and creates confusion concerning the outcomes that the profession is striving to produce. In the so-called "age of educational accountability" it seems foolhardy for physical educators to suggest that they can produce outcomes that available research indicates are unlikely. It seems unwise as well for our field to spread its limited resources across a lengthy list of objectives, several of which may not carry much weight with society.

A Contemporary Mission for Physical Education

In our view, physical education will not come to be or be seen as a successful enterprise until it tracks out meaningful, realistic goals and then documents their attainment. To be useful, the aim of the profession must meet certain criteria:

1. *The aim must be seen by society as very important.* An aim that is seen as just "worthy," "desirable," or "beneficial" will not suffice. Society will not invest vast resources in a school program that is "nice." It *will* invest such resources in programs that are seen as truly critical to the current and future well-being of youngsters.

2. *The aim must be realistic.* Ideally, there should be good evidence that a properly expended investment will result in attainment of the aim. At least, there must be strong evidence that a proper investment will attain specific objectives that could logically be expected to contribute to attainment of the aim.

3. *The aim must be understandable both to professionals and to the lay public.* Esoterica will not help and will only further confuse the issue.

4. *The aim must be widely accepted among professionals.*

Of these criteria, viewing the aim as critical may be the most important. Therefore, in identifying an aim, we think it wise to consider the opinions of credible organizations that have taken positions on physical education. In recent years several medical, health, and professional organizations have issued recommendations that pertain to school physical education (1,2,8,25). Figures 1 through 4 present excerpts from four of these.

In reviewing the statements presented in Figures 1 through 4, some common threads are apparent. First, there is a consistent expression of concern that existing physical education programs

- fail to provide youngsters with enough vigorous exercise,
- fail to adequately expose youngsters to the specific activities that are used by adults in our society to maintain fitness, and
- fail to place adequate emphasis on cognitive and affective learning objectives pertinent to lifelong activity and fitness.

Furthermore, in searching the statements in Figures 1 through 4 for information pertaining to the

---

Figure 1

Excerpt from a statement on *Physical Fitness and the Schools* issued by the American Academy of Pediatrics (1).

Because financial support for fitness programs in the schools is unlikely to increase in the foreseeable future, and television is unlikely to become less attractive, we must anticipate the probability that our children's degree of physical fitness will decline. Pediatricians must acquaint themselves with this problem and appeal to their local school boards to maintain, if not increase, the school's physical education program of physical fitness. School programs should emphasize the so-called lifetime athletic activities such as cycling, swimming, and tennis. Schools should decrease time spent teaching the skills used in team sports such as football, basketball, and baseball. Physical fitness activities at school should promote a lifelong habit of aerobic exercise. During anticipatory guidance sessions, pediatricians should encourage parents to see that all family members are involved in fitness-enhancing physical activities, so that these activities become an integral part of the family's life-style.

---

central mission of physical education, we perceive a common underlying theme: that physical education should prepare youngsters for a physically active adulthood. All four statements (Figures 1–4) call for curricular changes that would place more emphasis on "lifetime activities." The statements of both the American Academy of Pediatrics and the American College of Sports Medicine explicitly indicate that physical education should actively promote "lifelong exercise."

We believe that *the mission of physical education should be to promote in youngsters adoption of a physically active lifestyle that persists through adulthood.* This mission meets at least two of the four criteria cited herein, and the all-important first criterion is evidenced by its consistency with the statements in Figures 1 through 4. We believe that society regards sustained, lifetime physical activity as a very important health behavior. Furthermore, we should consider carefully the views of medical and public health authorities—not only because they come from knowledgeable and credible sources, but also because they come from outside the physical education profession. These organizations are in a sense speaking for society. If so, we may conclude that physical education needs to raise its sights and focus on the future physical activity behavior of the students it serves.

At present we are unable to evaluate the extent to which the proposed mission statement meets the second criterion. We think that physical education *can* promote lifelong physical activity, but relevant research is very limited (23), and unfortunately, we simply do not know much about the *long-term* effects of physical education (26). Nonetheless, it seems necessary that we act on the assumption that PE has the potential to promote adoption of active lifestyles, and we feel it is the only attractive option to meet that end.

Our mission statement meets the third criterion listed on page 3. We think that the public will understand, as well as appreciate, the message that physical education exists to promote *lifelong* physical activity behavior. The public seems to understand well that youngsters learn to read, write, and perform mathematical functions so that they will be able to use those skills throughout life. They understand that youngsters learn about world history and American culture so that they will carry with them throughout life an understanding and appreciation of the society in which they live. Purportedly, the public views education as preparation for a happy, healthy, and productive adulthood. Therefore, we think they are fully capable of understanding our mission statement, which suggests that PE provides youngsters with experiences, knowledge, and skills that promote lifelong adoption of an active lifestyle.

Of course, at the present time our proposed mission statement does not meet the fourth criterion (wide acceptance among professionals). Indeed, we have anything but a consensus on the mission of physical education and, in our view, this is a major problem for the profession. Given its history, it seems unlikely the profession will achieve that broad consensus in the near future. But we hope that a combination of forces acting on the profession from within and from without will move us toward consensus.

Figure 2

Excerpt from an opinion statement on *Physical Fitness in Children and Youth* issued by the American College of Sports Medicine (2).

It is the opinion of the ACSM that physical fitness programs for children and youth should be developed with the primary goal of encouraging the adoption of appropriate lifelong exercise behavior in order to develop and maintain sufficient physical fitness for adequate functional capacity and health enhancement. . . .

School physical education programs are an important part of the overall education process and should give increased emphasis to the development and maintenance of lifelong exercise habits and provide instruction about how to attain and maintain appropriate physical fitness. The amount of exercise required for optimal functional capacity and health at various ages has not been precisely defined. Until more definitive evidence is available, current recommendations are that children and youth obtain 20-30 minutes of vigorous exercise each day. Physical education classes typically devote instructional time to physical fitness activities, but class time is generally insufficient to develop and maintain optimal physical fitness. Therefore, school programs also must focus on education and behavior change to engagement in appropriate activities outside of class. Recreational and fun aspects of exercise should be emphasized. . . .

Physical fitness testing is a highly visible and important part of physical fitness programs. School, community, state, and national organizations must adopt a logical, consistent, and scientifically sound approach to physical fitness testing. The focus of physical fitness testing should be health-related rather than athletic-related. . . .

Educational programs designed to increase knowledge and appreciation of the role and value of exercise on physical fitness and health are virtually nonexistent in schools, although such programs are common at colleges and universities. Professional efforts need to be taken to develop, pretest, and publish educational materials suitable for use in schools. Training programs need to be developed and initiated to provide school teachers with the knowledge and skills to help their students achieve cognitive, affective, and behavioral skills objectives associated with exercise, health and fitness. Teachers also need assistance in ways to integrate other aspects of health promotion (good nutrition and not smoking, for example) into instruction about exercise and physical fitness. The educational components of testing, teaching physical fitness activities, and recognition through awards should be complementary and need to be coordinated for a comprehensive program. . . .

The ACSM recommends that physical fitness test scores be interpreted in relation to acceptable standards, rather than by normative comparison. It is illogical to declare that American children and youth are physically unfit as a group and then use group norms to interpret a student's fitness test scores. A standards approach establishes a desirable physical fitness score for each fitness component. Current research is inadequate to establish with scientific precision acceptable standards for all fitness components, but preliminary standards should be developed based on the best available evidence and professional opinion. Additional research to refine, modify, and validate standards is a crucial need. . . .

Awards systems that require excellent or exemplary performance on physical fitness tests are inadequate. Awards attainable only by students with superior athletic ability may discourage the majority of children and youth because they cannot qualify. A graduated awards system that rewards exercise behavior and achievement in relation to achievable physical fitness standards should be developed and implemented.

Figure 3

Selected physical activity and fitness objectives included in *Healthy People 2000, National Health Promotion and Disease Prevention Objectives* (25).

Objective *1.4*
   Increase to at least 20% the proportion of people age 18 years and older and to at least 75% the proportion of children and adolescents age 6 through 17 years who engage in vigorous physical activity (three or more days per week for 20 min or more per occasion) that promotes the development and maintenance of cardiorespiratory fitness.
Objective *1.6*
   Increase to at least 40% the proportion of people age 6 years and older who regularly perform physical activities that enhance and maintain muscular strength, muscular endurance, and flexibility.
Objective *1.8*
   Increase to at least 50% the proportion of children and adolescents in Grades 1 through 12 who participate in daily school physical education.
Objective *1.9*
   Increase to at least 50% the proportion of school physical education class time that students spend being physically active (preferably lifetime physical activities). *Note:* Lifetime activities are those that may be readily carried into adulthood because they generally need only one or two people. Examples include swimming, bicycling, jogging, and racquet sports. Also defined as lifetime activities are vigorous social activities such as dancing, whereas competitive group sports and activities like group games typically played only by young children are excluded.

Figure 4

Excerpt from the American Heart Association position statement, *Exercise Benefits and Recommendations for Physical Activity Programs for All Americans* (5).

Children should be introduced to the principles of regular physical exercise and recreational activities at an early age. Schools at all levels should develop and encourage positive attitudes toward physical exercise, providing opportunities to learn physical skills and to perform physical activities, especially those that can be enjoyed for many years. The school curriculum should not overemphasize sports and activities that selectively eliminate children who are less skilled. Schools should teach the benefits of exercise and the development and maintenance of exercise conditioning throughout life.

   Some studies demonstrate that such organized school programs are not only feasible but can also be successful. In addition, these programs can be used to promote proper nutrition and cigarette smoking prevention and cessation.

We sense that there is a growing momentum for change. In recent years authors of several major treatises, among them contributors to this book, have called for a fundamental change in direction for physical education (6,7,10-13,17-19). Although these authors disagree on the nature of the new direction, they express a philosophical consensus, which has been summarized by Sallis and McKenzie (19):

When physical education professionals and organizations develop programs and strategies to improve public health, they will be a significant force in the development of health-related physical education programs for the nation's youth. If the public health role and goal are resisted, those in the physical education community may not only lose a valuable opportunity to positively influence the health of the nation, they may also lose some control over their own field. Given financial pressures and the return to educational "basics," support for physical education programs could be lost altogether (American Academy of Pediatrics Committees on Sports Medicine and School Health, 1987). The increasing interest of the public health community in physical education is a golden opportunity to improve the effectiveness, status, and possibly funding of school physical education. The opportunity should be seized, and a solid, lasting partnership between public health and physical education should be cemented.

The Premise of This Book

This book is based on the proposition that school-based physical education, if appropriately designed and delivered, can successfully promote adoption of a physically active lifestyle during childhood *and* adulthood. Because direct scientific evidence is lacking, we can only assume that this aim is attainable. We think it is, and the authors of the ensuing chapters agree. Collectively we describe an approach to physical education that is today a reality in only a small percentage of schools. However, our belief is that physical education can change in a way described in this book. Furthermore, it is our belief that, in changing the primary emphasis of physical education to development of a physically active lifestyle, a greater percentage of youngsters will become adults who opt for activity.

The type of physical education described in this book—we label it *health-related physical education*—is a marked departure from both the status quo and the currently prevailing professional image of what constitutes an excellent physical education program. We describe a truly different approach yet do *not* call for replacement or abandonment of physical education. Health-related physical education is different but it is not foreign. Rather, it is a movement back toward the origins of the physical education profession—origins that are solidly rooted in a health promotion and disease prevention milieu. So, read on! We hope that you find excitement in *Health and Fitness Through Physical Education*.

References

1. American Academy of Pediatrics Committees on Sports Medicine and School Health. Physical fitness and the schools. Pediatrics 80:449-450; 1987.

2. American College of Sports Medicine. Physical fitness in children and youth. Med. Sci. Sports Exerc. 20:422-423; 1988.

3. Barron's profiles of American colleges—index of college majors. New York: Barron's Educational Series; 1986.

4. Barrow, H.M. Man and his movement: principles of his physical education. Philadelphia: Lea & Febiger; 1973.

5. Bucher, C.A. Foundations of physical education. St. Louis: Mosby; 1972.

6. Corbin, C.B.; Pangrazi, R.P. Are American children and youth fit? Res. Q. Exerc. Sport 63:96-105; 1992.

7. Freedson, P.S.; Rowland, T.W. Youth activity versus youth fitness: let's redirect our efforts. Res. Q. Exerc. Sport 63:133-136; 1992.

8. Fletcher, G.F.; Blair, S.N.; Blumenthal, J.; Caspersen, C.; Chaitman, B.; Epstein, S.; Falls, H.; Froelicher, E.S.S.; Froelicher, V.F.; Pina, I.L. Statement on exercise, benefits and recommendations for physical activity programs for all Americans. Circulation 86:2726-2730; 1992.

9. Frost, R.B. Physical education foundations—practices—principles. Reading, MA: Addison-Wesley; 1975.

10. Gutin, B.; Manos, T.; Strong, W. Defining health and fitness: first step toward establishing children's fitness standards. Res. Q. Exerc. Sport 63:128-132; 1992.

11. Haywood, K.M. The role of physical education in the development of active lifestyles. Res. Q. Exerc. Sport 63:151-156; 1991.

12. McGinnis, J.M.; Kanner, L.; DeGraw, C. Physical education's role in achieving national health objectives. Res. Q. Exerc. Sport 63:138-142; 1991.

13. Morris, H.H. The role of school physical education in public health. Res. Q. Exerc. Sport 63:143-147; 1991.

14. 1991-92 educational mailing lists and marketing guide. Shelton, CT: Market Data Retrieval; 1991.

15. Nixon, J.E.; Jewett, A.E. An introduction to physical education. Philadelphia: Saunders; 1974.

16. Oberteuffer, D.; Ulrich, C. Physical education: a textbook of principles for professional students. New York: Harper & Row; 1962.

17. Pate, R.R. The evolving definition of physical fitness. Quest 40:174-179; 1988.

18. Pate, R.R. Health and fitness through physical education: research directions for the 1990s. In: Park, R.J.; Eckert, H.M., eds. The academy

papers: new possibilities, new paradigms? Champaign, IL: Human Kinetics; 1991.

19. Sallis, J.F.; McKenzie, T.L. Physical education's role in public health. Res. Q. Exerc. Sport 63:124-137; 1991.

20. The shape of the nation 1993: a survey of state physical education requirements. Reston, VA: NASPE; 1993.

21. Siedentop, D. Introduction to physical education, fitness and sport. Mountain View, CA: Mayfield; 1990.

22. Siedentop, D.; Mand, C.; Taggart, A. Physical education: teaching and curriculum strategies for grades 5-12. Palo Alto, CA: Mayfield; 1986.

23. Simons-Morton, B.G.; Parcel, G.S.; Baranowski, T.; Forchbofer, R.; O'Hara, N.M. Promoting physical activity and a healthful diet among children: results of a school-based intervention. Am. J. Pub. Health 81(8):986-991; 1991.

24. Stephens, T.; Jacobs, D.R.; White, C.C. A descriptive epidemiology of leisure-time physical activity. Public Health Rep. 100:147-158; 1985.

25. U.S. Department of Health and Human Services Public Health Service. Healthy people 2000: national health promotion and disease prevention objectives. 1991. Available from: U.S. Government Printing Office. Washington, DC: (DHHS Pub. No. [PHS] 91-50213).

26. Vogel, P. Effects of physical education programs in children. In: Seefeldt, V., ed. Physical activity and well-being. Reston, VA: AAHPERD; 1986.

27. Zeigler, E.F. Physical education and sport philosophy. Englewood Cliffs, NJ: Prentice Hall; 1977.

Part I
Foundations of Health-Related Physical Education

In Part I the authors argue for a new direction in physical education by documenting the exercise–health relationship, giving its scientific basis, and by describing current school fitness programs. In addition, they present the fundamental principles of cognitive learning and mastery of behavioral skills in physical education.

Chapter 1

"The Exercise–Health Relationship: Does It Apply to Children and Youth?" by Steven N. Blair and Marilu D. Meredith indicates that adults engaging in even moderate physical activity show reduced risk for coronary heart and cardiovascular disease. They question whether the benefits of exercise accrue also for children, who generally do not suffer from heart disease. The authors contend that the physical education objective must be to help students acquire consistent exercise behavior that they will maintain into adulthood. The charge to physical educators is to create programs that assure children enjoy fitness activities enough to want to continue them in their adult lives.

Chapter 2

James G. Ross examines the results of the National Children and Youth Fitness Study I (NCYFS I) and Study II (NCYFS II), which measured enrollment and frequency of physical education, predominant physical education activities, and physical education and the promotion of fitness. Understanding how physical education is currently being taught, that is "The Status of Fitness Programming in Our Nation's Schools," will allow professionals to gauge progress and modify programs to reach the fitness goals outlined in Healthy People 2000: National Health Promotion and Disease Prevention Objectives.

Chapter 3

"Determinants of Physical Activity Behavior in Children," by James F. Sallis, describes the most promising theories of determinants of children's physical activity. Focusing on four models of these determinants, the chapter explores such personal and environmental variables as gender, age, obesity, knowledge of and barriers to physical activity, attitudes, seasons, days of the week, and peer, parental, and teacher modeling and support. After considering how these variables affect children's physical activity levels, Sallis makes 15 recommendations for physical educators to design programs that encourage participation.

Chapter 4

In "Principles of Cognitive Learning in Physical Education," Margaret E. Gredler reviews recent educational psychology studies of learning and how social and personal factors influence learning. Understanding how students comprehend, remember, and integrate information, skills, and procedures can have positive applications for physical educators. Instead of stressing content and teacher presentation, this chapter shows how teachers can focus on important capabilities that the student can use. The lesson's purpose becomes facilitating the student's personal progress, rather than enhancing a student's performance as measured against the performance of peers. The acquisition of beneficial skills can motivate students toward their personal fitness goals.

Chapter 1

The Exercise–Health Relationship: Does It Apply to Children and Youth?

Steven N. Blair
Marilu D. Meredith
Institute for Aerobics Research
Dallas, Texas

The natural state of human beings is to be physically active. Simple observation tells us that young children are spontaneously active. Watch a toddler for a few hours. He or she is constantly on the move, exploring the environment, playing, and moving apparently for the sheer joy of it. If you doubt that children are generally active, follow some around for a day and do everything they do. Objective measures of physical fitness confirm that children are, on average, the most physically fit group in our society. Unfortunately, as the legions of inactive adults prove, we are successful in engineering activity out of modern life; and we train children to be sedentary, even though we believe that regular exercise is good for us.

Although there is general agreement on the health benefits of regular exercise, there is much uncertainty about specific details. We do not know the precise dose–response relation between exercise and health, whether there is a minimum intensity threshold for benefits, if too much exercise is harmful to health, or if the health effects of exercise are comparable in different sociodemographic groups. In this chapter we review research that supports the value of regular physical activity as a good health habit for adults, and how much activity is needed to obtain health benefits, and we will discuss the role and contribution of physical education programs in developing and maintaining physical fitness.

Health Effects of Exercise in Adults

Most of the research on exercise and health has been done in adult populations. Some of the key studies are reviewed in this section, and implications of this work for children and youth are addressed later.

Physical Activity and Health

Several recent studies show the impact of regular physical activity on premature mortality.

Harvard Alumni Study

Paffenbarger and colleagues (16) have followed 16,936 men who entered Harvard College during the period 1916 to 1950. These men completed a mail-back questionnaire on their exercise and other lifestyle habits in 1962 or 1966 and were followed for mortality. There were 1,413 deaths in the study group during a follow-up interval of up to 16 years.

Physical activity in kilocalories (kcal) per week was estimated from the questionnaire responses, based on blocks walked, flights of stairs climbed, and participation in leisure-time sports. Age-adjusted death rates were calculated for each increment of 500 kcal per week of energy expenditure (see Figure 1.1). The all-cause death rate was 94 per 10,000 man-years of observation in men with less than 500 kcal per week in energy expenditure; in men with an energy expenditure of 3,000 to 3,499 kcal per week, the rate was only 43 per 10,000. There was a steady decline in death rates across the intervening categories of energy expenditure. Sedentary living habits were comparable to cigarette smoking, hypertension, and other well-known risk factors in impact on population death rates.

Multiple Risk Factor Intervention Trial

Leon et al. (14) evaluated the relation of leisure-time physical activity to the risk of all-cause mortality in 12,138 middle-age men who were at high risk for coronary heart disease (CHD). The men were assessed on self-reported leisure-time physical activity at baseline and were grouped into sedentary, moderately active, and highly active groups, with about a third of the men in each group. There were 488 deaths during a 6-year follow-up. Age-adjusted, all-cause death rates and coronary heart disease death rates are shown in Figure 1.2. Death rates were lower in the more active men, and these results held after adjustment for other risk factors for CHD. An important finding from this study was the apparent value of moderate physical activity. In fact, in this population, being in the most active group yielded no more advantage than being in the moderately active group.

Comprehensive Review of Physical Activity and CHD

Powell et al. (20) reviewed all the studies published in English on the relation of physical activity to CHD. In 47 comparisons of sedentary to physically active groups, 32 (68%) showed a lower CHD rate in the more active individuals. An innovative feature of this review was the careful evaluation of the quality of the study methodology. The authors rated the physical activity assessment techniques, the measurement of CHD, and the epidemiologic methods for each study. In studies where two or three of these evaluation areas were considered "good," 82% found higher CHD death rates in the inactive groups. These findings strengthen the

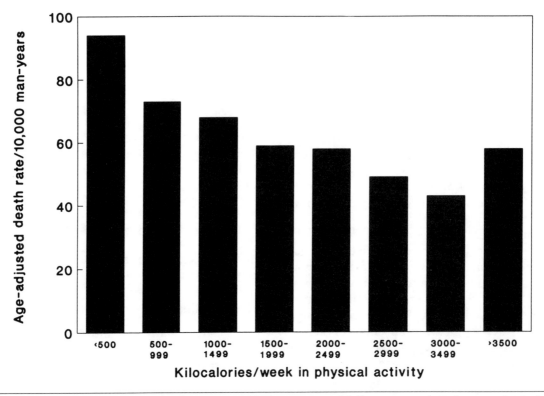

Figure 1.1 Age-adjusted, all-cause death rates per 10,000 man-years of follow-up are plotted across physical activity categories for 16,936 Harvard alumni followed for up to 16 years. (Adapted from reference 16.)

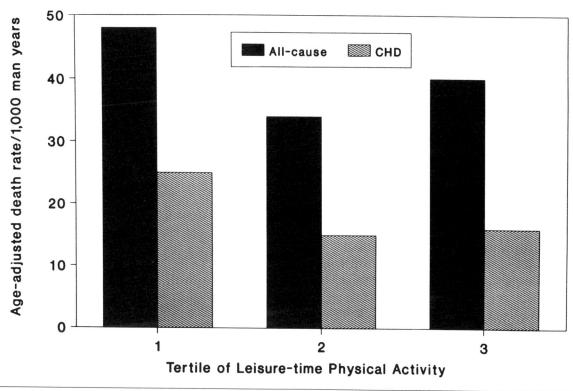

Figure 1.2   Age-adjusted, all-cause and coronary heart disease death rates are shown for tertiles of leisure time physical activity for 12,138 high-risk middle-age men in the Multiple Risk Factor Intervention Trial. (Adapted from reference 14.)

inference that physical activity protects against the development of CHD. This review shows that the risk of dying of CHD is approximately doubled in sedentary compared to physically active persons, and this increased risk is generally comparable to that for other well-known risk factors. Persons with high cholesterol or high blood pressure or who smoke cigarettes also have a risk of developing CHD 2 to 2-1/2 times higher than those without these risk factors.

Physical Fitness and Health

The studies we have discussed strongly support the hypothesis that sedentary habits increase the risk of premature death, primarily due to higher rates of cardiovascular disease. Habitual physical activity is difficult to assess with precision. Self-report of activity or estimates of activity from job classification may lead to inaccurate measurement of physical activity status, which could explain the results of studies that show no difference in death rates between active and inactive groups. The imprecise assessment of physical activity also leads to an underestimation of the importance of sedentary living as a risk factor.

An additional approach to studying the impact of inactivity on health is to examine the relation of physical fitness to disease and death rates. The primary determinant of physical fitness is physical activity, although heredity also makes a contribution. Thus, physical fitness can be used as a marker for physical activity level. The major advantage of using physical fitness in risk assessment is that it can be measured objectively, and therefore there is less misclassification of the exposure variable of interest.

Fitness and Heart Attacks in Los Angeles Public Safety Workers

Peters et al. (18) studied 2,779 policemen and firemen in Los Angeles County. All men were apparently healthy and had had no heart attacks at the time of their baseline examination. These men, 35 to 55 years old, were given a physical fitness test on a bicycle ergometer and participated in a health screen in which other risk factors were measured. Fatal (5) and nonfatal (31) heart attacks were recorded during follow-up (average follow-up time was 4.8 years) by review of death certificates and medical records.

The relative risk (RR) of developing a heart attack was approximately doubled (2.2) in men who were below the median on physical fitness. The RR of low fitness was comparable to that for other major risk factors: high cholesterol, 2.5; cigarette smoking, 2.8; and high blood pressure, 1.6. Low physical fitness in this study was more hazardous for men who were also at risk because of smoking, high cholesterol, or high blood pressure.

Lipid Research Clinics Study

Investigators from the Lipid Research Clinics program followed 3,106 healthy men who were 30 to 69 years old at baseline (10). Length of follow-up averaged 8.5 years. Each man was given a submaximal exercise test on a treadmill at the start of the study and received a medical examination and risk factor assessment. The men were assigned to one of four physical fitness groups (25% of the subjects in each group) based on their treadmill test performance.

There were 45 deaths due to cardiovascular disease during follow-up. The percent of men who died of cardiovascular disease (CVD) over the 8.5-year period declined across fitness categories (see Figure 1.3). The low-fit men were 8.5 times more likely to die of cardiovascular disease than

were the high-fit men. This study supports the hypothesis that the research on physical activity and cardiovascular disease may underestimate the effect of sedentary habits on death rates, presumably due to imprecise assessment and the resultant misclassification of the independent variable.

Aerobics Center Longitudinal Study

We have followed 10,224 men and 3,120 women who received at least one preventive medical examination at the Cooper Clinic during the interval 1970 to 1981 (2). Length of follow-up was slightly more than 8 years, which resulted in a total of 110,482 person-years of observation. None of them had a history of heart attack, stroke, diabetes, or hypertension, and all had normal resting and exercise ECGs at their baseline examination.

Physical fitness was assessed by a maximal exercise treadmill test at the clinic examination. The men and women were assigned to low-, moderate-, and high-fitness groups based on the treadmill test results. Twenty percent of the men and women were low-fit, the moderate-fitness group constituted the next 40%, and high fitness was assigned to 40% of the men and women.

There were 240 deaths in men and 43 deaths in women during the 8-year follow-up; 66 deaths in

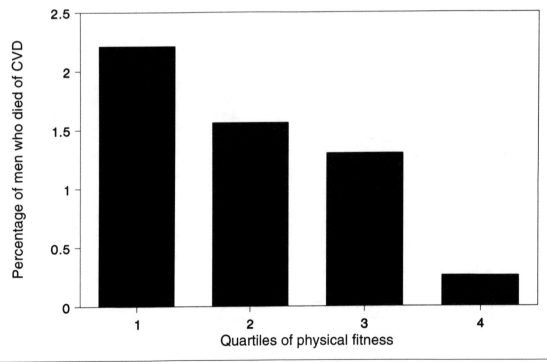

Figure 1.3 Cardiovascular disease death rates are plotted for quartiles of physical fitness as determined by a submaximal treadmill test for 3,106 men in the Lipid Research Clinics Study. (Adapted from reference 10.)

men and 7 deaths in women were due to cardio-vascular disease, and 64 deaths in men and 18 deaths in women were due to cancer. Age-adjusted death rates for each of these causes were calculated per 10,000 person-years of follow-up for low-, moderate-, and high-fitness groups. Results of these analyses are shown in Figures 1.4 through 1.6. It is obvious that there is a strong inverse relationship between physical fitness and risk of death from all causes, cardiovascular disease, and cancer. Note the much lower death rates in the moderate-fitness category compared to the low-fit group. This important finding suggests that an athletic level of physical fitness is not required for important health benefits.

The health value of being in the moderate-fitness category is perhaps the most important finding of this study. The moderate-fitness group consists of men and women falling between the 20th and 60th percentiles on the physical fitness distribution. Note that the high-fitness groups have lower death rates than the moderate-fitness groups. (However, the difference is not as great as that between the low- and moderate-fitness groups.) The high-fitness groups represent the top 40% of the fitness distributions, so they are not necessarily the "super fit." Too many people believe that very high levels of activity are necessary to benefit health, and this impression may put off many sedentary and unfit persons. The 55-year-old who has been sedentary for 40 years may not be able to imagine getting fit enough to run a marathon, so he or she does not even try to exercise.

Most people can achieve the amount of exercise required to move from the low to the moderate level of fitness. A brisk walk (3-4 mph or 15-20 min per mile) for 30 to 45 min on most days will develop and maintain moderate physical fitness. Furthermore, a recent study (6) suggests that the exercise session does not have to be continuous. Subjects who completed three 10-min workouts made almost the same improvement in fitness as persons who exercised continuously for 30 min. Surely even most busy individuals can find time to squeeze in three 10-min walks over the course of the day.

Health Effects of Activity and Fitness in Children

The major apparent health benefit of a fit and active way of life is reduced risk of developing several chronic diseases. Physical activity does not offer

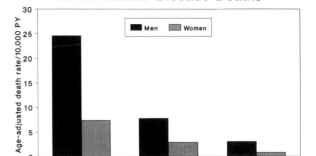

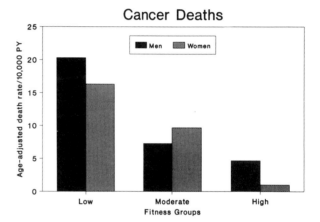

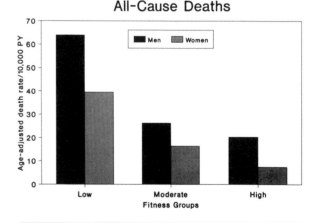

Figures 1.4-1.6   Age-adjusted cardiovascular disease (Figure 1.4), cancer (Figure 1.5), and all-cause (Figure 1.6) death rates are given for low, moderate, and high physical fitness categories for 10,224 men and 3,120 women in the Aerobics Center Longitudinal Study. (Adapted from reference 2.)

the same benefit, however, to children and youth, because they generally do not develop chronic diseases. The primary morbidities of children and youth are unwanted pregnancy, substance abuse, physical and sexual abuse, and anxiety disorders, and most deaths in this age group are due to violence. Physical activity and physical fitness are not likely to have an impact on many of these problems.

What then is the importance of physical activity for young people? Several contributions are possible. First, some medical problems, such as insulin-dependent diabetes and obesity and its attendant complications, can be alleviated by appropriate exercise. (This specific medical use of exercise intervention is beyond the scope of this chapter.) A second way physical activity may benefit young people is to help maintain proper growth. It is believed that a certain amount of exercise is necessary for growth, although the specifics are not known (15). Finally, the most important contribution children's physical activity can make is to influence their lifetime exercise patterns positively. Exercise and health interrelationships across the lifespan are illustrated in Figure 1.7. We have already reviewed the important impact that adult exercise can have on adult health, but there is not much evidence to support a hypothesis relating a direct benefit of childhood exercise to adult health (3,7,19).

If childhood exercise, however, can increase the likelihood that a person will maintain physical activity into and through adulthood, significant health benefits are possible. Unfortunately, it is difficult to study this issue. The optimum design would be to follow a group of children for several decades to see if the active children remain active as adults. Such data are not available, and the existing related studies (3,7,19) do not provide strong support showing a direct benefit of childhood exercise on adult health. For the moment we must

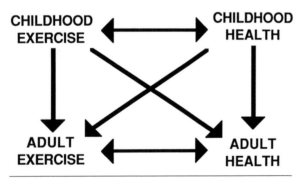

Figure 1.7 Conceptual model of how childhood exercise habits may affect health throughout life. Arrows indicate possible relationships.
Note. From Blair, S.N. et al. ''Exercise and Fitness in Childhood: Implications for a Lifetime of Health.'' In Gisolfi, C.V. and Lamb, D.R. *Perspectives in Exercise and Sports Medicine, Vol. 2. Youth Exercise and Sport* (p. 402). Indianapolis: Benchmark Press, 1989. Copyright © 1989 by Benchmark Press, Inc. Reprinted by permission of Wm. C. Brown Communications, Inc., Dubuque, IA. All Rights Reserved.

operate on faith that instilling good exercise habits early in life will have some positive carryover effect. This approach is similar to other areas of education; for example, we teach children to read and hope that they will enjoy literature as adults, and we hope that a civics class will produce better citizens.

It seems reasonable to identify children and youth who have substandard levels of physical activity and physical fitness and to implement interventions to correct these problems. This approach leads to the difficult issue of how to identify substandard levels of activity and fitness. Other chapters in this volume address this point.

School Physical Education: Contributions to Health

The school PE curriculum has undergone numerous changes over the years with redefinition of purpose and varied means of achieving program goals. Most notably, the emphasis has changed recently from skills acquisition and development to a focus on fitness for health, including concepts and routines for maintaining good health throughout one's lifetime.

Program Emphasis in Recent Decades

Trends come and go, but the predominant characteristic of 20th-century physical education in the United States has been to emphasize instruction in sports skills. We have two concerns about these characteristics of U.S. physical education programs. The emphasis on teaching sports skills presumes that if children become skilled they will remain active, especially if ''lifetime sports'' are taught. Recent estimates indicate that 50% or more of U.S. adults are either sedentary or irregularly active (4). Therefore, the sports skills approach to developing lifetime physical activity appears ineffective, at least for a large segment of the population. Also, there is something illogical about an emphasis on striving to develop high levels of physical fitness in children and youth when most are already active and fit. Instead, we recommend a focus on maintaining an active lifestyle into adulthood, in which case attention to behavioral and attitudinal factors becomes important.

Developing Physical Fitness in Physical Education

For years physical educators nationwide have used "the development and maintenance of physical fitness" not only as a primary program objective but as a major justification for the existence of PE programs. We agree that the fitness objective along with skill development are the two most important objectives in physical education. However, questions remain as to the specific nature of this fitness objective and what physical educators should attempt to accomplish in the area of physical fitness. Evidence supports the hypothesis that PE may positively impact physical fitness levels, the ultimate goal of physical education.

Is it realistic to think that school physical education can provide children with an adequate opportunity to develop physical fitness? The National Children and Youth Fitness Study (NCYFS I) (8,21) reported that two factors influence the physical fitness level of students in Grades 5 through 12: the variety of activities to which students are exposed and the weekly activity time in physical education. *Healthy People 2000: National Health Promotion and Disease Prevention Objectives* (22) suggests that youth should participate in vigorous activity 3 or more days per week, 20 min per session at a heart rate of at least 60% maximal heart rate for age. NCYFS I data indicate that only 52.5% of students in Grades 5 through 12 are in physical education 3 or more days each week (21). Koslow (12) speculated that a program containing adequate activity to develop cardiovascular capacity, muscle strength and endurance (4 exercises), and flexibility (11 exercises) would require 150 to 200 min of activity time per week. According to NCYFS I results, the average student in 5th- through 12th-grade physical education class only obtains a total of 141 min activity time per week for *all* activity—not just fitness development (21).

The Fitness Objective

Perhaps we should rethink the fitness objective for physical education. Obviously the limitation in instructional time is a factor for consideration. Of greater importance is the question, "What are we trying to accomplish with the fitness objective?" The primary objective is to equip children and youth with knowledge, attitudes, and skills for making healthy lifestyle choices—not only as children, but also as adults. There is little evidence

showing that development of high levels of childhood fitness is a factor in fitness development for adults. The key factor in being a physically fit adult is regular exercise during the adult years. Therefore, the most important fitness objective for physical education is to help students establish consistent exercise behavior patterns that will be maintained into adulthood.

In 1980 Bain (1) proposed that student enjoyment of movement participation be the central focus of physical education and that program decisions be based on that focus. Her proposal also encouraged program evaluation based on the degree to which students increased their voluntary participation in movement activities. Goals in physical education must be oriented to maintaining lifetime exercise (process) rather than short-term fitness improvement (product) (5,11). An important goal should be to ensure that each child enjoys the fitness activities enough to want to continue doing them. Programs should be fun, encourage activity that is intrinsically motivating, and instill competence and confidence by recognizing effort and process (5). Strategies for improving long-term activity patterns include teacher modeling, encouraging student responsibility, emphasizing the acquisition of exercise patterns at all levels of the program, and training teachers to provide students with experiences that encourage self-responsibility (13). Students also should be taught about the health benefits of regular activity, the principles of fitness development, and how to incorporate activity into their lives.

Definitive suggestions are not yet available for conducting a physical education program with the "development of fitness behavior" objective. Individual teachers and schools are beginning to experiment with new ideas and approaches, yet there are many unanswered questions. Major studies are underway in Project Go for Health (17) and Operation SPARK (J.F. Sallis, personal communication, December 15, 1989). The objective of developing lifetime fitness for all adults seems reason enough to change our focus in children's physical education from sports instruction and skills acquisition to an objective that more directly addresses the key ingredient in adult health: lifetime fitness through exercise.

Recommendations

Regular physical activity is a good health habit. Sedentary and unfit adults are more likely to develop chronic disease than their active and fit counterparts. Moderate levels of activity and fitness are associated with important health benefits. We believe that changes are needed in physical education programs where lifetime health habits may be introduced. The primary change that we recommend for promoting fitness is a de-emphasis on sports skills instruction, which presently consumes the bulk of time and resources in physical education. With less time spent in sports instruction and play, more time may be given to cognitive, affective, and behavioral components of physical activity. Teachers should strive to maximize the fitness development potential of each class session regardless of the activity being taught. If these changes can produce a more physically active adult population, many public health benefits and improved functional capacity will accrue to the population.

Acknowledgments

We thank Laura Becker for typing the manuscript and preparing the figures. Research was supported in part by U.S. Public Health Service research grant AG06945 from the National Institute on Aging, Bethesda, Maryland.

References

1. Bain, L.L. Socialization into the role of participant: physical education's ultimate goal. JOPERD 51:48-54; 1980.
2. Blair, S.N.; Kohl, H.W.; Paffenbarger, R.S.; Clark, D.G.; Cooper, K.H.; Gibbons, L.W. Physical fitness and all-cause mortality: a prospective study of healthy men and women. J. Am. Med. Assoc. 262:2395-2401; 1989.
3. Brill, P.A.; Burkhalter, H.E.; Kohl, H.W.; Blair, S.N.; Goodyear, N.N. The impact of previous athleticism on exercise habits, physical fitness, and coronary heart disease risk factors in middle-aged men. Res. Q. Exerc. Sport 60:209-215; 1989.
4. Caspersen, C.J.; Christenson, G.M.; Pollard, R.A. Status of the 1990 physical fitness and exercise objectives—evidence from NHIS 1985. Public Health Rep. 101:587-592; 1986.
5. Corbin, C.B. Fitness is for children: developing a lifetime fitness. JOPERD 57:82-84; 1986.
6. DeBusk, R.F.; Stenestrand, U.; Sheehan, M.; Haskell, W.L. Training effects of long versus short bouts of exercise in healthy subjects. Am. J. Cardiol. 65:1010-1013; 1990.
7. Dishman, R.K. Supervised and free-living physical activity: no differences in former athletes and non-athletes. Am. J. Prev. Med. 4:153-160; 1988.
8. Dotson, C.O.; Ross, J.G. Relationships between activity patterns and fitness. JOPERD 56:86-89; 1985.
9. Eaton, S.B.; Konner, M.; Shostak, M. Stone agers in the fast lane: chronic degenerative diseases in evolutionary perspective. Am. J. Med. 84:739-749; 1988.
10. Ekelund, L.; Haskell, W.L.; Johnson, J.L.; Whaley, F.S.; Criqui, M.H.; Sheps, D.S. Physical fitness as a predictor of cardiovascular mortality in asymptomatic North American men: the Lipid Research Clinics mortality follow-up study. New Engl. J. Med. 319:1379-1384; 1988.
11. Fox, K.R.; Biddle, S.J.H. The use of fitness test: educational and psychological considerations. JOPERD 59:47-53; 1988.
12. Koslow, R.E. Can physical fitness be a primary objective in a balanced PE program? JOPERD 59:75-77; 1988.
13. Lambert, L.T.; Barrett, M.L.; Grube, P.E. Reconceiving physical education: helping students become responsible for their physical activity. Phys. Educ. 45:114-119; 1988.
14. Leon, A.S.; Connett, J.; Jacobs, D.R.; Rauramaa, R. Leisure-time physical activity levels and risk of coronary heart disease and death. J. Am. Med. Assoc. 258:2388-2395; 1987.
15. Malina, R.M. Growth and maturation: normal variation and effect of training. In: Gisolfi, C.V.; Lamb, D.R., eds. Perspectives in exercise science and sports medicine. Vol. 2. Youth, exercise and sport. Indianapolis: Benchmark Press; 1989: p. 223-265.
16. Paffenbarger, R.S.; Hyde, R.T.; Wing, A.L.; Hsieh, C. Physical activity, all-cause mortality, and longevity of college alumni. New Engl. J. Med. 314:605-613; 1986.
17. Parcel, G.S.; Simons-Morton, B.G.; O'Hara, N.M. School health promotion of healthful diet and exercise behavior: an integration of organizational change and social learning theory interventions. J. Sch. Health 57:150-156; 1987.
18. Peters, R.K.; Cady, L.D.; Bischoff, D.P.; Bernstein, L.; Pike, M.C. Physical fitness and subsequent myocardial infarction in healthy workers. J. Am. Med. Assoc. 249:3052-3056; 1983.
19. Powell, K.E.; Dysinger, W. Childhood participation in organized school sports and physical

education as precursors of adult physical activity. Am. J. Prev. Med. 3:276-281; 1987.

20. Powell, K.E.; Thompson, P.D.; Caspersen, C.J.; Kendrick, J.S. Physical activity and the incidence of coronary heart disease. Annu. Rev. Public Health 8:253-287; 1987.

21. Ross, J.G.; Dotson, C.O.; Gilbert, G.G.; Katz, S.J. What are kids doing in school physical education? JOPERD 56:73-76; 1985.

22. U.S. Department of Health and Human Services Public Health Service. Healthy people 2000: national health promotion and disease prevention objectives. 1991. Available from: U.S. Government Printing Office. Washington, DC: (DHHS Pub. No. [PHS] 91-50213).

Chapter 2

The Status of Fitness Programming in Our Nation's Schools

James G. Ross
Macro International Inc.
Calverton, Maryland

Promoting physical fitness has long been acknowledged as a primary goal of school physical education programs. However, what typically occurs in physical education is more accurately characterized as "sport readiness" rather than fitness promotion. More recently, many national leaders in the field suggest that promoting fitness be the paramount goal of physical education. This suggestion has precipitated extensive debate over what a fitness-oriented curriculum would look like and how to balance time devoted to current fitness with time to promote lifelong fitness. This concerted effort to convert the rhetoric of fitness promotion into a programmatic reality has been impeded by a dearth of information about the determinants of physical fitness and physical activity during adolescence and, more important, throughout the life cycle. Unfortunately, little information is available about the current status of fitness programming in our nation's schools.

I describe here the status of fitness programming in schools, based primarily on the two National Children and Youth Fitness Studies (NCYFS) conducted during the 1980s and funded by the U.S. Department of Health and Human Services (16,17). These studies were the first to measure the health-related physical fitness of nationally representative samples of American youth. In addition, unlike earlier national studies of fitness, they gathered extensive information about the physical activity habits and other potential determinants of current fitness in the population under study. One product of the NCYFS data base is this description of the current status of fitness promotion in schools.

Background

From the moment today's "over-30 generation" was born, there have been periodic pronouncements of the "lamentable," "sorry," even "deplorable" physical condition of American youth. The media have picked up the message and helped to perpetuate a belief, largely unsubstantiated, that American youth are dismally unfit, are becoming less fit year after year, and are likely to pay the price in adulthood.

Emphasis on Daily Physical Education

A long-sought solution to the problem—for many publicists, *the* solution—has been daily physical education in school (1), considered important as a means for both incorporating fitness into the daily lives of students and for promoting sport readiness.

The singular importance of daily physical education as a means of reversing a suspected decline in fitness can be readily demonstrated. The 1980 study on disease prevention and health promotion objectives (23) set a single objective related to school physical education: that, by 1990, 60% of 10- to 17-year-olds would take physical education daily. In 1987 the American Alliance for Health, Physical Education, Recreation and Dance successfully sought and obtained a joint resolution from the U.S. Congress in support of daily school physical education. The President's Council on Physical Fitness also continues to promote daily physical education as a cornerstone of a sound school fitness program.

Quality Physical Education

Unfortunately, relatively little emphasis has been placed on how the content of physical education might determine the benefits students obtain from participation in PE, now and later in life (12). In other words, inadequate attention has been given to the quality of school physical education programs. Throughout the late 1980s, as efforts were made to redefine the national disease prevention and health promotion objectives for the nation and to target them to the year 2000, various concepts related to the quality of fitness programming were proposed and argued. These included (a) incorporating lifetime physical activities (those that readily carry over into adulthood) into physical education, especially during the high school years; (b) conveying awareness (if not acquisition) of a range of skills needed for participation in exercise, now and later in life; and (c) providing the immediate experience of regular, moderate to vigorous physical activity (and consequently cardiovascular fitness) to all students.

There have been signs of progress in shifting focus away from the *quantity* toward the *quality* of physical education programs:

• The new national disease prevention and health promotion objectives for the nation to be achieved by the year 2000 (22) include a new objective: that, during 50% of the time spent in PE, students will actively engage in moderate to vigorous physical activity (rather than sitting and listening or standing and watching). The objective also states that this activity will preferably involve lifetime physical activities (explained later in this chapter). The new objectives also include a more realistic target (50%) for the proportion of children and youth who will participate in daily PE (22).

• Physical educators may choose from several fitness testing protocols, but all current tests predominantly measure health-related fitness rather than sport readiness. In addition, several of the major fitness testing programs (Personal Best, FitnessGram, and Fit Youth Today) employ criterion-related fitness standards emphasizing minimal fitness levels for all children—rather than exclusive standards of excellence unattainable by most children (10).

• Professional preparation programs have increasingly stressed the importance of lifetime fitness for all children rather than the customary approach of stressing current participation in competitive athletics.

• Physical education departments have been forced to come to grips with limited time and resources for daily physical education. Declining school budgets and increasing demands given to other disciplines necessitate an emphasis on quality PE—a subject considered peripheral in many school systems (3).

• National organizations, such as NASPE, have de-emphasized the call for *daily* physical education in favor of *quality* physical education.

• Several states have developed lifetime fitness curricula to be taught in senior high school as a means of aiding the transition from high school and of improving the *quality* of carryover activities.

NCYFS I and II: Scope and Objectives

The two NCYFS broke precedent with prior normative studies of physical fitness in at least three important ways. First, as noted previously, they measured health-related fitness rather than sports readiness. Second, they gathered data about the physical activity habits of the same students whose fitness was under study, thereby allowing assessment of determinants of current fitness status. Third, they employed a sampling frame that included all students 6 to 17 years old (not just public school students). Prior to NCYFS II, no national study of the health-related fitness and exercise habits of 6- to 9-year-olds had been conducted.

Both studies were based on national probability samples, that is, nationally representative samples of students selected probabilistically, which gave each student an equal chance of being selected. NCYFS I (1984) involved collection of fitness and self-reported physical activity data from 8,800 students in Grades 5 through 12 (86% of the target sample) (8). In NCYFS II (1986), fitness data were collected from 4,678 students in Grades 1 through 4 (96% of the target sample) (9), as well as data from all of their physical education teachers and 95% of their parents. The data reported by parents included a description of their own physical activity habits and the extent to which they exercised with their children. Unlike most other reported fitness studies, the NCYFS I and II data, based on representative samples, can be generalized to the population at large.

The objectives of NCYFS I and II were specific:

1. Measure the health-related fitness of children and youth age 6 through 18 years.
2. Describe their physical activity habits, including participation in school physical education programs.
3. Assess the role of school physical education and other factors as determinants of their current physical fitness.

Due to differences between the older students (10–18-year-olds) and the younger students (6–9-year-olds), there were differences between the two studies in certain fitness measures (e.g., a modified pull-up for younger students and heavy reliance on parents as the source of data about younger children). Therefore, the findings of the two studies relating to school physical education will be reported separately.

Findings From NCYFS I

NCYFS I helped to answer questions about (a) what proportion of children age 10 through 18 years participate in PE daily (and with various lesser frequencies); (b) proper dress for a fitness-oriented physical education program and if students are provided with time and a place to shower afterwards; (c) whether or not the scope of physical education programs "expands beyond competitive sports" (as the *Objectives for the Nation* prescribe); and (d) to what extent physical education programs emphasize lifetime physical activity, especially at the high-school level (15). NCYFS I also sought to determine if the frequency or content of physical education affects the measured fitness of youth (7).

Enrollment in and Frequency of Physical Education

If daily physical education is an important objective, then two factors must be considered. The first is enrollment in PE and the second is the frequency of physical education class meetings. According to NCYFS I, nearly all students in Grades 5 and 6 are enrolled in physical education, however, rates of enrollment decline with each successive grade as students apparently complete requirements and elect other courses of study. The lowest rates of enrollment are for Grades 11 and 12. By Grade 12, only 56% of boys and 49% of girls take physical education. These figures may overstate actual enrollment in the upper grades, where response rates on NCYFS were lowest. It is likely that those refusing to participate in NCYFS were doing so to avoid having to run or participate in other vigorous testing activities; such students were also less likely to enroll in physical education in the upper grades, where physical education is normally an elective. The more recent Youth Risk Behavior Survey (1990), funded by the Centers for Disease Control, indicates that rates of enrollment in physical education approach 40% for both sexes in Grade 12—even lower than previously reported (6).

Among students taking physical education, most take it daily (more than any other frequency) in Grades 7 through 12; the modal frequency in Grades 5 and 6 was 1 and 2 days per week, respectively. In all, 36% of students in Grades 5 through 12 take daily physical education. The average frequency of physical education in Grades 5 through 12 is 3.6 times per week. The majority of students (53%, counting those who take no PE) take physical education 3 or more days per week. It is not yet established that 3 days of quality physical education per week is adequate to support the goals of a fitness-oriented physical education program.

Proper Dress and Access to Showers

Dress and showers may seem to be trivial issues, especially to an elementary physical educator. However, if students are to accept physical education as a means of promoting fitness, then appropriate conditions are required. Whether or not a school offers students time and a place to change clothes for physical education and to shower afterward might affect enrollment and participation. A student's decision to opt for PE as an elective in high school could be affected by availability of showers, and his or her ability to play hard at sports could be affected by attire and by knowing if there will be a chance to wash or clean up after vigorous activity.

NCYFS I showed that students in Grades 5 and 6 have little chance to shower (21%) or to change clothes (58%). The conditions are much better in the upper grades where greater than 60% have access to showers and approximately 90% are provided with time and a place to change clothes.

Predominant Physical Education Activities

The typical student spends the largest portion of time in PE on five activities listed in descending rank order: basketball, calisthenics/exercises, volleyball, baseball/softball, and jogging (distance running). The next 10 activities taking the greatest amount of time in the physical education curriculum are in descending order: kickball, running sprints, relays, dodgeball/bombardment, weight lifting or weight training, gymnastics (tumbling), aerobic dance, field or street hockey, gymnastics (free exercise), and swimming. Table 2.1 shows the relative popularity of 15 physical activities by grade and sex of the participants.

The relative predominance of the top activities varies between boys and girls and from one age group to another. Thus, to compile a list of 15 top activities for three age groups (upper elementary, junior high school, and senior high school) and for both sexes, a total of 25 activities were needed. Although many activities are done by both boys and girls, such as basketball and volleyball, a few activities entered the top-15 list for only one sex (aerobic dance for girls and wrestling for boys). Some activities virtually drop out of the picture as the student progresses through school. Activities like climbing ropes and monkey bars, relays, and tag are all major activities in physical education for both boys and girls in Grades 5 or 6, but not in the later grades. By senior high school, badminton, tennis, and swimming have taken a place in the physical education curriculum. Other activities remain part of the overall picture, but change in relative importance. For example, dodgeball or bombardment takes up a smaller portion of the physical education curriculum as the student progresses through school. In contrast, touch football, volleyball, and weight lifting take up a larger portion of the time as the student gets older.

NCYFS I concluded that the distribution of physical activity time in physical education mirrors the traditional reliance on relays and informal games

for the younger students and on competitive sports for the older ones. Such apportionment fails to support a key assumption in the *Objectives for the Nation* that "school-based programs will embrace activities which expand beyond competitive sports" (23). Competitive sports were still seen as the bread and butter of the physical education program.

Lifetime Physical Activity

A basic premise behind fitness-oriented physical education is the preparation of the student for a physically active lifestyle as an adult. Thus, many physical educators stress the importance of dedicating a major portion of the physical education curriculum to lifetime physical activities, especially in senior high school. Lifetime physical activities—such as swimming, walking, running, bicycling, racquet sports, aerobic dance, weight training, skiing, and rowing—are readily carried into adulthood because they generally need only one or two people. NCYFS I also cited vigorous social activities such as square dancing, but excluded group competitive sports (such as basketball, football, and soccer) and low-organized games typically played only by young children.

NCYFS I found that the average physical education student is exposed to 5.6 different lifetime activities over a year's time. A portion of the curriculum (48%) is dedicated to lifetime activities (45% for boys and 50% for girls) and tends to increase with age, ranging from 43% for boys in Grades 5 and 6 to 47% for boys in senior high school. For girls, the increase is somewhat steeper, from 45% to 55%.

The NCYFS I data suggested that teachers are trying to balance current student interests, which include competitive sports, with promoting lifetime physical activities. But they fall back heavily on the traditional competitive team sports with little carryover potential. Thus, even if physical educators succeed in conveying the importance of fitness, they may be failing to acquaint students with activities they can readily perform to stay fit throughout adulthood. NCYFS I concluded that inadequate effort is being made to convey the lifetime sports skills readily useful for active adults.

Physical Education and the Promotion of Fitness

Physical activity data, including information on participation in physical education, were analyzed

Table 2.1   NCYFS Rankings of the 15 Activities in Physical Education Class Taking the Largest Portions of Time

Physical activity	Boys			Girls		
	Grades 5 and 6	Grades 7, 8, and 9	Grades 10, 11, and 12	Grades 5 and 6	Grades 7, 8, and 9	Grades 10, 11, and 12
Badminton	*	*	10	*	*	9
Baseball and softball	6	3	3	6	5	4
Basketball	3	1	1	3	1	2
Calisthenics and exercises	1	2	5	1	2	3
Climbing ropes	13	*	*	15	*	*
Aerobic dance	*	*	*	15	9	6
Dodgeball or bombardment	5	9	15	9	13	*
Field hockey and street hockey	*	13	14	*	*	*
Football (tackle)	*	*	12	*	*	*
Football (touch)	11	4	6	13	8	7
Gymnastics–Apparatus	*	*	*	*	*	15
–Free exercise	*	*	*	13	15	13
–Tumbling	14	*	*	12	11	12
Jogging	2	5	7	2	4	5
Jumping or skipping rope	12	14	*	10	13	13
Kickball	4	12	*	4	7	15
Relays	7	10	*	5	11	*
Running sprints	9	8	13	10	9	*
Soccer	7	7	8	6	6	7
Swimming	*	*	9	*	*	15
Tag	15	*	—	*	*	—
Tennis	*	*	11	*	*	11
Volleyball	9	6	2	8	3	1
Weight lifting or weight training	*	10	4	*	*	9
Wrestling	*	14	*	*	*	—

Note. Activities marked with an asterisk (*) were performed but did not enter the top 15 for a grade or sex cell. Activities marked with a dash (—) were not performed by a grade or sex cell.

in NCYFS I to predict optimal, average, and below-average performance on each of five measured components of fitness (7). Although the nature of the relationships changed among tests, gender, and grade levels, several aspects of the physical education program either directly or in combination with other factors accounted for performance differences.

Starting in junior high school when enrollment in physical education begins to taper off, merely being enrolled helped to differentiate optimal from below-average performers, especially on sum of skinfolds, sit-ups, and chin-ups among girls. With few exceptions, students scoring in the optimal range reported exposure to a greater variety of physical activities in PE class than students scoring in the acceptable and below-average ranges. Furthermore, students scoring in the below-average range also reported lower weekly activity time in PE than students in the other two performance groups. Frequently, however, students at the optimal levels reported *less* activity time per week for physical education than students scoring in the acceptable range, suggesting that there may be a point of diminishing returns. Thus, NCYFS I suggests that *daily* physical education may not be the panacea it is thought to be.

NCYFS I was not designed to examine in greater depth the relationship between fitness-oriented physical education and measured fitness. The study did show that students scoring in the optimal range on cardiorespiratory endurance maintained a significantly higher level of involvement in high-intensity cardiorespiratory physical activities in the nonsummer months than students scoring in lower ranges. NCYFS I therefore may have helped to define a role for a fitness-oriented physical education program.

Findings From NCYFS II

NCYFS II sought to extend many of the analyses conducted in NCYFS I to the lower grades, while adding several analyses omitted from NCYFS I. NCYFS II sought to answer several questions:

1. How much physical education do younger students receive?
2. Who teaches physical education (i.e., whether or not the instructors have qualifications to teach)?
3. Where are physical education classes conducted?
4. Are appropriate fitness testing programs incorporated into physical education?
5. Are other sources of physical activity available at the elementary level?
6. What actually goes on in physical education (18)?

Like its predecessor, NCYFS II sought to determine if the frequency or content of physical education affected the measured fitness of children (14).

Enrollment in and Frequency of Physical Education

A major point of concern for elementary physical education is that classes are not held with adequate frequency. Although it was expected that most students would receive physical education of some type in Grades 1 through 4, it came as a pleasant surprise that the 97% enrolled in PE take classes an average of 3.1 times weekly, with 36% taking classes daily. However, it appears that a "have and have not" system has evolved in the early elementary grades. The "haves" take physical education daily; the "have nots" (37%) take physical education only 1 or 2 days per week. A similar bimodal distribution in the high school grades was found in NCYFS I, showing a split between those enrolled in daily physical education and those *not even enrolled*.

Teacher Credentials

A second major point of concern in elementary physical education is the belief that many students do not have the benefit of taking PE with a qualified specialist. That a high proportion of physical education classes are taught by specialists (79%) was also a pleasant surprise. However, this finding alone distorts the picture because many specialists (perhaps one third) do not hold valid certification in physical education; and because certification requirements vary widely, it is not known what standards are met by the two thirds who are certified (12).

A Place for Physical Education

A third point of concern is that, due to limited resources, many students in the early elementary grades may take physical education in surroundings that are unsuited to the purpose (e.g., an auditorium or regular classroom). NCYFS II showed that, in the majority of cases, elementary physical education is *not* taught in a gymnasium. In more temperate climates, the outdoors may be a more suitable location for many activities. And, indeed, students typically taking PE on the school grounds (rather than inside the school) have the benefit of 50% more class meetings per week. Still, there is concern that those schools not providing teachers who are specialists in physical education also appear unwilling or unable to support adequate teaching facilities.

Fitness Testing

Fitness testing serves several purposes, including educating students about the various components of physical fitness; tracking changes in fitness levels over time; providing students, parents, and teachers with information concerning the fitness of children (including areas in need of improvement); providing a basis for the development of personal exercise programs; and motivating students to improve their fitness levels and exercise habits. One of the *Objectives for the Nation* to be achieved by 1990 was that 70% of students would participate in fitness testing. No attempt was made to measure progress toward this objective in NCYFS I. However, NCYFS II did attempt to measure the extent to which elementary schools had adopted fitness testing programs, the type of program, and the extent of student participation.

An important finding in NCYFS II was that elementary schools have not adopted physical fitness testing programs on a broad basis. Fewer than half of students in Grades 1 through 4 attend schools that conduct some type of periodic fitness testing at their grade level. This came as no surprise because norms for children under age 10 years were first published only 6 years before the NCYFS II data collection in AAHPERD's Health-Related Physical Fitness Test Manual (4). As expected, when schools had adopted fitness testing programs, nearly all of them used tests from the Youth Fitness Test (YFT) (11), which has since been replaced (2).

Reward systems associated with fitness testing programs have been extensively debated in the late 1980s, when the abandonment of the YFT was accompanied by a proliferation of new test batteries. It was strongly argued that setting high standards of achievement for fitness test rewards, such as the Presidential Fitness Award, tended to reward only those students who were genetically gifted and who were already being rewarded through their participation in competitive sports. Feedback provided to parents, it was argued, would stimulate them to encourage activity among their children. NCYFS II found that reward systems varied widely and were not well thought out.

Other Opportunities for Physical Activity at School

Recess time is often viewed as a supplement to physical education in the elementary grades. The typical elementary student spends 30 min per day at recess and 35 min 3 days per week in PE. Based on NCYFS II, there is an inverse relationship between how much physical education time a child receives and the amount of recess received. This suggests that schools use recess to compensate for inadequate physical education programs, and that schools are willing to give only so much time to physical activity. Children who take a daily physical education class are thought not to need or be entitled to as much recess time. However, NCYFS II concluded that children need both structured time in PE and, like their teachers, discretionary time at recess. Recess can contribute in many important ways to the child's physical and mental well-being and should not substitute for physical education or vice versa.

NCYFS II also examined the possibility that sports teams and extracurricular physical activities at the elementary level can offer students additional exercise and the prospect of competition. If such programs encourage participation by students of widely varying skill levels, they can make an important contribution to the fitness of children. However, opportunities for extracurricular physical activities are offered at their grade levels to fewer than 20% of early elementary school students. NCYFS II concluded that more opportunities for children at the elementary levels may be necessary.

Predominant Physical Education Activities

How children actually spend their time in physical education class is the most important question in assessing the current status of fitness programming. Because NCYFS II was not an observational study, it was not possible to confirm or deny estimates from related studies of relatively small amounts of time (about 3 min each class period) spent in low to moderate physical activity (19). However, NCYFS II provided some revealing insights into the content of elementary physical education.

Listed are the five activities to which the largest percentages of children in Grades 1 through 4 were exposed: movement experiences and body mechanics (43%), soccer (32%), jumping or skipping rope (26%), gymnastics (25%), and basketball (21%). In addition, between 15% and 20% of students are exposed to throwing and catching activities, calisthenics and exercises, rhythmic activities, kickball, relays, running, and baseball and softball.

Not surprisingly, the relative rates of exposure to specific activities in physical education class vary from one grade to another (see Table 2.2). It is entirely appropriate that children's likes and dislikes change along with their aptitudes in the early elementary school grades as they develop greater attention spans, enhance their social skills, and mature physically. Therefore, physical education class activities should change as well. NCYFS II showed that from Grade 1 to Grade 4 a marked transition occurs in the activities conducted in physical education classes. The emphasis changes from movement education to fitness activities and sports skills. The dramatic shift toward team sports as early as Grades 3 and 4 gives cause for concern. As noted earlier in discussion of NCYFS I, a key assumption in the *Objectives for the Nation* was that "school-based programs will embrace activities which expand beyond competitive sports" (23). Like the first study, NCYFS II suggests that this important goal is not being met.

Table 2.2 Rank and Percent Reporting Top 10 Most Frequent Physical Education Class Activities by Grade

Physical activity	Grades							
	1		2		3		4	
	Rank	%	Rank	%	Rank	%	Rank	%
Baseball and softball		*		*	7	.20	6	.20
Basketball		*		*	5	.25	2	.40
Calisthenics and exercises	5	.22	8	.19	7	.20		*
Football		*		*		*	6	.20
Aerobic and running games	6	.21	4	.24		*		*
Low-organized games	10	.17		*		*		*
Gymnastics	7	.20	3	.25	4	.26	3	.28
Jumping or skipping rope	4	.24	2	.28	2	.27	5	.23
Kickball		*		*	6	.21	4	.26
Locomotor activities and basic skills	3	.26	6	.22		*		—
Movement experiences and body mechanics	1	.42	1	.36	2	.27		*
Relays	10	.17	8	.19		*	8	.17
Racing and sprinting	9	.18		*		*		*
Rhythmic activities	7	.20	8	.19	9	.18		*
Soccer		*	7	.21	1	.43	1	.54
Throwing and catching	2	.29	4	.24	10	.15		*
Track and field (not running)		*		*		*	10	.14
Volleyball		*		*		*	9	.16

Note. Activities marked with an asterisk (*) were performed but did not enter the top 10 for a grade. Activities marked with a dash (—) were not performed by a grade.

Physical Education and the Promotion of Fitness

As in NCYFS I, the NCYFS II data were analyzed to understand some of the determinants of fitness. Two aspects of fitness were studied: body composition and cardiorespiratory endurance. Multiple regression analyses were conducted on the data for students in Grades 3 and 4. Younger students in Grades 1 and 2 were excluded because they ran a shorter distance than students in Grades 3 and 4. These analyses showed that physical education programs, out-of-school physical activity habits, and parental physical activity have a significant impact on both components of fitness. However, the school factors apparently had weaker correlations with measured fitness than community or family factors. In fact, none of the physical education factors was related to body composition. The most noteworthy factor correlated with cardiorespiratory endurance was the percentage of classes taught by a physical education specialist.

Further analyses of the NCYFS II data have confirmed and extended the original analyses, suggesting there may be insufficient variation among physical education programs to produce corresponding measurable differences in fitness among children (13).

Summary and Conclusions

School physical education faces the complex task of satisfying apparently competing demands. Among them are maintaining or enhancing the current fitness status of students, introducing students to a range of sports and other physical activities meeting current interests as well as those likely to carry over into adulthood, and shaping attitudes toward the benefits of regular physical activity. Currently, many questions are being asked about the appropriate content of a fitness-oriented physical education program.

NCYFS I and II were designed to describe what is, not to measure what can or should be. Program goals may need redefinition in light of changing resources for education and other local government services. Promoting lifetime physical activity and fitness rests not on resources so much but rather on how physical education teachers approach the task, as well as the support they receive from school administrators to rethink how best to use physical education time and resources.

NCYFS I and II highlight several factors that physical educators can influence.

- First, they should familiarize themselves with the new national disease prevention objectives for the year 2000 (5, 21, 22), which may be found in *Healthy People 2000*, and join in the quest to define what *quality* physical education means.
- Second, they should select activities that are consistent with the developmental levels of students, the long-term commitment to lifetime physical activity, and the fitness-related year 2000 national health objectives (22).
- Third, physical educators can design classroom experiences that make the best of limited time and resources, balancing the need to provide both current experience of fitness and the sports skills needed to remain physically active later in life (20).
- Lastly, they can implement fitness testing programs that promote lifetime physical activity, motivate students to improve their fitness and exercise habits, reward students for their efforts, and keep parents aware of the fitness and exercise needs of their children.

The physical education teacher must remember that the goal of physical education, promoting physical fitness, contributes to the *full development* of each child and adolescent and that the ultimate payoff is an active lifestyle beyond the boundaries of the school.

Acknowledgments

NCYFS I was supported under a contract from the U.S. Department of Health and Human Services, Office of Disease Prevention and Health Promotion, Contract Number 282-82-0059.

NCYFS II was supported under a contract from the same agency, Contract Number 282-85-0053.

NCYFS I and II have been published as special inserts into *JOPERD*. Please see the January 1985 and November/December 1987 editions of *JOPERD*.

References

1. American Alliance for Health, Physical Education, Recreation and Dance. Fit to achieve through activity daily physical education: what you can do. Reston, VA: AAHPERD; 1990.
2. American Alliance for Health, Physical Education, Recreation and Dance. Personal best. Reston, VA: AAHPERD; 1988.
3. American Alliance for Health, Physical Education, Recreation and Dance. The shape of the nation: a survey of state physical education requirements. Reston, VA: AAHPERD; 1987.
4. American Alliance for Health, Physical Education, Recreation and Dance. AAHPERD health-related physical fitness test manual. Reston, VA: AAHPERD; 1980.
5. Allensworth, D.D.; Wolford, C.A. Achieving the 1990 health objectives for the nation: agenda for the nation's schools. In: American school health association. Bloomington, IN: Tichenor; 1988: p. 204-208.
6. Centers for Disease Control, unpublished data, 1990.
7. Dotson, C.O.; Ross, J.G. Relationship between activity patterns and fitness. JOPERD 56:86-90; 1985.
8. Errecart, M.; Ross, J.G.; Gilbert, G.G.; Ghosh, D.N. Sampling procedures. JOPERD 56:54-56; 1985.
9. Errecart, M.; Svilar, M.; Ross, J.G.; Gold, R.S.; Saavedra, P.J. Sample design. JOPERD 58:63-65; 1987.
10. Going, S.; Williams, D. Understanding fitness standards. JOPERD 61:34-38; 1989.
11. Hunsicker, P.; Reiff, G. Youth fitness test manual. Washington, DC: AAHPERD; 1976.
12. Pate, R.R.; Corbin, C.B.; Simons-Morton, B.G.; Ross, J.G. Physical education and its role in school health promotion. J. Sch. Health 57:445-450; 1987.
13. Pate, R.R.; Dowda, M.; Ross, J.G. Associations between physical activity and physical fitness in American children. Am. J. Dis. Child. 144:1123-1129; 1990.
14. Pate, R.R.; Ross, J.G. Factors associated with health-related fitness. JOPERD 58:93-95; 1987.
15. Ross, J.G.; Dotson, C.O.; Gilbert, G.G.; Katz, S.J. What are kids doing in school physical education? JOPERD 56:73-76; 1985.

16. Ross, J.G.; Gilbert, G.G. A summary of findings. JOPERD 56:45-50; 1985.

17. Ross, J.G.; Pate, R.R. A summary of findings. JOPERD 58:51-56; 1987.

18. Ross, J.G.; Pate, R.R.; Corbin, C.B.; Delpy, L.A.; Gold, R.S. What is going on in the physical education program? JOPERD 58:78-84; 1987.

19. Simons-Morton, B.G.; Baranowski, T.; O'Hara, N.M.; Parcel, G.S.; Huang, I.W.; Wilson, B. Children's participation in moderate to vigorous physical activities. Res. Q. Exerc. Sport; [in press].

20. Simons-Morton, B.G.; O'Hara, N.M.; Simons-Morton, D.G.; Parcel, G.S. Children and fitness: a public health perspective. Res. Q. Exerc. Sport 58:295-304; 1987.

21. Symons, C.W.; Gascoigne, J.L. The nation's health objectives—a means to school-wide fitness advocacy. JOPERD 61:59-63; 1990.

22. U.S. Department of Health and Human Services Public Health Service. Healthy people 2000: national health promotion and disease prevention objectives. 1991. Available from: U.S. Government Printing Office. Washington, DC: (DHHS Pub. No. [PHS] 91-50213).

23. U.S. Department of Health and Human Services. Promoting health/preventing disease: objectives for the nation. 1980. Available from: U.S. Government Printing Office. Washington, DC.

Chapter 3

Determinants of Physical Activity Behavior in Children

James F. Sallis
San Diego State University

Influences on Children's Physical Activity

Over the past 20 years we have learned a great deal about the various health benefits of regular activity. We see more clearly that physical activity and physical fitness do indeed provide important preventive health effects for adults (4) and children (42). Our task then becomes to learn how to promote healthful physical activity in the population. Some of the more important issues in physical activity today concern understanding and changing behavior to meet that end.

Behavioral research in physical activity addresses two key questions. First, what are the determinants of, or influences on, physical activity? Potential determinants are chosen for study on the basis of theoretical models of behavior, because it is impossible to study all conceivable influences. Hopefully, one outcome of determinants research will be to provide information that may be useful in the design of effective physical activity promotion programs.

The second question behavioral research addresses is what effects intervention programs have. School physical education is probably the most important intervention for promoting children's physical activity and fitness, making it an appropriate focus for this volume. However, children's physical activity can also be promoted through community agencies, youth sports organizations, public recreation programs, extracurricular school programs, the mass media, family interventions, the health care system, governmental policies and laws, and a variety of for-profit facilities and programs. Thus, school physical education is only part of an overall effort to promote desirable physical activity patterns in children.

In this chapter I summarize current knowledge of the determinants of children's physical activity. Rather than a detailed critical review of the literature, I have extracted from the existing studies and the most promising theories some recommendations for improving physical education and other types of physical activity promotion. I offer an introduction to the most common models of physical activity behavior that have guided research to date. Determinants are discussed in two separate sections. Biological and psychological characteristics, being personal factors, are distinguished from aspects of the social and physical environment. The chapter concludes with lessons for physical education and other intervention approaches that are derived from the physical activity determinants literature.

Theoretical Models of Determinants of Children's Physical Activity

Models are useful devices that encourage systematic thinking about a complex area of behavior.

Models attempt to focus attention on a small number of variables that are expected to be important determinants of physical activity. There are many models of physical activity determinants, and extensive reviews have been published (11,52), but most of them have been developed and tested with adults. No one model has been found to be either "correct" or markedly superior to the others. All models implicitly agree that physical activity is influenced by many factors, and there is no single "determinant" that explains physical activity. Each model has its own adherents and detractors, and models should be judged by their simplicity, their ability to be tested, their ability to "explain" physical activity behavior, and their relevance to the design of improved physical activity programs.

For present purposes, I have distinguished between models that emphasize only psychological influences and those that propose both psychological and environmental influences on physical activity. The oldest psychological model is the health belief model (3), which states that the likelihood of taking action regarding health is influenced by the cost-benefit ratio of taking action and the perceived threat of a specified disease. The overall threat of a disease is influenced by the perceived severity of the disease and one's perceived susceptibility. Another influential psychological model is the theory of reasoned action (1), which states that intentions are the primary determinants of voluntary behaviors, such as physical activity. Intentions are affected by two factors. The first factor is attitudes, which are based on the perceived consequences of the behavior. The second factor is subjective norms, which are based on perceptions about social influences. Both of these models are consistent with common sense, but they share a limitation that behavior is believed to be primarily determined by rational decisions.

Other theoreticians believe that, although personal decisions are important, they do not tell the whole story. There are forces outside the person that play a major role in influencing behaviors such as physical activity. Social cognitive theory emphasizes the important influence of social factors on behavior (2). We learn many of our attitudes and behaviors from role models, and the theory suggests that social pressures to be active or inactive will be difficult to resist. However, one's beliefs about the consequences of the behavior and/or the self-confidence to execute the behavior are also important. Gottlieb and Baker's (24) sociocultural model includes psychological variables, but it places particular emphasis on the role of cultural

and social influences. This model states that cultural norms, sex roles, laws, and policies are societal influences that are not obvious on a daily basis, but they can be important influences.

These various theories lead us to think broadly about the factors that might influence children's physical activity. Children's attitudes about activity may be important, but their attitudes are learned from those around them, such as parents, peers, and teachers. Furthermore children make daily decisions about what activities they will or will not do; however, their options are determined by policies governing their access to adequate facilities and programs. Thus, in thinking about various ways of promoting physical activity in children, it is not sufficient to consider only children's attitudes or their knowledge about the benefits of activity. We probably need to consider what role models they have for active lifestyles and whether or not they can realistically participate in after-school activity programs. No matter how good the school physical education program, it will never be sufficient to ensure that children will adopt active lifestyles, because there are many other influences on their activity levels.

Personal Factors: Biological and Psychological Influences on Physical Activity

Children's activity levels may be influenced by factors within them that can be broadly categorized as biological and psychological factors. Only a small number of the possible personal influences on physical activity have been studied in children.

Biological Factors

Gender is an important determinant of physical activity, although the difference may reflect cultural forces more than biological ones. Table 3.1

Table 3.1 Biological Factors and Children's Physical Activity

Variable	Relation to physical activity
Gender	Boys are more active.
Age	Activity declines with age.
Obesity	Unclear, conflicting findings. Obese children prefer low-intensity activities.

shows some biological influences on children's physical activity. From preschool (33,38) through adolescence (18,32,55,57) boys are usually more physically active than girls. This gender difference also persists throughout the adult years (53). There are increasing opportunities for women in sports and more acceptance of girls' physical activity, but these trends must be accelerated to provide females equal access and support for healthful physical activity. PE should include activities that are appropriate and acceptable for both boys and girls.

Children appear to be the most active segment of society; however, physical activity declines with age. At least three studies using objective heart rate monitors to estimate physical activity have shown its substantial decline from age 6 years to 18 years (44,49,57). The decline, steepest from childhood to young adulthood, continues during adulthood, and the elderly have very low levels of physical activity (53). This discouraging pattern presents a challenge to physical educators. The most effective method of promoting lifelong physical activity is probably to prevent a decline to low levels rather than trying to reinstate physical activity in those who have become sedentary. Because the decline begins in the elementary school years, physical educators bear some responsibility for halting the slide toward slothfulness. Furthermore, no other professional group is better prepared to prevent this or able to reach so many children for so many years.

Does lack of physical activity produce obesity, or are obese children particularly inactive because it is so hard for them to move around? Both factors are probably true, but the available studies are in conflict about whether obese children are less active than lean children (56). Two studies of preteen youngsters show that obese children and those with obese parents rate endurance activities more negatively than lean children and those with lean parents (14,60). If obese children experience less attraction to physical activity, they may need encouragement and even special programs to help them develop healthful habits. Physical educators can provide some support in class, but they should give it in a sensitive and positive way, so as not to stigmatize the obese child. Due to the increasing rate of childhood obesity (23), physical educators are encountering more and more children who have special needs for physical activity.

Consistent with obese children's preferences for sedentary activities are the findings of Epstein et al. (13) that obese children are more likely to maintain low-intensity rather than high-intensity activities. Two randomized studies have shown that obese children lose more weight if they are assigned low-intensity activities, such as walking, than if they are asked to do regular aerobic exercise (15,16). Nonobese children also may show a preference for lower intensity physical activity. Programs that promote moderate-intensity physical activity may be more effective at producing long-term behavior change and health benefits than programs that emphasize only vigorous exercise. Studies should be conducted specifically to address this question.

Psychological Factors

The relationship of variables derived from the health belief model (3) to physical activity and fitness in children and adolescents has been examined in four studies. In a study of obese and nonobese high school students, the following health beliefs were assessed:

- Knowledge of physical activity
- Severity of obesity
- Susceptibility to obesity
- Cues to exercise
- Benefits of physical activity
- Barriers
- Social support (36)

None of these variables was associated with the physical activity of *nonobese* adolescents, but cues to exercise and social approval of dieting were related to physical activity of *obese* adolescents. The same variables were measured in a separate sample of high school students, and they were studied in relation to cardiovascular fitness (9). Students classified as high- or low-fit had significantly different scores on all of the health belief variables except benefits.

The third study assessed barriers to physical activity (54). Of the nine barriers assessed, only "time" and "interest" barriers were significantly different between high- and low-activity groups of high school students. Finally, a study of children in Grades 6 to 8 found that benefits of exercise were correlated with current exercise, but attitudes toward physical activity and knowledge were not (17). Table 3.2 lists some psychological influences and their relationship to children's physical activity.

These studies appear to provide some support for the health belief model. When all questions were specifically related to physical activity, like in Desmond et al. (9), the model was supported. When the questions primarily revealed perceptions of physical activity in relation to the risk of

Table 3.2 Psychological Factors and Children's Physical Activity

Variable	Relation to physical activity
Knowledge of health effects	Not related
Knowledge of how to exercise	Related
Cues to be active	Related
Barriers to physical activity	Related
Perceived susceptibility to obesity	Not related
Intention to be active	Related
Attitudes about activity	Weakly related?
Subjective norms (perceptions of others' beliefs)	Weakly related?
Self-efficacy about activity	Related
Personality	Probably not related

obesity (see O'Connell et al., 36), health beliefs were not related to physical activity. Desmond et al. (9) show the following items most highly associated with fitness levels:

- Many of my friends regularly exercise.
- If my doctor told me to exercise I would do so.
- If I do not exercise I will get out of shape.
- People who exercise feel better about themselves.
- I do not have time to exercise.
- I do not exercise because I have to work.

The specific results of these studies provide clues about the design of intervention programs for young people. These findings suggest that physical activity promotion programs should enhance peer support for physical activity as well as appeal to the adolescents' desires to stay in shape, look good, and feel better about themselves. Physician encouragement to be physically active may be an effective approach with teens. Studies by both Desmond et al. (9) and Tappe et al. (54) indicate that high school students complain about lack of time to exercise, much like adults do (12).

Several studies were based explicitly on the theory of reasoned action. In an important confirmation of the theory, intention to exercise was significantly correlated with exercise behavior (17,21, 27). In one study, attitude and subjective norms (perception of others' beliefs) showed low but significant correlations with both intention and reported exercise behavior (21), and a similar study

found no correlations (27). Both of these studies indicate that the theory of reasoned action is a weak model for explaining either intention to exercise or actual physical activity in adolescents. Therefore, changing specific beliefs about the consequences of physical activity through education is unlikely to be an effective change strategy.

The interpretation of subjective norms is more complex. Subjective norms, as perceptions of what others want you to do, are very indirect measures of social support, which can take the form of role modeling, exercising with the child, or providing verbal encouragement to be active. In one study a child's perceptions of whether or not parents and friends wanted him or her to exercise were weakly related to reported activity habits, but perceptions about teachers' desires were not related (19). Because subjective norms involve the child's perceptions of someone else's desires, a much more direct measure of social influence would reflect what significant others actually say and do. Social influences are discussed more in the next section.

Self-efficacy for exercise is confidence in one's ability to be physically active, and it was tested in the only longitudinal study of high school students (39). Self-efficacy was a significant predictor of physical activity 4 months and 16 months later in both boys and girls. This result supports social cognitive theory and indicates that adolescents can predict their own physical activity behavior by rating their self-efficacy. Other tests of social cognitive theory variables are described in the next section.

Many health education efforts over the years have been based on the theory that increased knowledge will create behavior change. It has been assumed that if children know how good exercise is for them, they will start exercising. Although most studies have shown that such knowledge is not related to physical activity (17,36), conversely, a few studies have found knowledge to be significantly related (9,25).

Knowledge about *how* to be physically active is probably more important than knowledge about *why* to be active, and Desmond et al. (9) support this interpretation. Some knowledge may be necessary to start exercising, but it is rarely sufficient to change a sedentary person to an active one. It is often believed that physical activity can reduce feelings of stress, and that stress can interfere with physical activity. Although rated stress did not predict physical activity in high school students (39), there is some evidence that physical activity is an effective method of reducing the stress of adolescence (5).

Other psychological factors have been studied in relation to children's physical activity, and a variety of approaches for measuring physical activity attitudes have been reported (51). But attitudes are usually found to be weak correlates of physical activity at all ages (12), as well as during adolescence (8), and they do not provide much guidance about how to improve intervention programs.

There has been some interest in the relationship of personality to physical activity in children (7). The many dimensions and theories of personality have not been extensively investigated in children. However, the small correlations in adults (12) suggest this is not a fruitful area of inquiry with children. All of the models of physical activity determinants emphasize that the major influences are dynamic and subject to change, even though personality is by definition stable over time.

A psychological factor that may influence physical activity in adolescents is the fear of obesity. This is a particularly common fear among adolescent girls (34) that may lead not only to stringent dieting, but also to excessive exercise. Because overexercise can cause injuries and amenorrhea, physical educators should recommend moderation in physical activity and counsel underweight students who appear overly committed to exercise.

The available research does not permit a conclusion that one model or one group of psychological variables explains physical activity behavior better than the others. However, a commonsense approach to interpreting the theories and research can be helpful. The health belief model suggests that a child who perceives a health threat from a sedentary lifestyle is more likely to become active. Such an interpretation could lead to an emphasis on fear-based approaches that may be counterproductive. The positive social and emotional effects of physical activity are powerful motivators for children, and these should be stressed.

Self-efficacy can be increased by using a gradual approach to build mastery of physical skills. Increasing children's self-efficacy through their own experience with physical activity is more effective than verbal persuasion or pep talks to improve attitudes (2). Improving knowledge, attitudes, intentions, and self-efficacy may all play a role in promoting physical activity, but physical educators should consider what changes are likely to be necessary and sufficient to help a child become physically active on a regular basis.

Environmental Factors: Social and Physical

Just as researchers have explored personal factors and their influence on physical activity, so too have they studied some social and physical environmental factors that may influence the level of physical activity.

Social Factors

Social influences are included in virtually all behavioral models applied to the study of physical activity, but they are central to social cognitive theory (2) and the sociocultural model (24). These models emphasize that we live in a social world and depend upon other people to help us learn values, attitudes, and behaviors that are appropriate in society. There are many sources of social influence on children, and the importance of these sources changes as the child develops. Parents and siblings are clearly dominant influences in all areas of children's lives, but during adolescence peers become more important sources of learning and support (6). Teachers, coaches, physicians, and other adults can make an impact on children's lives. The actions and words of any of these people can be determinants of children's physical activity (see Table 3.3).

Greendorfer and Ewing (26) found that preteen boys and girls in different racial groups rated different people as more influential on their participation in sports. White children rated their fathers as the most important influence, whereas black children rated brothers as the most important. Teacher influence was given an intermediate rating by most subgroups, and peer influence was not rated. In a study of high school students the combined influence of friends and family members predicted subsequent physical activity (39).

Unfortunately, no studies could be located that specifically documented the influence of peers on physical activity or compared the influence of

Table 3.3 Social Factors and Children's Physical Activity

Variable	Relation to physical activity
Peer modeling and support	Probably related
Parent modeling and support	Related, but probably weaker in adolescence
Teacher modeling and support	Unknown

peers, family members, and teachers. It is widely believed that peers are very important determinants of children's physical activity. If most of their friends hike, go on bike rides, play basketball, or jog, there is strong pressure on children to join in those activities. Children and adolescents do most of their activities and sports in group settings, so there is built-in social influence. In studies of adults, the number of friends who exercise is a strong correlate of exercise (45). Thus, one might surmise that for youth, peers are very powerful determinants of physical activity, especially among adolescents, but the research has not yet shown this to be true.

Many more studies have addressed the question of family influence on physical activity, and the findings are convincing that families can exert strong influence on children's physical activity in a number of ways. Parents can be role models for physical activity. Several studies have shown that the children of physically active parents also tend to be active, which is true for both young children (47,59) and young adolescents (25,48). The influence of family modeling on physical activity may be weaker in adolescence (22) as the child develops independence from the family (6). In an interesting study with preschoolers, 5-year-old children were more active when their mothers were in the room than when they were absent (43)—a powerful indication of parents' influence on their children's physical activity. Furthermore, there is some evidence that the physical activity levels of siblings also are correlated (48).

Besides their presence and their activity level, parents can influence their children through their words. Parents can encourage children to go outside and play tag or they can prompt children to sit still and be quiet. At least two studies of young children have documented that parental encouragement and discouragement have immediate effects on the youngster's activity levels (29,31).

A physical education teacher may be one of the most influential adult figures promoting physical activity. Many articles have been written about the importance of teachers setting good examples and encouraging physical activity in their students. However, I found no studies that examined the association between teachers' and students' physical activity. From one study we can infer a teacher's potential to influence students' behavior (58). Preteen children were asked to teach a sport skill to a younger peer. Half the student-teachers received preliminary instruction in the skill from their PE teacher, along with many encouraging statements—the other half received no instruction. The

first group, despite no specific suggestions on how to teach, gave three times as many encouraging statements to their younger peers, compared to the student-teachers who had received no instruction or encouragement. It appears that children learn more from teachers than just the specific content skills being taught. Teachers model many types of behavior, so it is likely that physical educators who are active and enthusiastic about teaching will be more successful in stimulating their students' enjoyment of physical activity.

Another important adult role model influencing physical activity is the physician. Even where physicians are seen infrequently, they are regarded as very influential persons. Healthy adults felt their physicians wanted them to exercise, and they were highly motivated to comply with that advice (20). There is little reason to believe that children would value their physician's advice less. Fortunately, substantial numbers of pediatricians advise children to be physically active (35), and a few pediatricians are developing specific programs as a part of their practice that promote physical activity (41). The impact of physician advice is not known, but their contact with virtually all children could have an important effect.

The Physical Environment

The physical environment is a broad term that incorporates setting (indoor, outdoor), weather (cold, hot, rainy), time factors (night, day, weekday, weekend), availability of organized teams or programs, and access to facilities such as parks, gymnasia, and swimming pools. Any or all of these factors may promote or hinder physical activity (see Table 3.4). The environmental factors are probably more important in determining physical activity outside of school, because physical education

Table 3.4 Physical Environment Factors and Children's Physical Activity

Variable	Relation to physical activity
Day of week	Probably more active on weekend
Season	Most active in summer, least active in winter
Setting	More active outdoors
Organized programs	Related
Television and video games	Probably related

programs are usually designed for local climate and resources. Because the vast majority of physical activity takes place outside of school (40), it is important to study environmental factors and their effects that have the potential to facilitate activity.

Weekend and weekday differences in physical activity were studied in Canadian children age 10 to 12 years (50). Students who were receiving 1 hr each day of vigorous PE in school were more active on weekdays; but students who were not in the experimental program were consistently more active on the weekends. If these results can be generalized, then children are possibly more active during the weekends, even though they have no organized physical education and watch more television. One likely reason for the lower levels of physical activity during weekdays is that children are required to sit in class for 4 to 6 hr each day, limiting the opportunity and time available for activity.

The most careful analysis of seasonal differences in physical activity was carried out as part of the National Children and Youth Fitness Studies (40). Boys and girls at all age levels were most active in the summer and least active in the winter—a pattern easy to understand. In summer, most children do not attend school all day, there are more daylight hours, the weather facilitates outdoor play, and there are more organized youth activity programs in operation. Even in cold winter climates there are many vigorous activities available. However, more preparation is required before the child can go outside, parents are likely to have additional restrictions on activity, and the weather discourages both outdoor recreation and transportation to appropriate facilities.

Time spent outdoors appears to be an important determinant of physical activity, at least in young children. Klesges, Eck, Hanson, Haddock, and Klesges (30) reported that time outdoors was the strongest correlate of physical activity in preschool children. In many urban environments there are few safe and appropriate places for children to play, and in the interests of safety many parents restrict their children from spending time outdoors. Parents worry less about their children when they are playing video games at home that when they are playing basketball somewhere in the neighborhood. These impediments to children's physical activity are probably very serious, and physical educators should be involved in developing ideas to overcome these barriers.

Children and adolescents do most of their physical activity in the context of organized programs (40). The types of organizations used most frequently by youth are sports teams, parks and recreation departments, private organizations (e.g., boys' and girls' clubs and health clubs), and religious organizations. Over one third of youth participated in each of these types of organizations (40). YMCAs and YWCAs, Scouts, farm clubs, and parents' employers played a smaller role in providing youth with physical activity. Access to organized programs and appropriate facilities by poor and minority youth is an issue that must be addressed by those who seek to promote youth physical activity.

Youth organizations would enhance their achievement of the public health goal of regular physical activity for children and adolescents if they all were committed to promoting physical activity in all children. The emphasis of many organizations on competitive sports ensures that only elite athletes benefit from the resources of the organization. Most youth service organizations should be judged by the number of children involved in sports and exercise, not on their won–lost record. There are many school, community, and national opportunities for truly gifted athletes to receive rewards for physical activity, but the average child receives limited encouragement or support to be physically active.

No discussion of the determinants of children's physical activity would be complete without mention of television. Even though strong associations between television viewing and physical activity have not been documented, it is clear that time spent watching TV is time that cannot be spent in physical activity. Dietz and Gortmaker (10) presented convincing evidence from national samples of children age 6 to 17 years that television viewing is strongly associated with obesity. The rate of obesity increased 2% for each additional hour of television viewed per day.

The 24 hr of television watched per week by the average child is consuming very significant amounts of time that could be devoted to other pursuits, including physical activity and sports. Although a few programs and videos, like *Mousercise*, encourage physical activity, the vast majority of children's television programs promote sedentary and passive behavior. Reduced activity may be one mechanism for the link between television viewing and obesity, but television programs and commercials also promote dietary habits that are associated with obesity (10).

A closely related sedentary behavior, which is becoming more popular, is playing video games. Although Nintendo and other games may enhance fine motor skills, they are absolutely incompatible with physical activities that are required for health-related fitness. The appeal of these games is very strong, and physical educators must meet the challenge of competing with these forces that seek to promote sedentary behavior. Lest the supposed connection between sedentary pursuits, like watching television and playing video games, be overstated, keep in mind it is possible to play outdoors for an hour or two and still watch television for 3 hours before the child's bedtime.

Summary of Current Knowledge of Influences on Children's Physical Activity

What can we make of all this information about the influences on children's physical activity?

It can be seen as discouraging, because there are so many factors that have to be changed in order for a program to be effective. It can also be seen as encouraging, because there are so many approaches that one could take to promote children's physical activity. Some key points must be made before summarizing the review. First, no one program can be so comprehensive as to address all the known influences; and no one institution, not even the school, can by itself guarantee that children will be active enough to achieve optimal health.

Second, there are many powerful forces working against our efforts to promote children's physical activity. A great deal of money is spent by the television industry to entice children to sit for hours on end. The spread-out designs of suburbs make it difficult for children to walk from place to place. Crime in the inner-city and elsewhere prompts parents to keep children indoors or very close to home. Decreased funding for public recreation programs creates further disadvantage for the poor. Strong incentives for viewing popular televised sports lead children into passive concentration on games such as baseball and football.

The third key point is that (despite the first two) it is possible to effectively promote children's healthful physical activity. However, comprehensive community-based programs require the participation of several sectors of society, with interventions taking place at the personal, interpersonal, organizational, environmental, institutional, and legislative levels (28). Educational programs by themselves may not be very effective

unless conducted in a supportive social environment (where there are people with whom to be active) and are encouraged by meaningful policies (e.g., after-school activity programs supervised on the school grounds). Thus, we should optimistically pursue the development of physical activity promotion programs, but we should be realistic about the constraints faced by educational programs.

It is clear that the biological variables of age and gender are strongly related to children's physical activity, but they are not subject to change in an intervention program. Although it is suspected that low or insufficient physical activity plays a role in the development of childhood obesity, physical activity is known to be an essential part of effective treatment.

Some psychological variables are strongly related to physical activity. For example, self-efficacy, the intention to be active, barriers to activity, and cues to be active are important influences. Weakly related may be knowledge about physical activity, attitudes, and subjective norms. Finally, such general variables as knowledge about the effects of physical activity and personality appear not to be directly related to physical activity.

The importance of social influences should not be underestimated. Even if children are highly motivated, they are unlikely to be active unless their social environment is supportive. Parental influences are strong, but as children enter adolescence, parental effects can be expected to decrease as peer influences increase. The influence of teachers, even physical educators, on children's physical activity has not been thoroughly studied.

The effects of the physical environment on children's physical activity, though rather obvious, are often ignored. Children tend to be more active on the weekends when they are not sitting in school for 6 hours or more. They are more active in the summer, suggesting they need assistance to stay more active in the winter. They are more active if they are outdoors, so a possible intervention against inactivity is keeping children occupied outdoors and away from the television set. Finally, most children engage in activity as part of organized programs, so we need to make appropriate programs available to large numbers of children.

Implications for Promoting Children's Physical Activity

One of the major reasons for studying determinants of children's physical activity is to identify factors that may be important to target in physical activity promotion programs. In taking current theory and research in the field of determinants of children's physical activity and applying them to the field of physical education, we define PE broadly to include not only formal classes but other efforts and programs that physical educators could implement to promote regular physical activity with the goal of improving the health of children and adolescents. The following ideas should not be taken as facts. Rather, they are interpretations of how current research can be useful in guiding the development of approaches to physical education that might enhance its public health impact.

1. The age-related decline in physical activity suggests that physical educators in elementary schools should adopt the goal of maintaining current age levels of physical activity for most children, whereas teachers in secondary schools may need to adopt increased physical activity as their primary goal. School physical education must take some responsibility for halting the age-related decline in activity, because no other institution or program devoted to physical activity can reach the entire population of children and adolescents (46).

2. High school and college students must be prepared for the transition to adult life that is associated with further declines in physical activity. Assisting students to begin personal programs of exercise or to join attractive community programs while in school may help them continue to be active after graduation despite the loss of structured activities provided by school.

3. Determinants almost certainly differ in strength by age. Young children are likely to be motivated by the enjoyment, companionship, and adult approval of physical activity and sports. Adolescents may be more motivated by the ability to demonstrate self-control, to improve body shape, and the possibility of controlling stress. Parental influence decreases and peer influence increases as children grow up. Interventions should be developmentally matched to the target group.

4. Because girls appear to be less active than boys (and are more likely to become obese) special efforts are needed to motivate girls and young women to be physically active and to make available programs and resources that will support them in doing so.

5. There may be gender differences in determinants of physical activity for boys and girls, but these have not been identified by research. Barriers to physical activity, for example, could be different. Boys who are not elite athletes may be embarrassed by exercising in groups. Girls may dislike sweating and may prefer spending their time socializing. Perceptive teachers may be able to motivate boys and girls in gender-appropriate ways.

6. Girls and obese children require more support to be physically active, but that support should be so given that it is perceived as helpful and not stigmatizing.

7. Knowledge and attitudes about health are weak and inconsistent determinants of physical activity in children, and the possibility of improved health in late adulthood does not motivate many children and teens. There are many benefits in the here and now that are more appealing to youth. Important reasons to be active include a desire to look fit and trim, a desire to emulate peer role models, and a desire for improved self-esteem as a result of exercise. Physical educators can point out students that have lost weight and improved their body shapes through appropriate physical activity, being careful not to inadvertently encourage overexercise, severe dieting, or anabolic steroid use. A teacher can publicly recognize and encourage students with healthful physical activity patterns. Having students share with the class the psychological and physiological benefits they have received from physical activity may be more effective than anything the teacher can say.

8. Self-efficacy, or confidence in one's ability to exercise regularly, is enhanced most effectively by making sure students are successful at physical activity. Building skills gradually, choosing games in which students compete with themselves, and rewarding participation rather than winning, are methods by which the physical education teacher can improve self-efficacy in all class members.

9. Physicians are highly credible sources of health information, so physical educators should work with physicians to promote children's physical activity. Physicians could visit classes to state the health benefits of physical activity. Physical educators could work with physicians through professional organizations to ensure that both groups are giving consistent messages.

10. Parents and siblings are important role models and sources of support for physical activity, but physical educators rarely consider methods of increasing family involvement in children's physical activity programs. Families can be reached through student-parent homework and newsletters. Parents can be volunteer aides during PE, they can be invited to attend special family events

at the school in the evenings, or family exercise classes can be organized at the school. Teachers need to explore creative ways of family involvement. Family influence is most critical for younger children, but families remain important even for high school students.

11. Teachers who are themselves physically active and talk positively about their experiences are more likely to be effective than those who disclose their dislike for being active.

12. Even elementary school students may need some assistance finding time for physical activity outside of school. Many children have tutoring, music lessons, church activities, chores, specific homework time, and babysitting duties after school. These factors, along with instructions to stay indoors (not to mention the presence of television) make it difficult for children to be active on school days. Physical education class could provide instruction to help students schedule activity or help them get assistance from parents.

13. Crime in the streets, high-density housing with little open space, and working parents with little time for outdoor supervision all conspire to keep modern children indoors after school playing video games instead of outdoors playing tag or soccer. There may be little that physical education teachers can do about these problems, but teachers can be sensitive to the difficulties children have getting adequate amounts of physical activity and work toward developing such opportunities.

14. Children may prefer low- rather than high-intensity activities, and research with adults indicates that moderate-intensity activities such as walking have substantial health benefits (37). However, most physical activity promotion programs for youth, including physical education, mainly emphasize high-intensity activities or vigorous sports. Public health goals may be better served if children are given the option of choosing less intensive activities, which they are more likely to maintain.

15. One of the barriers to promoting children's physical activity is that facilities and programs are not available to all children. Affluent children not only have access to many more resources, but their parents may be more likely to encourage them to participate in physical activity or sport programs. In contrast, poor children do not have membership fees or transportation to facilities outside their neighborhood. They may not have bicycles to ride or money to buy balls and other equipment. Parents of poor teens may instruct the youth to go to work or baby-sit rather than play sports or go for

a run. Even when public recreation programs are available for poor youth, they are not going to be as comprehensive or as attractive as private programs. The physical education teacher can bypass the resource gap by promoting activities that can be done with little or no equipment or special facilities. Walking, running and running games, Frisbee games, and jump rope may fall into that category. Teachers should be sensitive to the needs of children who differ by income, race, and ethnic background.

This section has highlighted some ways in which physical education teachers can promote children's overall physical activity level. This assumes that teachers are willing to take some responsibility beyond what happens during class time or on the school field. Merely encouraging a talented child to join a scholastic sports team is inadequate, because it does not address the physical activity and health needs of the 98% of students who are not athletically gifted.

Summary

In this chapter I have described the theories of behavior that have been applied to understanding physical activity, summarized studies that examined influences on physical activity in youth, and suggested how these results can be translated into more effective programs for promoting physical activity. Physical activity influences can be categorized as biological, psychological, social, and environmental. All of these factors are associated with children's physical activity, so effective interventions must operate on multiple levels. No single approach is likely to be effective, and children's needs change with age. Special attention should be devoted to girls and to adolescents, because their activity levels are relatively low, and to economically disadvantaged youth, because they have access to fewer facilities and programs. Based on the results of the determinants research, 15 recommendations were made for physical educators who hope to be successful in promoting physical activity in their students.

I challenge teachers to define physical education as more than "letting the kids blow off steam" or teaching basic movement skills. I believe physical education should prepare children for a lifetime of physical activity, just as other teachers prepare children for a lifetime of learning and work. Children should not become dependent on PE for their physical activity. They should understand the need to develop a habit of being regularly active outside of school (46). If physical education teachers accept some responsibility for promoting physical activity in youth, then determinants research may provide some direction as to how to promote physical activity most effectively.

Acknowledgment

Preparation of this chapter was supported by NIH grant HL44467.

References

1. Ajzen, I.; Fishbein, M. Understanding attitudes and predicting social behavior. Englewood Cliffs, NJ: Prentice Hall; 1980.
2. Bandura, A. Social foundations of thought and action. Englewood Cliffs, NJ: Prentice Hall; 1986.
3. Becker, M.H.; Maiman, L.A. Sociobehavioral determinants of compliance with medical care recommendations. Med. Care 13:10-24; 1975.
4. Bouchard, C.; Shephard, R.J.; Stephens, T.; Sutton, J.R.; McPherson, B.D., eds. Exercise, fitness, and health: a consensus of current knowledge. Champaign, IL: Human Kinetics; 1990.
5. Brown, J.D.; Siegel, J.M. Exercise as a buffer of life stress: a prospective study of adolescent health. Health Psychol. 7:341-353; 1988.
6. Buhrmester, D.; Furman, W. The development of companionship and intimacy. Child Dev. 58:1101-1113; 1987.
7. Buss, D.M.; Block, J.H.; Block, J. Preschool activity level: personality correlates and developmental implications. Child Dev. 51:401-408; 1980.
8. Butcher, J. Socialization of adolescent girls into physical activity. Adolescence 18:753-766; 1983.
9. Desmond, S.M.; Price, J.H.; Lock, R.S.; Smith, D.; Stewart, P.W. Urban black and white adolescents' physical fitness status and perceptions of exercise. J. Sch. Health 60:220-226; 1990.
10. Dietz, W.H.; Gortmaker, S.L. Do we fatten our children at the television set? Obesity and television viewing in children and adolescents. Pediatrics 75:807-812; 1985.
11. Dishman, R.K.; Dunn, A.L. Exercise adherence in children and youth: implications for adulthood. In: Dishman, R.K., ed. Exercise adherence: its impact on public health. Champaign, IL: Human Kinetics; 1988:p. 155-200.
12. Dishman, R.K.; Sallis, J.F.; Orenstein, D.R. The determinants of physical activity and exercise. Public Health Rep. 100:158-171; 1985.
13. Epstein, L.H.; Koeske, R.; Wing, R.R. Adherence to exercise in obese children. J. Cardiac Rehabil. 4:185-194; 1984.
14. Epstein, L.H.; Valoski, A.; Wing, R.R.; Perkins, K.A.; Fernstrom, M.; Marks, B.; McCurley, J. Perception of eating and exercise in children as a function of child and parent weight status. Appetite 12:105-118; 1989.
15. Epstein, L.H.; Wing, R.R.; Koeske, R.; Ossip, D.; Beck, S. A comparison of lifestyle change and programmed aerobic exercise on weight and fitness changes in obese children. Behav. Ther. 13:651-665; 1982.
16. Epstein, L.H.; Wing, R.R.; Koeske, R.; Valoski, A. A comparison of lifestyle exercise, aerobic exercise, and calisthenics on weight loss in obese children. Behav. Ther. 16:345-356; 1985.
17. Ferguson, K.J.; Yesalis, C.E.; Pomrehn, P.R.; Kirkpatrick, M.B. Attitudes, knowledge, and beliefs as predictors of exercise intent and behavior in school children. J. Sch. Health 59:112-115; 1989.
18. Fuchs, R.; Powell, K.E.; Semmer, N.K.; Dwyer, J.H.; Lippert, P.; Hoffmeister, H. Patterns of physical activity among German adolescents: the Berlin-Bremen study. Prev. Med. 17:746-763; 1988.
19. Godin, G.; Shephard, R.J. Normative beliefs of school children concerning regular exercise. J. Sch. Health 54:443-445; 1984.
20. Godin, G.; Shephard, R.J. An evaluation of the potential role of the physician in influencing community exercise behavior. Am. J. Health Prom. 4:255-259; 1990.
21. Godin, G.; Shephard, R.J. Psychosocial factors influencing intentions to exercise of young students from grades 7 to 9. Res. Q. Exerc. Sport 57:41-52; 1986.
22. Godin, G.; Shephard, R.J.; Colantonio, A. Children's perception of parental exercise: influence of age and sex. Percept. Mot. Skills 62:511-516; 1986.
23. Gortmaker, S.L.; Dietz, W.H.; Sobol, A.M.; Wehler, C.A. Increasing pediatric obesity in the United States. Am. J. Dis. Child. 141:535-540; 1987.

24. Gottlieb, N.H.; Baker, J.A. The relative influence of health beliefs, parental and peer behaviors, and exercise program participation on smoking, alcohol use, and physical activity. Soc. Sci. Med. 22:915-927; 1986.

25. Gottlieb, N.H.; Chen, M.S. Sociocultural correlates of childhood sporting activities: their implications for heart health. Soc. Sci. Med. 21:533-539; 1985.

26. Greendorfer, S.L.; Ewing, M.E. Race and gender differences in children's socialization into sport. Res. Q. Exerc. Sport 52:301-310; 1981.

27. Greenockle, K.M.; Lee, A.A.; Lomax, R. The relationship between selected student characteristics and activity patterns in a required high school physical education class. Res. Q. Exerc. Sport 61:59-69; 1990.

28. King, A.C. Community intervention for promotion of physical activity and fitness. Exerc. Sport Sci. Rev. 19:211-259; 1991.

29. Klesges, R.C.; Coates, T.J.; Moldenhauer, L.M.; Holzer, B.; Gustavson, J.; Barnes, J. The FATS: an observational system for assessing physical activity in children and associated parent behavior. Behav. Assess. 6:333-345; 1984.

30. Klesges, R.C.; Eck, L.H.; Hanson, C.L.; Haddock, C.K.; Klesges, L.M. Effects of obesity, social interactions, and physical environment on physical activity in preschoolers. Health Psychol. 9:435-449; 1990.

31. Klesges, R.C.; Malott, J.M.; Boschee, P.F.; Weber, J.M. The effects of parental influences on children's food intake, physical activity, and relative weight. Int. J. Eating Disord. 5:335-346; 1986.

32. Kraft, R.E. Children at play: behavior of children at recess. JOPERD 60:21-24; 1989.

33. Kucera, M. Spontaneous physical activity in preschool children. In: Binkhorst, R.A.; Kemper, H.C.G.; Saris, W.H.M., eds. Children and exercise XI. Champaign, IL: Human Kinetics; 1985:p. 175-182.

34. Moses, N.; Banilivy, M.M.; Lifshitz, F. Fear of obesity among adolescent girls. Pediatrics 83:393-398; 1989.

35. Nader, P.R.; Taras, H.L.; Sallis, J.F.; Patterson, T.L. Adult heart disease prevention in childhood: a national survey of pediatricians' practices and attitudes. Pediatrics 79:843-850; 1987.

36. O'Connell, J.K.; Price, J.H.; Roberts, S.M.; Jurs, S.G.; McKinley, R. Utilizing the health belief model to predict dieting and exercising behavior of obese and nonobese adolescents. Health Educ. Q. 12:343-351; 1985.

37. Paffenbarger, R.S.; Hyde, R.T.; Wing, A.L.; Hsieh, C. Physical activity, all-cause mortality, and longevity of college alumni. New Engl. J. Med. 314:605-613; 1986.

38. Poest, C.A.; Williams, J.R.; Witt, D.D.; Atwood, M.E. Physical activity patterns of preschool children. Early Child. Res. Q. 4:367-376; 1989.

39. Reynolds, K.D.; Killen, J.D.; Bryson, S.W.; Maron, D.J.; Taylor, C.B.; Maccoby, N.; Farquhar, J.W. Psychosocial predictors of physical activity in adolescents. Prev. Med. 19:541-551; 1990.

40. Ross, J.G.; Dotson, C.O.; Gilbert, G.G.; Katz, S.J. After physical education . . . physical activity outside of school physical education programs. JOPERD 56(1):35-39; 1985.

41. Rowland, T.W. Motivational factors in exercise training programs for children. Phys. Sportsmed. 14:122-126; 1986.

42. Rowland, T.W. Exercise and children's health. Champaign, IL: Human Kinetics; 1990.

43. Routh, D.K.; Walton, M.D.; Padan-Belkin, E. Development of activity level in children revisited: effects of mother presence. Dev. Psychol. 14:571-581; 1978.

44. Sallis, J.F.; Buono, M.J.; Roby, J.J.; Micale, F.G.; Nelson, J.A. Seven-day recall and other physical activity self-reports in children and adolescents. Med. Sci. Sports Exerc. 25:99-108; 1993.

45. Sallis, J.F.; Hovell, M.F.; Hofstetter, C.R.; Faucher, P.; Elder, J.P.; Blanchard, J.; Caspersen, C.J.; Powell, K.E.; Christenson, G.M. A multivariate study of exercise determinants in a community sample. Prev. Med. 18:20-34; 1989.

46. Sallis, J.F.; McKenzie, T.L. Physical education's role in public health. Res. Q. Exerc. Sport 62:124-137; 1991.

47. Sallis, J.F.; Patterson, T.L.; McKenzie, T.L.; Nader, P.R. Family variables and physical activity in preschool children. J. Dev. Behav. Pediatr. 9:57-61; 1988.

48. Sallis, J.F.; Patterson, T.L.; Buono, M.J.; Atkins, C.J.; Nader, P.R. Aggregation of physical activity habits in Mexican-American and Anglo families. J. Behav. Med. 11:31-41; 1988.

49. Saris, W.H.M.; Elvers, J.W.H.; van't Hof, M.A.; Binkhorst, R.A. Changes in physical activity of children aged 6 to 12 years. In: Rutenfranz, J.; Mocellin, R.; Klimt, F., eds. Children and exercise XII. Champaign, IL: Human Kinetics; 1986:p. 121-130.

50. Shephard, R.J.; Jequier, J.C.; Lavallee, H.; LaBarre, R.; Rajic, M. Habitual physical activity: effects of sex, milieu, season, and required

activity. J. Sports Med. Phys. Fitness 20:55-66; 1980.

51. Smoll, F.L.; Schutz, R.W. Children's attitudes toward physical activity: a longitudinal analysis. J. Sport Psychol. 2:137-147; 1980.

52. Sonstroem, R.J. Psychological models. In: Dishman, R.K., ed. Exercise adherence: its impact on public health. Champaign, IL: Human Kinetics; 1988:p. 125-153.

53. Stephens, T.; Jacobs, D.R.; White, C.C. A descriptive epidemiology of leisure-time physical activity. Public Health Rep. 100:147-158; 1985.

54. Tappe, M.K.; Duda, J.L.; Ehrnwald, P.M. Perceived barriers to exercise among adolescents. J. Sch. Health 59:153-155; 1989.

55. Tell, G.S.; Vellar, O.D. Physical fitness, physical activity, and cardiovascular disease risk factors in adolescents: the Oslo youth study. Prev. Med. 17:12-24; 1988.

56. Vara, L.; Agras, S. Caloric intake and activity levels are related in young children. Int. J. Obes. 13:613-617; 1989.

57. Verschuur, R.; Kemper, H.C.G. Habitual physical activity in Dutch teenagers measured by heart rate. In: Binkhorst, R.A.; Kemper, H.C.G.; Saris, W.H.M., eds. Children and exercise XI. Champaign, IL: Human Kinetics; 1985: p. 194-202.

58. Westcott, W.L. Effects of teacher modeling on children's peer encouragement behavior. Res. Q. Exerc. Sport 51:585-587; 1980.

59. Willerman, L.; Plomin, R. Activity level in children and their parents. Child Dev. 44:854-858; 1973.

60. Worsley, A.; Coonan, W.; Leitch, D.; Crawford, D. Slim and obese children's perceptions of physical activities. Int. J. Obes. 8:201-211; 1984.

Chapter 4

Principles of Cognitive Learning in Physical Education

Margaret E. Gredler
University of South Carolina, Columbia

Physical education teachers face at least two major challenges unique to the principles of cognitive learning. First, they must integrate the development of motor skills with the learning of essential knowledge for informed decision making. Second, and more difficult, is the challenge of motivating students to take an active, lifelong role in maintaining personal physical fitness.

Currently, three major developments in educational psychology provide useful information for addressing these challenges:

1. Robert Gagné's conditions of learning
2. information-processing theory
3. Bernard Weiner's attribution theory

Gagné's instructional model describes the different kinds of learning outcomes that represent the range of human skills and the key essentials for effective classroom instruction for each type of learning. Gagné's model also provides guidelines for integrating motor and cognitive skills in planning instruction.

Complementing Gagné's model are the contributions of information-processing theory. Briefly summarized, information-processing principles describe the ways that individuals perceive and process information for later use. In other words, learning is not a passive experience. Instead, effective learning requires several steps by the learner that include interacting with the new knowledge in particular ways.

Also important are recent developments in motivational research. Specifically, Bernard Weiner's attribution theory addresses the role of learner beliefs about personal success and failure in achievement-related situations. These beliefs are important because they influence the learner's subsequent behavior. That is, motivation for particular tasks or subject areas is influenced by the student's particular cognitive conclusions about his or her relative success or failure.

This chapter presents an overview of the major points in each of these three theories and applies them to physical education. The discussion is presented in three sections: (a) selecting and organizing information and skills to be learned, (b) implementing appropriate instructional methods, and (c) social and personal factors that influence learning.

Selecting and Organizing Information and Skills to Be Learned

Planning typically focuses on the content and activities to be presented by the teacher. However, planning instruction for *effective* learning, according to Gagné (11,12), begins with identifying the new capabilities or skills that students will be able to execute at the end of the lesson. Therefore, planning in Gagné's model is guided by (a) the capabilities that students are to acquire by the end of the lesson and (b) the activities and interactions in which the *students* will engage to become proficient in those capabilities. In other words, simply naming a few skills does not contribute to an effective instructional plan. Instead, the selection of learning outcomes should be part of a coherent framework that also indicates the essential requirements for student achievement during instruction.

The analyses of human learning undertaken by Gagné were conducted for the purpose of identifying key elements of instruction. Of course, learning the definition of the term "butterfly stroke" and learning to execute the stroke are accomplished in quite different ways. However, Gagné sought to identify the specific differences between various kinds of learning and to organize these differences in terms of requirements for effective instruction. Therefore, the analyses conducted by Gagné began with the question, "What are the various kinds of learned activities and performances that humans execute in their daily lives?" In other words, what are the similarities and differences among reciting the Pledge of Allegiance, balancing one's checkbook, organizing information to write a term paper, and executing the butterfly stroke?

The result was the identification of five distinct categories of learning outcomes. In addition to motor skills and attitudes, three of the categories describe cognitive learning. Summarized in Table 4.1, they are verbal information, intellectual skills, and cognitive strategies (12,13). These learning outcomes (like motor skills and attitudes) are independent of subject area, age, grade level, and educational setting.

Each of the categories in Table 4.1 reflects a unique capability or skill with particular requirements for successful learning. Verbal information, for example, involves only the recall of stated information. Learning definitions, reciting chemical formulas, and paraphrasing bodies of information, such as the Bill of Rights, are examples.

Although important, definitions and facts are not the ultimate goals of instruction. Instead, intellectual skills, which are the capabilities executed by competent members of society, are important classroom lesson outcomes. Examples of intellectual skills used in daily life include balancing a checkbook, using the rules of grammar in speaking and writing, and selecting food menus to provide a balanced diet. Unlike verbal information, intellectual skills involve decision making and the application of knowledge. The capabilities in intellectual skills, from simple to complex are

- discriminating (same and different),
- identifying examples (of a concept),
- predicting results or outcomes (by applying rules), and
- generating problem solutions (by manipulating sets of learned rules).

As indicated in Table 4.1, learning a definition requires hearing or reading the definition in a meaningful context. However, if the learning outcome is that of discriminating between the terms *strength* and *endurance*, then merely hearing or reading the definition is insufficient. Instead, students must be informed of the particular criteria that differentiate the two terms, and they must also be given opportunities to identify typical examples of each. Pictures of students engaged in various activities, such as lifting a pile of books or completing a long hike, may be used as situations for student identification.

In contrast, learning a concept means that students have acquired the finer points of the category that the concept represents. In other words, students can correctly categorize both obvious *and* subtle examples of the concept. This skill is more complex than that of simply differentiating between two terms. Effective instruction for concept learning, therefore, should include opportunities for the student to interact with a variety of situations from the most easily recognized examples to the more difficult ones.

For example, acquiring the concepts of endurance and strength also involves understanding the relationships between the two. When shown a picture of a child who is unable to execute even one sit-up, the student should be able to identify the root cause as a lack of strength of the abdominal muscles. In other words, the student's acquisition of the concept *strength* means clearly understanding that it involves the largest amount of force one can put forth at one time and identifying the role of that characteristic in a variety of situations.

Rule learning, the third capability in Gagné's progression of intellectual skills, is more complex than learning a concept. First, a rule states a relationship between two or more concepts. Second, learning involves demonstrating or applying the rule to new situations. It does *not* refer to merely stating a rule (the skill of verbal information). An

Table 4.1 Major Characteristics of Gagné's Categories of Cognitive Learning

Category	Capability (skill)	Major instructional requirements	Examples
Verbal information	Acquiring labels, facts, and organized bodies of knowledge	Provide a meaningful context for the new information and assistance in processing.	1. Define "cardiovascular." 2. Describe "health-related physical fitness."
Intellectual skills	Manipulating symbols and concepts in the application of knowledge	Assist in recall of prerequisite skills. Provide varied concrete examples and rules. Provide opportunities for interacting with examples in a variety of ways and give feedback.	1. Discriminate between pictures that illustrate "strength" and those illustrating "endurance" (**discrimination learning**). 2. Categorize written descriptions of activities as those that develop (a) strength, (b) endurance, or (c) both strength and endurance (**concept learning**). 3. Given data related to inactivity of different individuals, predict future health-related problems (**rule learning**). 4. Restructure high-calorie and high-fat menus to meet specified standards (**problem solving**).
Cognitive strategies	Efficiently managing one's own learning, remembering, and thinking	Assist in recall of essential intellectual skills. Provide opportunities for students to organize and monitor their thinking with support and feedback.	1. Select and organize information essential to planning a personal fitness program.

example is predicting the changes in physical indicators (such as pulse rate) for various levels of activity.

Problem solving, the most complex of the four intellectual skills, requires that the student generate a solution to a stated problem. Generating a problem solution requires that the student select from memory the set of rules appropriate for the situation and then apply the rules in the correct sequence. As indicated in Table 4.1, an example is restructuring high-calorie and high-fat menus to meet specified goals.

One purpose of the category of intellectual skills is to assist teachers in selecting the highest level intellectual skill for the focus of a lesson and then identifying the related subskills to be taught. A curriculum goal, for example, may state that the students are to understand sound nutritional practices related to physical fitness. Using the category of intellectual skills, the teacher determines if problem solving, rule learning, or concept learning

is to be the focus of the lesson on food characteristics. That is, are the students to be able to identify high-calorie and high-fat foods (concept learning), or are they to be able to restructure poorly designed menus (problem solving)?

In addition to intellectual skills, the category of cognitive strategies is also important in school learning. However, little is known at present about the most effective ways to teach these capabilities. Unlike verbal information and intellectual skills—which directly apply to definitions, concepts, and rules—cognitive strategies refer to the learner's own thought processes. Organizing information to write a term paper is an example. In physical education, a cognitive objective for students might be selecting and organizing appropriate information for evaluating one's personal fitness status.

Table 4.1 describes the major characteristics of Gagné's categories of cognitive learning. Some capabilities that are learned, however, are organized sets of skills that include both intellectual skills and motor skills. Gagné (12,13) refers to such sets of skills as *procedures*. Examples include writing a check and parallel parking. The motor skills in parallel parking, for example, include positioning the vehicle properly, backing in slowly, and straightening the wheels after the turn (12,13). The intellectual skills include identifying the correct angle of approach, identifying alignment with the other car, and so forth. Learning a procedure, therefore, involves learning to perform the discrete motor skills as well as the essential concepts or rules.

An example of a simple procedure in physical education is determining one's pulse rate. The capabilities involved are learning the definition of pulse (verbal information), identifying appropriate locations of the body where the pulse may be obtained (discrimination learning), positioning the fingers correctly (motor skill), counting the pulse beats for 10 sec (rule learning), and determining the rate per minute (rule learning).

The categories of learning identified by Gagné assist the teacher in identifying important capabilities to be learned. Textbooks and other materials often are composed of items of information that reflect important developments and findings in a subject area. However, they are not designed to identify or organize important guideposts in learning a subject. In planning a lesson, therefore, the instructor should first ask, "What should the student be able to do at the end of this lesson?"

In physical education, the questions are more specific:

1. What problems should the student be able to solve at the end of the lesson, or what rules should the student be able to apply?
2. What procedures should the student be able to execute?
3. What new motor skills should the student be able to execute?

The answers to these questions identify the instructional goals for the lesson. Then, using Table 4.1, the instructor identifies the essential subskills for any intellectual skills identified as the end point of instruction for the lesson. For example, the lesson objective may be for the student to calculate resting heart rate, maximum heart rate, and target heart rate range. Supporting subskills include taking one's pulse (procedure) and identifying the similarities and differences between resting heart rate, maximum heart rate, and target heart rate range (concept learning).

Table 4.2 summarizes the planning steps for instruction. First determine the skill that is the lesson objective, then determine the nature and type of the skill, and lastly, identify the supporting subskills that also must be learned.

Table 4.2 Steps in Planning Instruction

1. Identify the important lesson outcomes.
   - Are students to learn a procedure, to apply rules or solve problems, or to execute a motor skill?
   - Write a learning-outcome statement for each end-of-lesson skill.
2. Determine supporting skills for the lesson outcomes.
   - If a problem-solving outcome, what are the supporting rules, concepts, and discriminations?
   - If a procedure, what are the subskills, concepts, and discriminations?
   - If a motor skill, what are the subskills?

Implementing Appropriate Instructional Methods

Fitness concepts may be introduced during activity and then expanded in a classroom setting or they may be introduced in a classroom lesson. Regardless of setting, instruction should facilitate the student's processing and later recall of the new learning.

Of importance in selecting instructional methods are the findings of the information-processing research conducted since the 1970s. Briefly summarized, this research indicates that cognitive learning (whether verbal information, intellectual skills, or cognitive strategies) requires several stages of internal processing by the student. The four major stages required for the storage of new learning in long-term ("permanent") memory are illustrated in Figure 4.1.

A large number of the continuous stream of physical signals received by the sensory registers (ears, eyes, and skin) are not processed further and are lost to us. For effective instruction students must be attentive to the stimuli associated with the new learning so that the stimuli are selected for further processing. An important first step in instruction is to direct students' attention to important learning. For example, the teacher may say, "Today, we are going to learn why joint flexibility is important." The importance of directing student attention to the goal of the lesson should not be underestimated, particularly for younger students. Research reported by Peterson (19) indicates that

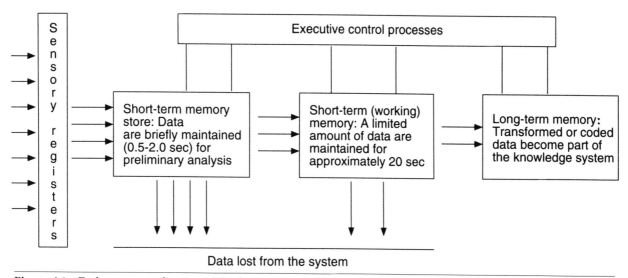

Figure 4.1   Early conceptualization of the human memory as a structural system. (Adapted from reference 17.)

most elementary school students are unable to determine the skills and concepts to be learned in their lessons. Typically, they report that the goal is simply to get through the material or to finish a particular task.

Information that is received by the sensory registers is then retained for up to 2 sec in the short-term store (see Figure 4.1). If selected for further processing, the signals proceed to short-term or *working memory*. Here they may be processed for immediate use and then forgotten, or they may be processed for long-term storage and later recall. After looking up a telephone number, for example, we may repeat the number a few times until the call is completed and then forget it. In contrast, a physical education student who is expected to learn the definition of *cardiorespiratory endurance* seeks to process the information so that it may be stored in long-term memory.

The process by which information is processed for storage in long-term memory is referred to as *encoding*. Of primary importance is the way information is treated during encoding, because this process has major consequences for the value of the information at a later point in time (9). That is, the information either is forgotten, is stored as an isolated fragment, or becomes integrated within some larger framework. For example, reciting information over and over—such as names, dates, and definitions—leads to fragmented learning and only temporary recall. In other words, this method of processing does not contribute to conceptual understanding, and the information is quickly forgotten.

Effective encoding for long-term storage by the student involves transforming the new learning in

some way so that it is more easily recognizable. Two effective processing activities are

- associating the new learning with familiar images and/or letter codes,
- relating the new learning to the student's existing store of knowledge and skills.

These activities are referred to as *elaborative* because they involve the construction of relationships between the new learning and prior knowledge.

For verbal information, associations may take the form of mnemonic cues, visual images, or a combination of the two. An example of a mnemonic strategy is the construction of a sentence, "Every good boy does fine," to remember the musical notes in the treble clef that are on the staff lines (E,G,B,D,F). An example of visual association for the term *cardiorespiratory endurance* would be to imagine a heart and a pair of lungs in track shoes running down the street. Recall of the visual image facilitates the recall of the key elements in the definition.

By contrast, in learning the terms *vein* and *artery*, one may use either a visual or mnemonic elaboration. Veins may be visualized as thin spaghetti strips with a group of CO_2s sitting on them. The CO_2s visually represent the vein's function of carrying carbon dioxide. Arteries may be visualized as thick, round rubber tubes that stretch like rubber bands with bubbles of O_2s passing through them. A mnemonic strategy for differentiating arteries from veins is to recall the sentence, "*Art(ery)* was *thick* around the middle so he wore pants with an *elastic* waistband'' (6) (see Table 4.3). The advantage of the visual image is that it may be easier to remember and it also incorporates the functions of arteries and veins.

In contrast to learning verbal information, acquiring intellectual skills may require different kinds of opportunities for the students to interact with the subject matter in making decisions and relating criteria and conditions to prior knowledge. For example, suppose that the lesson objective is to select activities that develop muscular strength, muscular endurance, and cardiorespiratory endurance. First the students are taught the basic definitions (verbal information). Then a picture (or a description) of an appropriate activity for each type of endurance may be presented by the teacher along with the reasons why each picture is appropriate for a term. Lastly, students select from a group of activities those that are appropriate for each term and discuss the rationale for their choices. The discussion assists each student to relate the correct choices to his or her existing store of knowledge and to correct misconceptions. Then students may be asked to think of other activities seen on television or in other settings that are appropriate for each type of endurance.

Asking students during a lesson to describe examples that they have observed or read about is important because this strategy makes use of their store of knowledge. Referred to as *schemas*, these organized stores provide a guide for interpreting new information. For example, if a friend tells you

she has a big dog named Brutus, you infer that the animal has four legs and fur, barks, and likely is protective of his home territory. Schemas also prevent the mental chaos that would result from random, erroneous associations. For example, in reading about John Dean in *All the President's Men*, one does not confuse him with King John, Pope John, or a former classmate, John (1).

In teaching concepts and rules, the new learning should be related to the student's existing schema whenever possible. Comparisons and contrasts and the recall of related or similar events in the student's life are ways both to establish links to existing knowledge and to facilitate later recall. In addition, when the subject matter is new to the student, such as health-related fitness, instruction should include establishing meaningful links among important concepts and relationships in the subject. One useful approach is to structure lessons so that some fitness concepts are integrated into the performance of an activity. For example, an activity such as rope jumping may be halted temporarily so that the students may take their pulse. Such efforts at integration, even if pulse taking was previously learned, help students construct an integrated schema of knowledge.

Social and Personal Factors That Influence Learning

Among the developments of the 1980s is research indicating the types of relationships between social and personal factors and school learning. These relationships are particularly important to physical education because a major goal is for students to adopt a healthy lifestyle. Therefore, positive attitudes toward physical fitness and a receptivity to both cognitive and motor skill learning is crucial.

Key organizational (social) factors that influence students' perceptions of themselves and their motivation for learning are both the task and the reinforcement structure of the classroom. The two types of goal structure recently identified in the research literature are performance-oriented classrooms and learning- or mastery-oriented classrooms. The focus in the performance-oriented goal structure is on looking good compared to others, whereas the focus in the mastery-oriented classroom is on learning new skills (see Table 4.4).

The two different goal orientations have distinct effects on students' learning strategies and motivation. In one group of 176 secondary school students, the mastery-oriented students preferred

Table 4.3 Types of Elaborative Learning Strategies

Strategy	Example
Associating new learning with familiar images	Cardiorespiratory endurance: image of a heart and pair of lungs in track shoes running down the street
Associating new learning with letter codes	''Art(ery) was *thick* around the middle so he wore pants with an *elastic* waistband'' (Bransford et al., 1989).
Relating the new learning to existing knowledge and skills (schema)	After students have learned the basic food groups and guidelines for calories and fat, they can learn to critique daily menus.

Table 4.4 Comparison of the Performance–Goal and Learning–Goal Orientation

	Performance–goal orientation	Mastery- or learning–goal orientation
Definition of success	Appearing to outperform others with little effort; attaining high grades or scores in comparison with others	Learning new skills; mastery of new tasks; improvement and progress in learning new skills
Teacher orientation	How are students performing?	Are the students learning?
Student focus	How can I best obtain external verification of my performance?	How can I best acquire this skill or master this task?
Reasons for effort	High grades; performing better than others	Learning something new
Views of errors	Anxiety-eliciting; symbols of failure	Signals to redirect effort and to change strategy
Classroom characteristics	Stable learning groups, written assignments graded from A to F; only "A" or mostly correct papers displayed on bulletin boards; frequent tests with letter grades; positive and negative feedback—often in a public context	Flexible instructional groups; variations in assignments according to the students' skills levels; discouragement of normative comparisons; encouragement of peer assistance; frequent group projects

challenging tasks and held a more positive attitude toward class than the performance-oriented students (2). The problem with a performance goal orientation is that it sets up a win–lose situation that has detrimental effects on students. Children in several performance-oriented kindergartens, for example, rated their competence lower than children in learning-oriented kindergartens (21). Even more important, the effects of past successes can be erased by a single comparative judgment (10,18). When goals consistently emphasize social comparison, the win–lose nature of the situation generates anxiety and, in the long term, hampered ability to learn (10).

The implications for the physical education classroom are clear. These findings support Corbin (8) who states that fitness test performances should not be overemphasized. Specifically, fitness testing should not be determined by meeting performance criteria that are based on arbitrary normative standards (8). Grading based on performance abilities in particular activities defeats the basic purpose of physical education. Some students will achieve adequate scores, but the majority are likely to be turned off to exercise for lifetime fitness.

Classrooms that emphasize performance, whether physical or cognitive, also set in motion undesirable cognitive processes. Specifically, when students perceive that a class is organized on a success-or-failure basis, they begin searching for the major causes of their perceived successes or failures.

Research conducted by Weiner has identified the major causes of success and failure outcomes selected by students. They are ability, effort, task difficulty, and luck (22,23,25). Success attributed to ability and/or effort generates pride and an expectancy for future success. Conversely, failure attributed to lack of ability or effort contributes to a negative self-image. Failure attributed to a lack of ability generates feelings of embarrassment, disgrace, humiliation, and/or shame. In addition, failure is likely to be anticipated in similar situations. Failure attributed to lack of effort, on the other hand, tends to generate guilt feelings that may lead to withdrawal or retribution (25). Both situations, in other words, exert a debilitating influence on future achievement-related behavior.

In a performance-oriented classroom, where the focus is on comparative judgments, teacher behaviors often send signals to students about their ability. Excessive sympathy to particular students for poor performance is one cue that signals low ability (14,15,16), another is unsolicited help. Unrequested help, for example, is often extended when a student's difficulty is the result of factors beyond his or her control, such as lack of ability (24). Thus, unsolicited aid may lead the student to conclude that the teacher perceives his or her ability to be low. Further, excessive criticism of wrong answers and excessive praise for marginal and correct answers also send lack-of-ability messages, because both patterns are in excess of the criticism and praise received by others (7).

In a learning- or mastery-oriented classroom, by contrast, the emphasis is on learning new skills. Therefore, the focus is on treating errors as information for changing strategies rather than as failures. The focus on learning also reduces the problem of students attempting to "psych out" the causes of success or failure. That is, in the learning-oriented classroom, success is defined as either doing something new today that the student did not know how to do yesterday or as improving at an important personal fitness skill. Because a major goal in PE is motivating students to maintain a healthy lifestyle, a learning-oriented classroom is of utmost importance. In other words, progress toward *personal* fitness goals, rather than comparative or normative grading, is essential. An important side-benefit of gearing instruction to cognitive strategy objectives (e.g., devising one's own personal fitness program) is that the emphasis is directed toward learning for a personal goal.

The long-term benefit of a learning- or mastery-goal orientation is the development of the student's sense of *self-efficacy*. It is the belief in one's capability to execute a required behavior successfully (3,4,5)—a self-judgment about one's capabilities. Individuals with high self-efficacy persist longer at difficult tasks than those with low self-efficacy. Therefore, over the long term, they tend to become involved in a variety of activities and experiences. An important factor in the development of self-efficacy is the kind of school experiences that the student undergoes. Authentic mastery experiences contribute to a judgment of high self-efficacy (5). Success tends to raise the judgment of efficacy, whereas repeated failure lowers the judgment.

One of the challenges for the physical education teacher involves self-efficacy in the low-fit child. These children often exhibit low self-worth and a lack of confidence. Because they lack self-efficacy, they may slip to the back of the line and avoid taking a turn or they may bring an excuse when high-exertion activities are to be attempted. Of particular importance in improving both fitness level and self-efficacy for the low-fit child is the selection of appropriate physical activities. Personal goals for improved fitness should be established and activities within the child's range of accomplishment that contribute to improved fitness should be selected. Two other factors also are important. One is that progress toward the goal should be noted and the child complimented for his or her attainments. The second is the presence of models, who through their views and activities, demonstrate the continued benefits of personal fitness.

Summary and Implications

The developments presented in this chapter each assist the physical education teacher in different ways to meet the challenge of today's classroom or gymnasium. Gagné's conditions of learning assist the teacher in establishing an instructional framework for integrating cognitive and motor skills in instruction. The model provides a set of five unique types of capabilities and their associated requirements for learning. They are verbal information, intellectual skills, cognitive strategies, attitudes, and motor skills. Students in PE also learn procedures, which are sets of sequential skills composed of both motor skills and rule application.

Once the end-of-lesson capabilities are identified, the teacher can then identify the supporting subskills for problem solving and rule learning using the model. This crucial step ensures that important prerequisite skills are not omitted. Also of primary importance in the Gagné model is the focus on *planning*, which is shifted from content and teacher presentation, to *important capabilities that the student can execute*. Thus, the emphasis in instruction is on the interactions between the student and the new learning that will lead to proficiency in the skill.

Complementing Gagné's model are the essential interactions between the student and the new learning that are identified by information-processing theory. Specifically, unless new learning is actively processed by the student, relating it to already acquired information and skills, it will not be stored in long-term memory. Imagery, mnemonic strategies, and relating information to one's existing knowledge store are important processing strategies for learning. Collectively, these strategies are referred to as encoding strategies because they transform the new learning so that it is meaningful to the student.

Finally, the cognitive processes that students undertake to analyze their performance in the classroom stem from repeated achievement-related situations that are evaluated by their school program as success or failure. The conclusions students reach about their performances compared to their peers' and the reasons for their success or failure influence their future effort, their attitudes about fitness, and their self-concept. The research undertaken by Weiner identifies a variety of conclusions that students reach and some of the problems arising from performance-oriented classrooms. Other researchers, such as Dweck (10) and

Stipek and Daniels (21) confirm the importance of mastery-oriented classrooms for both teachers and students.

Typically, planning for instruction emphasizes steps to be taken by the teacher and to be made by the teacher. In contrast, the focus in each of the developments in this chapter is on the student. The transition from teacher-focused plans to student-focused plans may require some practice. Therefore, it is recommended that teachers consider the following questions when planning instructional activities:

1. Why have I included particular activities in the lesson? What new skills or attitudes will the students acquire from these activities, or are they included because this lesson is traditionally presented in this way?

2. Do the activities require that students learn to apply rules and to solve problems, or will the students only be demonstrating recognition and rote recall of information? How can activities be restructured to emphasize student skills in addressing issues and problems?

3. Does the lesson address the learning of prerequisite skills? Have I ensured that essential prerequisites are taught during the lesson or have they been previously learned?

4. In what ways can I integrate the learning of intellectual skills and motor skills in the classroom and in physical activity? How will the integration enhance encoding and memory for later use?

5. Which visual and/or verbal associations were most effective during instruction? Have I included sufficient opportunities for students to identify new examples in the learning of new concepts?

6. In what ways does the lesson provide opportunities for students to relate activities and skills in class to those in which they have participated or observed in other settings?

7. Is the goal structure of my classroom that of mastery? That is, are errors treated as information for learning rather than indicators of failure? What remnants of competitive organization and/or assessment remain that should be altered?

8. Do the unobtrusive signals in the classroom indicate that all students can enhance their skills, or are the signals primarily those of success/failure?

In summary, a focus on individual progress and the acquisition of particular beneficial skills can motivate students to develop personal fitness goals and to take pride in their accomplishments.

References

1. Adams, M.J. Thinking skills curricula. J. Educ. Psychol. 24(1):25-77; 1989.
2. Ames, C.; Archer, J. Achievement goals in the classroom: students' learning strategies and motivational processes. J. Educ. Psychol. 80(3):260-267; 1988.
3. Bandura, A. Social learning theory. Englewood Cliffs, NJ: Prentice Hall; 1977.
4. Bandura, A. The self and mechanisms of agency. In: Suls, J., ed. Psychological perspectives on the self. Vol. 1. Hillsdale, NJ: Erlbaum; 1982.
5. Bandura, A. Social foundations of thought and action. Englewood Cliffs, NJ: Prentice Hall; 1986.
6. Bransford, J.D.; Vye, N.; Adams, L.T.; Perfetto, G. In: Lesgold, A.; Glaser, R.; eds. Learning skills and the acquisition of strategies. Hillsdale, NJ: Erlbaum; 1989:p. 199-249.
7. Brophy, J. Teacher praise: a functional analysis. Rev. Educ. Res. 76:146-148; 1981.
8. Corbin, C.B. The fitness curriculum—climbing the stairway to lifetime fitness. In: Pate, R.R.; Hohn, R.C., eds. Health and fitness through physical education. Champaign, IL: Human Kinetics; 1994.
9. DiVesta, F.J. The cognitive movement and education. In: Glover, R.; Ronning, R., eds. Historical foundations of educational psychology. New York: Plenum; 1987:p. 203-233.
10. Dweck, C.S. Motivation. In: Glaser, R.; Lesgold, A., eds. The handbook of psychology and education. Vol. 1. Hillsdale, NJ: Erlbaum; 1989:p. 187-239.
11. Gagné, R.M. Domains of learning. Interchange 3(1):1-8; 1972.
12. Gagné, R.M. The conditions of learning. 3rd ed. New York: Holt, Rinehart & Winston; 1977.
13. Gagné, R.M. The conditions of learning. 4th ed. New York: Holt, Rinehart & Winston; 1985.
14. Graham, S. Can attribution theory tell us something about blacks? J. Educ. Psychol. 23(1):3-21; 1988.
15. Graham, S. Communicating low ability in the classroom: bad things good teachers sometimes do. In: Graham, S.; Folkes, V.S., eds. Attribution theory: applications to achievement, mental health, and interpersonal conflict. Hillsdale, NJ: Erlbaum; 1990:p. 17-26.
16. Graham, S.; Weiner, B. Some educational implications of sympathy and anger from an attributional perspective. In: Snow, R.; Farr, M.,

eds. Aptitude, learning, and instruction. Vol. 3. Cognitive and affective policy analysis. Hillsdale, NJ: Erlbaum; 1983:p. 199-221.

17. Gredler, M.E. Learning and instruction: theory into practice. 2nd ed. New York: Macmillan; 1992.

18. Jagacinski, J.M.; Nicholls, J.G. Competence and affect in task involvement and ego involvement: the impact of social comparison information. J. Educ. Psychol. 79:107-114; 1987.

19. Peterson, P.L. Selecting students and services for compensatory education: lessons from aptitude–treatment interaction research. J. Educ. Psychol. 23(4):313-352; 1988.

20. Pintrich, P.R.; Blumenfeld, P.C. Classroom experiences and children's self-perceptions of ability, effort, and conduct. J. Educ. Psychol. 77:646-657; 1985.

21. Stipek, D.J.; Daniels, D.H. Declining perceptions of competence: a consequence of changes in the child or in the educational environment? J. Educ. Psychol. 80(3):352-356; 1988.

22. Weiner, B. Theories of motivation from mechanism to cognition. Chicago: Markham; 1972.

23. Weiner, B. A theory of motivation for some classroom experiences. J. Educ. Psychol. 71:3-25; 1979.

24. Weiner, B. The role of affect in rational (attributional) approaches to human motivation. J. Educ. Res. 9:4-11; 1980.

25. Weiner, B. An attributional theory of achievement motivation and emotion. Psychol. Rev. 92(4):548-573; 1985.

26. Weiner, B. Human motivation. New York: Springer-Verlag; 1985.

Part II
Curriculum and Methods

Part II contains several chapters dedicated to the curricular and methodological aspects of health-related physical education. The spectrum of issues discussed is broad, ranging from presentation of the major curricular goals of health-related physical education to analysis of the pertinent teaching techniques appropriate for children with health impairments. Collectively, these chapters present the core of a successful, health-related physical education program.

Chapter 5

Charles B. Corbin's "The Fitness Curriculum—Climbing the Stairway to Lifetime Fitness" presents a five-step progression as a model for physical education curricula. Corbin offers nine specific recommendations for elementary school physical educators and seven recommendations for secondary school physical educators to help guide students up the fitness staircase. His program has the goals of making people not only physically fit but healthy, self-motivated, and self-sufficient physical activity consumers.

Chapter 6

In "Fitting Fitness Into the School Curriculum" Judith E. Rink explores how fitness goals can be a

part of the total physical education curriculum. She considers alternative ways to implement and integrate these goals into the curriculum. In planning fitness goals teachers should differentiate programs for each grade. They can use school time outside of physical education class to teach fitness, approach fitness as a health maintenance behavior, integrate fitness instruction with motor skill instruction, design PE instruction to facilitate vigorous activity, and integrate fitness goals with a health curriculum.

Chapter 7

Robert P. Pangrazi argues in "Teaching Fitness in Physical Education" that because fitness is a lifetime *process*, physical educators must focus on teaching it as a fun experience, rather than focusing on the *product*, or outcomes, of physical activity. This chapter offers teachers 6 strategies for helping students develop positive attitudes toward activity, 8 suggestions for helping motivate children to maintain physical fitness, and 11 guidelines for implementing fitness programs in the elementary school.

Chapter 8

James R. Whitehead's "Enhancing Fitness and Activity Motivation in Children" has two main parts. The first is an account of pertinent motivation theory, primarily the concept of intrinsic motivation. It offers a short review of studies that support the theory. The second part presents some guidelines for enhancing fitness and activity motivation.

Chapter 9

In "Physical Fitness Education and Assessment: Addressing the Cognitive Domain," Clayre K. Petray notes that students are ultimately responsible for their fitness. Petray favors a comprehensive plan that establishes values and objectives, provides preinstruction fitness testing, helps students set personal goals, carefully implements activities designed to help students achieve those goals, encourages self-testing and postinstructional testing, recognizes achievements in the process of physical fitness, and properly evaluates students. In this way the physical education program can provide children with learning experiences that will enable them to achieve and maintain optimal personal fitness for life.

Chapter 10

"Exercise for Children With Special Needs," by Dianne S. Ward, indicates that physical impairments can rob children of fulfilling the fundamental need to be physically active. The health-related components of physical fitness (cardiovascular fitness, muscular fitness, flexibility, and body composition) should be emphasized to improve a child's capacity for exercise. Ward recommends assessment, goal setting, and individualization of training for each child, based on the impairment, and modifying the learning environment. Children with special fitness needs often may be accommodated within the regular physical education program, but in many cases specially adapted physical education programs are necessary. Increasing habitual physical activity is the ultimate goal of the physical education program; this goal becomes even more important when the child is limited by a health condition.

Chapter 11

Patricia J. McSwegin addresses "Fitness Programming and the Low-Fit Child." Low-fit children should be identified and helped to deal with limitations imposed by their specific fitness problems.

Whenever possible the low-fit child should participate in peer activities, but with modifications that increase the likelihood of successful participation. Certain characteristics of activities signal a need for modification for low-fit children, including speed, strength, and movement of the entire body weight. The underlying causes of low-fitness levels include inadequate knowledge, poor fitness skills, and poor attitudes, as well as the more obvious ill effects of overweight, minimal strength, lack of endurance, and muscle tightness. Teachers have a major responsibility to implement a systematic plan that offers low-fit children emotional support and sound physiological guidance.

Chapter 12

In "Fitness Testing: Current Approaches and Purposes in Physical Education," Russell R. Pate notes the controversy surrounding physical fitness testing during the past decade. Fitness testing methods have changed dramatically, and the most current testing programs (e.g., AAHPERD's Physical Best, FitnessGram, President's Challenge, YMCA Youth Fitness Test, and the Chrysler Fund-AAU Physical Fitness Test) emphasize health components that are important across the lifespan. This chapter reports that fitness tests have been used for various purposes, not all of which are realistic and pedagogically sound. It also suggests how to incorporate fitness testing into a physical education curriculum so that it contributes to cognitive and affective learning.

Chapter 13

Kirk J. Cureton's "Physical Fitness and Activity Standards for Youth" reports that in recent years criterion-referenced standards for youth have been developed that estimate the minimal levels of physical fitness and activity consistent with good health and performance of daily tasks. These have replaced normative standards as the principal means for evaluating and interpreting individual fitness and activity levels in youth. The standards are tentative, and additional research is needed to validate them against health outcomes. Several different tests and sets of standards exist, and consensus on a single set of fitness and activity-referenced standards is needed.

Chapter 14

"Implementing Health-Related Physical Education," by Bruce G. Simons-Morton, presents a case study involving implementation of elementary school health-related physical education (HRPE) and discusses the conditions required for the broad diffusion of HRPE in American schools. Emphasizing lifetime participation in moderate to vigorous physical activity for most students as a means of promoting fitness and health, such curricula usually feature frequent physical education classes. HRPE teachers stress effective class management, keep group instruction and demonstration to a minimum, maximize the number of practice trials, and provide frequent individual feedback, instruction, and reinforcement.

Chapter 15

Thomas A. Ratliffe points out in "Teaching Fitness in the Elementary School: A Comprehensive Approach" how a comprehensive fitness curriculum develops in small steps. Although some aspects of the new curriculum can be implemented immediately, others may take years. Long-range planning, such as a 5-year plan, can help teachers decide how and when to integrate fitness into an elementary physical education curriculum. This long-range plan should include many of the strategies the chapter discusses—practical presentations, varied instructional methods, exercise that is both fun and challenging, and homework activities—all to help children experience, understand, and value fitness as essential to their lives.

Chapter 16

"Super Active Kids: A Health-Related Fitness Program," by Melissa A. Parker and colleagues, describes a collaborative project between a university and a public school. Super Active Kids (SAK) is a health-related fitness program for elementary school children. Supported by school administrators, physical education teachers, teachers' aides, parents, and students, the SAK program has accomplished positive goals. With four program components (noonday program, after-school program, fitness corners, and fitness knowledge), the program meets North Dakota's time recommendation for physical activity, increases spontaneous play, promotes good playground behavior, and enhances children's knowledge about health and physical activity.

Chapter 17

"A Health Fitness Course in Secondary Physical Education: The Florida Experience," by Dewayne J. Johnson and Emmanouel G. Harageones, details the formation and implementation of a personal fitness course. Passing this standardized course became a requirement for high school graduation as a result of education reforms enacted by the 1983 Florida Legislature. Working with Florida's Department of Education, physical education professionals conducted teacher training activities and worked through eight distinct implementation strategies. After discovering and resolving implementation problems, they fashioned a program with a positive impact on principals, teachers, and—most importantly—students.

Chapter 18

In "Moving to Success: A Comprehensive Approach to Physical Education" elementary school physical educators Jenifer J. Steller and Dan B. Young describe Moving to Success, a comprehensive fitness program at the Woodland Heights Elementary School in Spartanburg, South Carolina, that successfully blends the school staff, families, and community. Classroom teachers are directly involved in PERK (Physical Exercise Revives Kids), 5 min of music broadcast over the school's PA system in the early morning to which students perform a choreographic routine. Teachers also DUCK Walk (Discover and Understand Communities, Kids, by Walking) with their students, accumulating class miles that they equate to an imaginary walk through South Carolina, learning along the way about the culture of the communities they have "walked to." This school's PE program goes beyond the gymnasium to involve the entire school, providing students with creative learning experiences.

Chapter 5

The Fitness Curriculum—
Climbing the Stairway
to Lifetime Fitness

Charles B. Corbin
Arizona State University

According to national polls, the number of adult Americans participating in regular exercise has increased dramatically in recent years. Although there is disagreement as to how many American adults are active enough to reap the optimal benefits of exercise, opinion polls have consistently reported that about 60% of American adults consider themselves active. As professionals, we may view this as bad news because it means that 40% are inactive and that some of the active 60% are probably not active enough to attain the full health benefits of exercise. Seen in a different context, the current level of activity among adults may be viewed more positively. Considering that the first Gallup poll in 1960 showed that only 24% of American adults were active, 60% is a good improvement. American adults have become considerably more active in recent decades, but there still is a long way to go. Recent estimates indicate that only 22% of American adults do as much as 30 minutes of activity 5 days a week and as many as 24% do no leisure time physical activity. The federal government's goal seems worthy—namely raising the number of highly active Americans from 22% to 30% and decreasing the number of totally inactive people from 24% to 15% (17).

Kinesiology and physical education professionals have contributed significantly to the increased level of activity among Americans through the development of new knowledge and through the increased provision of opportunities for regular exercise among adults. Much of what we now recognize about the health benefits of exercise and fitness was unknown in 1960. Being less informed then, many adults were not convinced of the value of regular exercise for good health. Today most adults accept that regular exercise is important to a healthy life, a realization that has helped change the social norm in our society. Being active is socially popular. Our profession, once limited mostly to schools, has adapted and now provides educational opportunities for people of all ages both in and outside the school environment. The opportunities for activity are much more numerous now than they were 30 years ago.

If reports in the popular literature are correct, our success in persuading youth about fitness and exercise is not nearly so spectacular as it has been with adults. Dr. George Sheehan, a leading adult fitness leader, once said, "There is a fitness movement in the United States; unfortunately it is passing physical education by." His statement apparently was based on the widely held notions that our youth are considerably less active and fit than they should be and that schools are not providing the fitness education necessary for a lifetime of activity. Although he and I would probably agree that we must place more emphasis on physical education *and* fitness education in the future, I am not a doomsayer about the fitness of American youth.

My years of research and teaching in the area of physical fitness lead me to several conclusions at odds with people who believe that all American children are inactive and unfit and becoming more so with each passing year. A summary of conventional wisdom on youth fitness and my "alternative wisdom" is presented in Table 5.1. The alternate conclusions in Table 5.1 are based on results of national fitness surveys (1,2,3,9,10,14) in addition to the literature about youth fitness published in the last 30 years (7,12). The philosophy and fitness objectives for school programs in this chapter are also derived from this literature.

The Fitness-for-Life Philosophy

The philosophy presented here provides the basis for a sound fitness education program primarily

Table 5.1 The State of Youth Fitness in America

Conventional wisdom	Alternative wisdom
1. Most American youth are inactive and unfit.	1. Youth are more active than adults as a group. Still, many are less active than they should be.
2. The level of youth fitness is considerably lower now than in previous years.	2. With the exception of having more body fat, youths are probably no less fit now than 30 years ago. Fit children may be more fit, and unfit children less fit, than in previous decades.
3. The best way to improve youth fitness is to create programs that require youth to exercise at levels known to produce fitness.	3. The best way to improve youth fitness is to convince children that exercise is something they can enjoy and to educate them to be informed exercise and fitness consumers.

for school programs. Note, however, that it could also provide direction for a comprehensive fitness program for people of all ages. Fitness education is a part of physical education that is devoted principally to the physical fitness objective. It is not a substitute for a comprehensive physical education program but a central part of a sound program.

The Fitness-for-Life philosophy builds from four basic assumptions. These assumptions provide the basis for the HELP philosphy.

H = Health
E = Everyone
L = Lifetime
P = Personal

First, the philosophy is based on the notion that fitness for good *health* is paramount. Regular exercise in an appropriate amount yields many known health benefits. No matter who you are, these benefits are available to you within the limits of your heredity. Beyond good health, regular exercise can also enhance performance and skill-related physical fitness. Although a sound fitness education program enhances performance, a desirable goal, these performance benefits are secondary. Being an outstanding performer may be a worthwhile goal, but outstanding performance in sports or fitness tests is not necessary for a healthy and fruitful life.

The second assumption is that fitness is for *everyone*. Few people will disagree with this assumption. Yet teachers, coaches, fitness leaders, and school administrators who speak of their commitment to "fitness for everyone" by their actions reveal a lack of commitment. For example, recent research raises questions about national fitness testing programs that profess to be for all children but reward only a select few (4). Acting on the commitment to fitness for all is the key. Lip service is not enough!

The third assumption, fitness for a *lifetime*, is one that many people preach but do not practice. Fitness is a transient state of being. You use it or you lose it. To promote programs that build fitness for now while discouraging lifetime fitness through enjoyable exercise betrays the true Fitness-for-Life philosophy. Using exercise as a form of punishment illustrates this point.

Personal is the word that characterizes the final assumption of the HELP philosophy and that is the basis for Fitness-for-Life programs. There is no one best activity for all people. That lifetime activity is personal is illustrated by the results of national surveys that show a wide variety of participation activities among American adults ranging from aerobic fitness to walking.

It is my belief that a sound fitness curriculum is based on these four assumptions, and the objectives for fitness education that follow are organized around this philosophy.

Objectives for Fitness Education: The Stairway to Lifetime Fitness

The Stairway to Lifetime Fitness presented here is a description of hierarchical objectives for a fitness education program (Figure 5.1). I will provide a general outline of the steps in the stairway, then suggest ways in which the objectives can best be carried out in elementary and secondary schools. The stairway provides a basis for fitness education from the lowest to the highest level. Young children, because they are beginners, are dependent on us as experts. For this reason they will focus on the lowest level objective, the first step in the stairway. As students grow older and progress educationally they will gradually focus more attention on the higher order objectives, Steps 2 through 5 in the stairway. At all levels of learning, some attention will be given to each of the five fitness objectives (steps). The focus on a particular objective will change as the learner proceeds up the stairway to lifetime fitness.

• Step 1: *Exercise*. If you exercise, and do it properly, fitness will follow. At an early age the focus on fitness and fitness test scores is not necessary.

Most children naturally love exercise. Our job should be to foster this love. Involving kids in activity and helping them to enjoy it should be our primary program focus in the early years.

• Step 2: *Achieving fitness*. Good fitness contributes to good health. It helps youth feel good, look good, and enjoy life. However, fitness is temporary. If children achieve fitness without a love of exercise, maintaining fitness for life will not be accomplished. We have *not* achieved our fitness goals when our students are fitter than "average" or even "super fit" if we have not promoted a love of activity and a commitment to fitness for life. Our job is not complete (indicated by the dotted line above Step 2 in the stairway) (Figure 5.1) when Step 2 is reached. If our students are to be fully educated we must progress up the stairway to Steps 3 through 5.

• Step 3: *Fitness patterns*. When children are young we try to involve them in a wide variety of activities. We want them to experience as many different activities as possible. Some they will enjoy, others they will not. At some point youth will be able to make decisions about *personal* exercise patterns that are best for them. What is best for one person is not best for another. The key is for each individual to find some form of vigorous activity that he or she enjoys and will do for a lifetime. We as educators must begin to relinquish the decision-making process to our students. We must help them make personal activity choices that are sound and realistic.

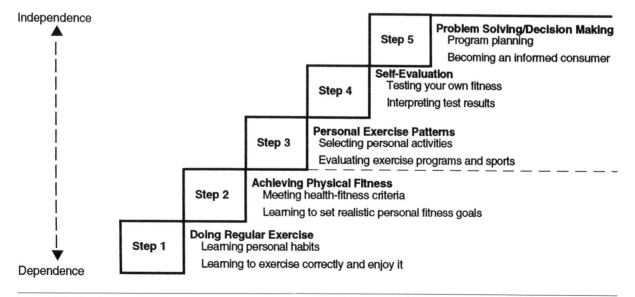

Figure 5.1 Stairway to lifetime fitness.
Note. From *Fitness for Life: Teachers Annotated Edition* (3rd ed.) (p. T9) by C.B. Corbin and R. Lindsey, 1993, Glenview, IL: Scott, Foresman. Copyright 1993 by Scott, Foresman. Adapted by permission.

• Step 4: *Self-evaluation.* As youth progress in our fitness education programs they have experienced enjoyable exercise, have known what it is like to achieve fitness levels necessary for good health, and have begun to establish personal habits and patterns of lifetime exercise. To be fully educated people, older students must be able to assess their own fitness, having a basis for making informed decisions about lifetime fitness. By learning self-evaluation they can revise their own fitness programs as needed, hopefully resisting the false information perpetuated by the multitude of questionable health and fitness prescriptions. Contrary to what some might think, this is an attainable objective for most youth.

• Step 5: *Problem solving.* Every high school graduate should have a good grasp of the essential facts about exercise and fitness. He or she should be able to plan a personal fitness program now and for a lifetime. Students should know the facts about each of the essential components of health-related fitness and should know the value of different forms of exercise in promoting fitness. Information such as this will help each individual to become an informed consumer.

It is my view that fitness education has often focused exclusively on Steps 1 and 2 of the stairway. I hope that I can convince you as professionals to dedicate yourselves to the promotion of all five steps in the stairway so that students using this program will move from dependence on us as instructors (Step 1) to fitness independence (Step 5). Though even the well-educated person will need to consult an expert such as a physical educator or a physician from time to time, a truly educated person is an independent problem solver capable of making sound choices. In the following sections I will make some specific recommendations concerning changes that we can make in physical education to help youth to achieve fitness independence (the top of the stairway).

Elementary School Fitness Education

I believe that the following guidelines and recommendations can help us fulfill the fitness-for-life philosophy and meet the appropriate objectives on the fitness stairway. The list is not meant to be all-inclusive, but it does list factors critical to moving children up the stairway.

1. *Focus programs of fitness education for young children on activities that both promote fitness and teach a love of activity.* Most children already enjoy activity, and every attempt should be made to keep activity fun. Programs that create the perception that exercise is work should be avoided.

2. *Accompany fitness education for young children with a quality program of skill education.* Basic skills (such as reading and motor skills) are very difficult to learn later in life; they must be taught and learned in elementary schools. People who are skillful and feel competent in physical activity are more likely to enjoy and benefit from it. Skill education is not a substitute for fitness education and vice versa. Elementary school children need ample time for skill instruction and additional time for activity designed to meet fitness objectives. In addition to physical education, children need some free time during the school day. Children are designed to be physically active. Corporate America provides breaks for adults; children also need that free time during their day.

3. *Do not use exercise as punishment.* Exercise as punishment may achieve an immediate goal, but it does not help in the long-term quest of fitness for life. It teaches people to hate exercise, not enjoy it.

4. *Do not deny children fitness or skill education because of lack of performance in other subjects.* Classroom teachers should not be allowed to withhold participation in PE because of behavior in other classes.

5. *Do not overemphasize fitness test performances.* Fitness achievement is only one step in a long-term educational process. Too much emphasis on performance can turn kids off to exercise and fitness. Because heredity plays a significant role in fitness test performance and because it takes considerable time to build fitness through regular exercise, special care should be used when interpreting test results. Personally, I do not advocate the use of fitness test scores in student grading.

6. *Place special emphasis on helping those who are low-fit to reach appropriate health fitness standards.* Although we do not want to neglect those who are already fit, there is evidence that fit children are more likely to find opportunities for exercise outside of school and are likely to stay fit over time. Those who are low-fit tend to become less fit with time and may drop out (6,11). These youth especially need our help.

7. *Take special care not to undermine self-esteem in fitness education programs.* Most young children feel competent and confident in physical activity.

They believe us when we say "you are good." By the middle to upper elementary school years, many students begin to realize that they are not as good as the best; and the number of youths who feel competent and confident in activity begins to decrease. We must do everything possible to help all kids feel "exercise is for me."

8. *Expose upper elementary school and middle school children to the many activities of our culture.* Students need to see what choices of activity are available for enjoyment in later life. Emphasis should be on enjoying the activities, regardless of ability. Grading based on performance should be minimized, if not eliminated.

9. *Focus fitness testing on meeting health criteria rather than performance criteria based on arbitrary normative standards.* Both parents and students should be educated concerning the meaning of test results. Self-evaluation can begin early in the schools. Awards should be based on sound educational concerns and should promote the process of exercise rather than high-level fitness performance (5,8).

Secondary School Fitness Education

By the time students reach secondary school many elements of their lives have become well established, including regular patterns of activity or inactivity. Students will have skills in some activities and not others. They will have definite feelings about which physical activities they like and which they dislike. Some will feel competent in physical activity, but many will not. The relatively homogeneous group of children who entered school will now be very heterogeneous, making our task of teaching more difficult. At this point, the P (personal) in the HELP philosophy becomes very important. The following recommendations are offered not as final solutions to problems of fitness education but as possible aids in helping youth reach the top of the lifetime-fitness stairway.

1. *Make every effort not to threaten the self-esteem of teenage students in fitness education.* Take care to keep the locker room, the gym, and other experiences from making students feel incompetent. Locker and shower rooms can become places where some students are physically intimidated and less physically mature students are taunted. At this age feelings of incompetence can result in

withdrawal from situations that are threatening to self-esteem, including many types of physical activity.

2. *Recognize that physical appearance is critical to teenagers.* When PE classes keep students from looking how they want to look, all PE is perceived as unattractive and to be avoided. Be responsive to your students' need to look attractive, including allowing enough time to groom after activity and providing adequate facilities and equipment (e.g., hairdryers, mirrors) to accommodate them.

3. *Offer students a variety of activities from which to choose.* The third step in the stairway to lifetime fitness is exercise patterns. The goal is to help students choose lifetime activities they enjoy. By secondary school most youth have had the chance to sample a variety of activities. Forcing them to perform activities they do not enjoy is counterproductive. Programs that allow students to choose the activities in which they will participate are encouraged.

4. *Give all secondary school students a class teaching the facts about fitness and exercise, including fitness self-evaluation and program planning.* The class should include both gymnasium and classroom activities designed to help all students become good fitness and exercise consumers and effective problem solvers. A sample of class content is included in Table 5.2. Such a class should be required for high school graduation.

5. *After a required basic fitness education class (see Item 4 in Table 5.2), have all students participate in a required elective physical activity program.* One period of daily activity should be required, but students who have completed a basic problem-solving class should be able to choose the activities in which they participate. Many choices should be available from a list of activities that do not require a high level of skill and are known to be popular choices for great numbers of adults (swimming, walking, jogging, cycling, aerobic dance, home calisthenics, weight training, etc.).

6. *Modify school facilities to accommodate sound fitness education programs.* Facilities should include well-equipped classrooms and student labs, weight rooms, dance and general exercise rooms, running tracks, bike trails, and other facilities that accommodate the most popular adult activities in our culture. Fitness educators must be involved in facility planning and in making modifications in existing facilities—too often designed for team and athletic activities for spectators rather than participants. Such facilities would accommodate the educational needs of students in sound fitness education classes as well as the needs of adults in the

Table 5.2   Content for a High School Fitness-for-Life Class

1. Introduction to physical fitness
   - The parts of health-related physical fitness
   - The parts of skill-related physical fitness
   - Fitness attitudes
2. Exercising safely
   - Being medically prepared
   - Exercise-related injuries
   - Exercise and the weather
   - Harmful exercises
3. Preparing for exercise
   - Warm-up
   - Workout
   - Cool-down
4. How much exercise is enough?
   - Overload principle
   - Progression principle
   - FIT (frequency, intensity, and time) formula
   - Specificity
   - Personal fitness and exercise goals
5. Exercise and good health
   - Hypokinetic conditions
   - Hyperkinetic conditions
   - Risk factors and exercise
   - Posture and back care self-evaluations
6. Cardiovascular fitness
   - The cardiovascular system
   - Exercise and cardiovascular health
   - Cardiovascular FIT formula
   - Building and self-evaluating cardiovascular fitness
7. Strength
   - Muscle system
   - Strength and good health
   - Strength FIT formula
   - Building and self-evaluating strength
8. Muscular endurance
   - Your body and muscular endurance
   - Muscular endurance and fitness
   - Muscular endurance FIT formula
   - Building and self-evaluating muscular endurance
9. Flexibility
   - Flexibility and good health
   - Flexibility FIT formula
   - Building and self-evaluating flexibility
10. Exercise and fat control
    - Body fatness and good health
    - Optimal levels of fatness
    - Body fatness FIT formula
    - Gaining and losing body fatness
    - Myths about exercise and fatness

11. Skill-related physical fitness
    - The parts of skill-related fitness
    - Benefits of skill-related fitness
    - Improving skill-related fitness
    - Learning sports skills
    - Self-evaluating skill-related fitness
12. Nutrition and exercise
    - Nutrients and body needs
    - Facts about exercise and nutrition
    - FIT formula and nutrition
    - Eating disorders
    - Analyzing food choices
13. Living with stress
    - Defining stress
    - Good and bad stress
    - Stress management, fitness, and good health
    - Getting help
    - Evaluating stress levels
14. Making consumer choices
    - The meaning of "quackery"
    - Health and fitness quackery
    - Evaluating books and articles
    - Consumer organizations
15. Evaluating exercise programs
    - Planned exercise programs
    - General exercise programs
    - Evaluating programs
16. Fitness and sports
    - Lifetime sports
    - Sports for fitness
    - Fitness for sports
    - Choosing lifetime sports
17. Planning your exercise program
    - Deciding what to do
    - Planning the program
    - Evaluating the program
18. Fitness and your future
    - Lifelong attitudes
    - Planning for future fitness
    - Planning for future exercise
    - Realistic goal setting

Note. From *Fitness for Life: Teachers Annotated Edition* (3rd ed.) (pp. iii-vii) by C.B. Corbin and R. Lindsey, 1993, Glenview, IL: Scott, Foresman. Copyright 1993 by Scott, Foresman. Adapted by permission.

community who could and would use them if they were made available.

7. *Design fitness testing largely for self-evaluation.* Students should learn to self-administer tests and interpret their own results. To ensure meaningful results, I do *not* recommend that fitness test results be used in student grading, especially at this level.

The Process Versus the Product

As we try to meet the five objectives represented in the stairway to lifetime fitness, it is most important to remember the importance of the lifetime process of exercise. Step 1 of the stairway represents activity for now; we hope this activity will become a permanent habit for a lifetime. Step 2 of the stairway represents fitness for now; we hope it will become a lifetime state of being. Steps 3 through 5 promote knowledge, attitudes, and behaviors that will result in both exercise and fitness for a lifetime. In the final analysis, however, it is the *process* of exercise that is most important. If we can get people to do correct exercise for a lifetime (the process), the *product* (physical fitness) will follow. We will have met our objectives when the process becomes a regular, permanent part of a person's lifestyle. Fitness and good health will follow to the extent that an individual's heredity will allow.

Extending the Curriculum

The focus of this chapter has been school fitness education. However, fitness education is not something that can be done by the school alone. Schools cannot "do fitness to kids"—kids must undergo the process of exercise to become fit. Fewer than half of our elementary school youths have PE more than 3 days a week, and the average time spent in a class is 33-1/2 min (13,16). In these classes, skill and fitness education are only two of the program objectives. With limited time and many different objectives, how is it possible to devote enough time to exercise to produce adequate fitness? Often, it is not possible. Certainly, physical education can be part of a total exercise program for youths, but schools cannot do it by themselves.

Families and communities must get more involved. They can begin by arguing for more physical education time in the schools. Until this is accomplished there are other things that can be done. Parents can exercise with their children. Although this seems to be a reasonable suggestion, approximately 60% of parents of primary grade children report that they do not exercise with their children in the typical week. Children of active parents are more likely to possess good fitness if their parents are physically active, suggesting that the example of the parent can be important in promoting fitness among children (15). Parents must come to the aid of the child if youth fitness is to improve.

Nearly all young children are involved in some type of community activity program at least 1 day a week. However, most of the activities in which they participate are organized sport programs, often team sports (15). Also, participation is often seasonal. If we are to increase the number of youths who participate in physical activity regularly, communities and agencies within the community must make special efforts to provide opportunities for all children. It is my view that many youths opt out of organized programs, especially organized sports, because they feel threatened in these programs. This is true especially in the preteen and teenage years. Alternatives to organized sport should be provided for youth who do not choose this kind of involvement. After-school activities other than school sports should be offered if we are to honor the commitment to fitness for everyone.

A good fitness education program, based on the philosophy and objectives discussed in this chapter, can do much to encourage involvement in family and community activities. No matter how effective the school program, involvement in these activities will not occur if the programs are not available. Parents and communities must help us if we are ever to accomplish our fitness goals for all youngsters.

Summary

Having been involved in fitness work for more than 35 years as a community recreation leader, an elementary school PE teacher, a professional youth sports coach, a parent-volunteer youth sports coach, a college teacher and researcher, and an advocate for youth fitness, I express concern about fitness and exercise for all Americans. I believe that youths are not as inactive and unfit as many would lead us to believe and that the level of fitness and exercise among adults is improving as knowledge and attitudes toward fitness improve. But I am not satisfied.

We, the fitness educators of America, can do much to change things as we set new goals for the year 2000. From 1960 to 1990 we operated on "an old strategy" based on scaring the American public with claims of deteriorating youth fitness, often followed by programs to get youth fit now, but at the expense of lifetime fitness and exercise goals. This chapter proposes a philosophy and set of objectives that can establish "a new strategy," one that takes on the challenge of helping all people achieve acceptable levels of health-related physical fitness through a lifetime of exercise. The focus is on the process of lifetime exercise rather than the achievement of arbitrary fitness standards that characterized the old strategy. We can accomplish this if we establish a clear philosophy and meaningful objectives for school fitness education and implement programs consistent with them. With a concentrated effort to put into practice some of the suggestions in this chapter and to recruit parents and community agencies in partnership, I think the future is bright. This new strategy will result in a more active and fit America by the year 2000.

References

1. American Alliance for Health, Physical Education and Recreation. Youth fitness test manual. Washington, DC: AAHPER; 1958.
2. American Alliance for Health, Physical Education and Recreation. Youth fitness test manual. Washington, DC: AAHPER; 1965.
3. American Alliance for Health, Physical Education, Recreation and Dance. Youth fitness test manual. Reston, VA: AAHPERD; 1975.
4. Corbin, C.B.; Lovejoy, P.Y.; Steingard, P.; Emerson, R. Fitness awards: do they accomplish their intended objectives? Am. J. Health Prom. 4:345-351; 1990.
5. Corbin, C.B.; Pangrazi, R.P. Teaching strategies for improving youth fitness. Dallas, TX: Institute for Aerobics Research; 1989.
6. Corbin, C.B.; Pangrazi, R.P. A five year study of the body fatness of children. Paper presented to the American College of Sports Medicine. Salt Lake City, UT; 1990 May.
7. Corbin, C.B.; Pangrazi, R.P. Are American children and youth fit? Res. Q. Exerc. Sport 63(2): 96-106; 1992.
8. Corbin, C.B.; Whitehead, J.; Lovejoy, P. Youth physical fitness awards. Quest 40:200-218; 1988.
9. Office of Disease and Health Promotion. Summary of the findings from national children and youth fitness study. JOPERD 56:43-90; 1985.
10. Office of Disease and Health Promotion. The national children and youth fitness study II. JOPERD 58:51-96; 1987.
11. Pangrazi, R.P.; Corbin, C.B. A longitudinal study of the flexibility of school children. Paper presented to the AAHPERD national convention. New Orleans, LA; 1990 April.
12. Pangrazi, R.P.; Corbin, C.B. Physical fitness: questions teachers ask. JOPERD 64:14-19; 1993.
13. Pate, R.R.; Ross, J.G. Factors associated with health-related fitness. JOPERD 58:93-96; 1987.
14. Reiff, G.; Dixon, W.; Jacoby, D.; Ye, G.; Spain, C.; Hunsicker, P. The president's council on physical fitness and sports national school population fitness survey. Ann Arbor: University of Michigan; 1986.
15. Ross, J.G.; Pate, R.R.; Caspersen, C.J.; Damberg, C.L.; Svilar, M. Home and community in children's exercise habits. JOPERD 58:85-92; 1987.
16. Ross, J.G.; Pate, R.R.; Corbin, C.B.; Delpy, L.A.; Gold, R.S. What is going on in the elementary physical education program? JOPERD 58:78-84; 1987.
17. U.S. Department of Health and Human Services Public Health Service. Healthy People 2000: national health promotion and disease prevention objectives. 1991. Available from: U.S. Government Printing Office. Washington, DC: (DHHS Pub. No. [PHS] 91-50213).

Chapter 6

Fitting Fitness
Into the School Curriculum

Judith E. Rink
University of South Carolina, Columbia

Although the school physical education program is not the only means to develop fitness objectives with youth, it is certainly a primary avenue. The major issue of our time is not if we should have fitness goals in physical education. Rather, the concern is what those fitness goals are and, more importantly, how to implement them within the curriculum of the school program.

Fitness has been a major focus of recent conferences and professional literature. Most of the dialogue has concentrated on issues related to whether fitness should be a primary curriculum focus. Practical ideas on how to develop fitness with the school population are beginning to emerge in the professional literature. Although it is helpful to give PE teachers ideas that can be used directly and immediately with students, it is more important to understand clearly fitness goals and their place in the total program—apart from what you do with students next week.

From my perspective, the major problem with its attempts to integrate fitness into the school program has been the failure of our profession to define long-term program goals and to develop long-term plans for the implementation of those goals. Such planning in an educational program requires curriculum development, the process through which we define comprehensively our goals and objectives and then consider alternative ways to accomplish them over the length of a program. This is accomplished not in a month, in a

year, or during a grade level, but in a K-12 program. Failure to look at long-term goals condemns a profession to actions based on trivial pursuits, which yield short-term accomplishments and long-term failure.

This chapter is divided into two parts. First, I explore the question of fitness goals from the perspective of the total physical education curriculum. Second, I consider alternative ways to implement and integrate these goals within the physical education curriculum.

Fitness Goals and Physical Education

The outcomes committee of the National Association for Sport and Physical Education recently drafted their definition of a physically educated person (7). There are five components to the definition, followed by several more specific and descriptive outcomes (see Table 6.1).

The traditional goals of physical education programs are reflected in the outcomes statements. The motor skill development component (Component 1) assumes the development of competence in at least a few forms of activity, and the fitness component (Component 2) assumes the development of the skills to assess, achieve, and maintain

Table 6.1 National Association for Sport and Physical Education: Definition of a Physically Educated Person

A physically educated person

1. **Has learned skills necessary to perform a variety of physical activities.**
   - Moves using concepts of body awareness, space awareness, effort, and relationship
   - Demonstrates competence in a variety of manipulative, locomotor, and nonlocomotor skills
   - Demonstrates competence in combinations of manipulative, locomotor, and nonlocomotor skills performed individually and with others
   - Demonstrates competence in many different forms of physical activity
   - Demonstrates proficiency in a few forms of physical activity
   - Has learned how to learn new skills

2. **Is physically fit.**
   - Assesses, achieves, and maintains physical fitness
   - Designs safe, personal fitness programs in accordance with principles of training and conditioning

3. **Participates regularly in physical activity.**
   - Participates in health-enhancing physical activity at least three times a week
   - Selects and regularly participates in lifetime physical activities

4. **Knows the implications and the benefits of involvement in physical activities.**
   - Identifies the benefits, costs, and obligations associated with regular participation in physical activity
   - Recognizes the risk and safety factors associated with regular participation in physical activity
   - Applies concepts and principles to the development of motor skills
   - Understands that wellness involves more than being physically fit
   - Knows the rules, strategies, and appropriate behaviors for selected physical activities
   - Recognizes that participation in physical activity can lead to multicultural and international understanding
   - Understands that physical activity provides the opportunity for enjoyment, self-expression, and communication

5. **Values physical activity and its contributions to a healthful lifestyle.**
   - Appreciates the relationships with others that result from participation in physical activity
   - Respects the role that regular physical activity plays in the pursuit of lifelong health and well-being
   - Cherishes the feelings that result from regular participation in physical activity

fitness. The other three components (3-5) deal directly with participation in physical activity. Students are expected to participate in physical activity at least three times a week, to know the benefits of participation, and to value the contributions it can make to a healthful lifestyle.

The definition of a physically educated person is important because it clearly identifies the integration of motor competence, the development and maintenance of fitness, and the important role that knowledge and effort play in the long-term success of our programs. The goal is to develop participants who maintain an active, healthy lifestyle. Some educators suggest that a fitness focus should replace a motor skill one in physical education. This would be short-sighted and might even endanger the very goal for which programs have been designed. Most leaders in our field recognize the integral relationships and importance of all components outlined in Table 6.1 to the goal of an active lifestyle. Programs that neglect any of these components are not likely to accomplish the major goal of physical education programs, which is a physically educated individual.

Alternative Fitness Goals

One of the most important decisions program planners have to make is the specification of program goals. Although the primary and unique psychomotor goals of physical education are usually divided into motor skill emphases and fitness emphases, the dichotomy may be a false one in view of long-term and ultimate goals. The overriding concern should be education for an active lifestyle, which would maintain health and add to the quality of life.

Current research on fitness supports the belief that the health benefits of activity are achieved through regular, moderate levels of activity (2). We need to move people from the "couch potato" set—without expecting results seen in the category of the highly conditioned athlete—in order to maintain the health benefits of activity. Although PE programs have a tremendous potential to effect this objective, the question of an active lifestyle is a bigger issue. Active lifestyle is more related to the affective outcomes that are part of the purpose and goal of schooling, the end result of the total school curriculum.

Active people are not so much active because of what they know, but because they have some sense of being in charge of their lives; they feel competent, they feel responsible, and they feel in control.

They seek activity in much the same way as they seek participation in other aspects of their lives, whether this is cognitive, social, or emotional participation. Educators use terms like *locus of control*, *high self-esteem*, and *independent, self-initiating people* (4). Television commercials give us terms like *the Pepsi generation, gusto,* or *just do it.* The point is that attention to fitness goals and developing an active lifestyle is part of a society's much more comprehensive effort to empower people to take charge of their lives. An active lifestyle includes sport and fitness activities within a broader rubric than just physical education. In fact, a person can have an active lifestyle without ever engaging in sport or activity designed specifically for fitness benefits.

Physical education can make a major contribution to this goal, but we deceive ourselves if we think that fitness educators have a monopoly on the idea of a healthy lifestyle. The goals related to the development of self-esteem, self-direction, and a sense of responsibility for self and others, which we share with all educational programs in the school, may actually have more of an impact on maintaining an active lifestyle than our unique contribution in motor skills and fitness.

How to go about establishing program objectives from this shared goal depends on your ideas for meeting the present needs of youths (1,3,6,10) and preparing them for an active adult lifestyle in the context of a physical education program. Although research, experience, and other factual kinds of information all can help you make this decision, the program objectives you decide on largely will be value decisions—what I call *I believe* issues (9).

Fitness Through Motor Skills

The development of motor skills is one of the most pervasive program goals in today's physical education programs. A motor skill orientation to fitness assumes that people who lead an active lifestyle really participate in vigorous physical activity. They seek out activity they find enjoyable because they have achieved a reasonable amount of success at it. According to this perspective, active participants (those active enough to develop and maintain the health benefits of activity) evolve primarily through the development of competence in motor skills. Indeed, students should develop enough success in motor skills to enable them to participate in the physical activities of their culture. More importantly, they must want to participate. The term *motor skills* is interpreted largely to mean

sport skills, but motor competence makes an important contribution to all phases of life.

At the elementary school level the development of fundamental motor abilities is critical (5,10). Elementary school children who have not developed fundamental motor patterns enough to be successful at them often do not choose to be active or to place themselves in learning situations in which they risk failure. There is some support for the idea that the self-concept of elementary-age students is in part determined by their success in motor skills (4). The content of secondary programs (oftentimes complex sport skills) is largely out of reach to students who have not developed some success in fundamental abilities and who no longer are willing to try.

To make the development of motor and sport skills the primary route to accomplishing health-related fitness, programs would have to be redesigned to ensure both competence in several or more activities before graduation and a more positive attitude toward participation than what most students have now. An essential aspect of programs that aspire to develop fitness through learning the skills for an active lifestyle is making activity a positive experience.

Recent publications on high school physical education strongly suggest the use of a selective program (11). Let kids choose and give them enough time and good instruction to acquire competence at something. The very students who need high levels of activity are the ones who opt not to participate in the programs we now conduct. In practice, relatively few programs produce competence or are a positive experience for large numbers of participants. If we are to contribute to an active lifestyle through motor skill competence, we will have to do a much better job of developing competence in a way that encourages, rather than discourages, positive attitudes toward activity.

Fitness as a Primary, Unique Goal

A second alternative to developing an active lifestyle through physical education is to make fitness a primary and distinct program goal apart from the development of motor skills. Programs that choose this route generally combine some of the following ideas:

1. The development of fitness
2. The maintenance of fitness
3. Concepts related to fitness (including the why, the how, and effects of fitness on the body)

4. Attitude or affective concerns related to fitness

Of all the objectives in physical education, we know most about how to develop fitness. What has changed are our notions about what level of fitness is necessary to obtain the health benefits of physical activity. Although basic principles of duration, intensity, and frequency have long guided training in this area, we know the health benefits of activity are achievable without striving for high levels of training. We also know that fitness training limited to jogging and traditional calisthenics may be counterproductive in terms of attitudes toward PE and physical activity for the adolescent.

Another major problem with specifically focusing on fitness in youth is that high levels of fitness are hard to maintain. Unlike the acquisition of motor skills, unless you do something to maintain fitness, you lose it. From a curricular standpoint this means that a 6-week unit to develop fitness is insufficient. You have to think in terms of regular levels of at least moderately vigorous activity as the goal of a lifetime, and those practices need to begin in adolescence. Students will associate fitness with something they do during class, without it making an impact on their lives unless programs either maintain fitness through a broad range of activities or foster attitudes and skills that enable students to maintain fitness through their school and home life.

The real challenge of the physical education program is the integration of all of these critical components of the fitness goal. To accomplish this you must help students develop at least a health-related level of fitness, help them maintain it through continuous levels of moderately vigorous activity, give them the knowledge needed for self-direction in this area, and teach them to value fitness to the extent that they will want to continue to be active both as youth and later as adults. Most importantly, this should be done in a way that develops a "take charge" attitude in their lives. How to best meet these goals over a K-12 program is really a curriculum question.

Curriculum Planning for Fitness Goals

Almost all physical education teachers value fitness and want to incorporate fitness goals into their programs. When asked how their programs

are incorporating fitness, most physical education teachers respond with one of the following:

1. We work on fitness through a 5-min warm-up every class period.
2. I give the blankety-blank fitness test every year.
3. I have a 3-week fitness unit with each of my classes each year.
4. I don't have time to develop fitness so I do "concepts."
5. I teach motor skills because the effects of learning at least are enduring.
6. We do Jump Rope for Heart.

When pursued further, "concepts" usually means how to take your heart rate and, in a conscientious program, how to deal with the concept of target heart rates. There is little differentiation between skills taught in one grade or another. In some programs a student might "learn" to take his or her heart rate every year for 12 years.

All of these ideas are well intentioned but none of them in and of themselves are likely to contribute to major goals related to the physically educated or to the "take charge" person. They are not well thought through, nor are they part of a comprehensive and long-term program perspective. Our failure to be effective in this area is largely a failure to come to grips with comprehensive planning over the entire school program. By nature we are much more comfortable with quick fixes even if our efforts do little more than take students through the motions.

If we begin to consider ways to accomplish these primary program goals in the K-12 curriculum rather than looking at what we can do with each of our classes in limited program time, we begin to ask different questions. Instead of trying to do everything in one grade, we begin to ask where certain program objectives are better placed throughout the K-12 physical education program and in other dimensions of the school program as well. If we are to impact the goal of an active lifestyle through physical education programs we will need to begin thinking about K-12 perspectives on curriculum and the many alternatives recommended for fitness.

Differentiate Programs for Each Grade

Many of our programs do not have a great deal of time for physical education. The most common arrangement is probably 2 days a week in elementary school, varied patterns in middle school, and as little as 1 year of PE in high school. Many programs try to accomplish everything in each of the years with no difference between what each grade does, and nothing is really accomplished. Program time allotted to different objectives is generally too short to accomplish anything other than exposure to ideas quickly forgotten or to skills without enough time to learn them. An alternative would be to focus on fitness a substantial part of designated years (e.g., fourth and eighth grades). Taking more time to seriously assess, develop, and work with the knowledge, skills, and attitudes students need in fitness at these critical points in the curriculum, we would probably be more effective than with the common "shotgun" approach to our objectives. In the same total program time, learning in this area would likely be more effective. Table 6.2 describes in general terms how a K-12 fitness plan might sequence and concentrate fitness objectives into several large blocks of time.

Programs that use fitness concepts and short fitness units without ever fully developing the fitness of students may not be successful in encouraging students to develop and maintain fitness on their own. Furthermore, programs that are limited in the amount of time devoted to PE may try to justify spending all their program time in the pursuit of obtaining or maintaining fitness, thus considerably limiting the scope of their program.

Table 6.2 Sample Fitness Sequences in a K-12 Program

Grade 4 (10-15 class periods)	• Introduction to fitness components • Assessment, achievement, and reassessment of basic fitness components • Personal programs for the year—teacher-directed and designed with activity choices for each component
Grade 8 (20 class periods)	• Body composition and weight control • Health-related issues • Assessment, achievement, and reassessment of fitness components • Evaluating activities
Grade 10 (25 class periods)	• Designing and conducting personal programs • Assessment and reassessment of basic fitness components • Lifestyle issues

Targeting grades for particular goals allows time to develop those goals avoiding the use of all the K-12 time for one aspect of the program. Targeting fitness as a major program goal for several grades does not mean neglecting fitness in the other years. Rather, each grade's program should reinforce fitness ideas and provide high levels of activity, but focus mainly on other program goals. The state of Florida's required high school fitness program is an example of one that requires a concentrated amount of time to work on a program goal that has some chance of being successful. Unfortunately, the same attention has not been given to other program goals.

Use School Time Other Than Physical Education Instruction Time

Integrating fitness goals into the school experience could be accomplished by using school time other than physical education instructional program time. There have been many examples of this approach in schools that have identified fitness as an all-school objective. These programs appear in both elementary and secondary programs, but differ in their design, depending on the source of the support and commitment for the program and the alternatives open within each setting.

Usually in the elementary schools the classroom teacher plays a major role in all school fitness programs with the support of the principal, though program responsibility and administration lies with the physical educator. In the secondary schools programs are usually computer-based and individualized with facilities available for students during lunch periods, free periods, and before and after school. Generally speaking, the major emphasis of the all-school programs is the assessment, development, and maintenance of a designated level of fitness, focusing largely on cardiorespiratory fitness. In most cases it is difficult to sustain these programs beyond the initial enthusiasm without constant teacher involvement and monitoring of students or a major attempt to personalize programs and create student ownership.

Approach Fitness as a Health Maintenance Behavior

Many, although not all, programs designed to maintain fitness rely primarily on cardiorespiratory exercise to train or maintain a level of fitness. Although most program leaders make an effort to maintain the interest level of participants through the use of a variety of forms of cardiorespiratory exercise, many are not concerned with variety. The main thrust of these programs is largely to encourage the view that vigorous activity on a regular basis is a health maintenance behavior similar, for example, to brushing your teeth. It is just something you do. You don't necessarily have to like it or feel like doing it. You do it because it is good for you and essential to maintain health. Programs using this approach educate participants from a different perspective than those programs attempting to make physical activity enjoyable.

Integrate Fitness With a Motor Skill Emphasis

There are many ways in which fitness objectives can be integrated in the curriculum along with a motor skill emphasis. A primary way selects content of the program on the basis of its potential to contribute to fitness objectives. Usually fitness is interpreted to mean cardiorespiratory endurance, but it should not be limited to this. Activities selected for their cardiorespiratory contribution are those that require a high level of endurance, such as soccer, cross-country, and running and chasing activities (in the elementary school). These would be selected rather than activities such as archery, softball, and volleyball, which do not require a great deal of vigorous activity.

This approach, however, has several problems. First, in many sport activities high levels of vigorous activity are required only when they are played by skilled participants. Beginning players tend to stand around a lot because they lack the skills to keep a game continuous. And second, many of the activities young people select for cardiorespiratory value are the ones adults avoid. Although it is tempting to consider vigorous large muscle activity as the overriding criterion for selecting a sport, doing so may be shortsighted in terms of realizing the goal of an active lifestyle throughout adulthood.

Design Instruction to Facilitate Vigorous Activity

Perhaps more important than the selection of the activity is how the activity is taught. Technically speaking it is possible to teach any activity in a manner that maintains high levels of vigorous activity, if that is your objective. We could invent ways to teach archery to maximize vigorous activity, for example, by running to retrieve the arrows or providing vigorous activity for those students in line to shoot. Certainly there are ways to keep students vigorously active during basketball units. Although maintaining vigorous activity is important, and we don't do enough of it, our enthusiasm to make vigorous activity the overriding concern in the way we teach sport must be tempered with the realization that other objectives are not always best reached in an environment of high vigorous activity. For instance, students at beginning levels of motor skill learning require simplified conditions during practice. In some cases this means practicing skills in stationary positions. Likewise, many of the cognitive objectives we have for fitness may best be taught in classroom environments.

Teachers must determine the objective for a class before deciding how best to achieve it. An overriding concern should be to design and conduct learning experiences in PE that are vigorous in nature if this does not have a negative effect on the accomplishment of other program objectives—whether short-term or long-term goals of the K-12 program. Teachers often vacillate in approach because they have failed to come to grips with program goals, the big picture. They spend little time looking at alternative ways to accomplish lesson objectives that would balance vigorous and not-so-vigorous experiences within a lesson. There is no professional conflict between fitness and motor skill acquisition in terms of program goals. When vigorous activity becomes an obsession and the single criterion for conducting PE lessons, it may conflict with other program objectives.

Integrate Fitness Goals With the Health Curriculum

Another choice for the placement of fitness in the school curriculum is the assignment of some fitness objectives to the health program. Many professionals would say that most of the cognitive content in this area legitimately belongs in the health curriculum. It does not make a lot of difference where the content is taught, only that it is taught. Coordinating efforts of physical education teachers and health teachers would avoid overlap. The goals of physical education are broader than those of health in this area. Placement of the content related to exercise and health is primarily situational, depending on state curriculums, amount of program time devoted to health and physical education, interests of the teachers involved, and other factors.

Affective Concerns

The most important curricular factors related to fitness are often the most neglected and are affective in nature. Long-term studies of work in fitness curriculum suggest very strongly that the most important factor determining ownership of the values related to fitness and behavior that maintains fitness is the degree to which programs have been personalized and conducted with the goal of self-direction (8). Developing fitness is relatively easy from an instructional perspective. By contrast, designing fitness experiences for students that have a lasting effect on their behavior, helping them take charge and be responsible for the quality of their lives, is far more difficult.

In most schools, an entirely different instructional approach is required to accomplish objectives if the ultimate goal is for students to be self-directed in this area. Clearly, having expectations that students achieve levels of fitness without any efforts to lead the student to ownership is ineffective (8). Helping students to value fitness to the extent that it strongly influences the way in which they conduct their lives requires carefully thought through curricular and instructional decisions.

Instructional Issues

Effective instruction that both personalizes objectives and develops competence takes time and an instructional environment conducive to learning. It has been my experience, also supported by research, that we do not allow enough instructional time in what we teach for learning to occur (9). Many physical education teachers are more interested in exposure than learning. This is true regardless of whether or not we teach fitness or motor skills, or try to develop self-initiating behaviors. It is important that teachers know how to teach for learning and value learning in a physical education setting. Many concepts basic to effective teaching are violated on a continuous basis. Rarely do you see any attempt at repetition and review, which are critical to learning whether using the direct or indirect teaching style. These principles are continuously violated by the design of our curricula, and our instructional methods render any claim to meeting program objectives questionable.

Summary

The inclusion of fitness into a comprehensive program of physical education requires that teachers carefully think through the nature of the ultimate goal of their physical education program, lest we win the battle but lose the war.

This chapter has explored how fitness goals can be *part* of the total physical education curriculum and has considered alternative ways in which these goals can be implemented and integrated into the physical education curriculum. In planning for fitness goals we can differentiate programs for each grade, use school time other than physical education instruction time to teach fitness, approach fitness as a health maintenance behavior, integrate fitness instruction with motor skills instruction, design physical education instruction to facilitate vigorous activity, and integrate fitness goals with the health curriculum. Incorporating fitness into our lessons is easy. Intentionally placing curricular experiences in a long-term, K-12 plan to accomplish total program goals is far more difficult.

References

1. Bar-Or, O. A commentary on children and fitness: a public health perspective. Res. Q. Exerc. Sport 58:304-307; 1987.
2. Blair, S.; Clark, D.; Cureton, K.; Powell, K.E. Exercise and fitness in childhood: implications for a lifetime of health. In: Gisolfi, C.V.; Lamb, D.L., eds. Perspectives in exercise science and sports medicine. Vol. 2. Youth exercise and sport. Indianapolis, IN: Benchmark Press; 1989.
3. Corbin, C.B. Youth fitness, exercise and health: there is much to be done. Res. Q. Exerc. Sport 58:303-314; 1987.
4. Fox, K.R. The self-esteem complex and youth fitness. Quest 40(3):230-246; 1988.
5. Haywood, K.M. The role of physical education in the development of active lifestyles. Res. Q. Exerc. Sport 62(2):151-156; 1991.
6. Lee, A.M.; Carter, J.C.; Greenockle, K.M. Children and fitness: a pedagogical perspective. Res. Q. Exerc. Sport 58(4):321-325; 1987.
7. National Association for Sport and Physical Education. The physically educated person. Draft copy of material presented at the AAHPERD national convention; 1990.

8. Philip, A.; Piland, N.; Seidenwurm, J.; Smith, H. Improving physical fitness in high school students. J. Teach. Phys. Educ. 9(1):58-73; 1989.

9. Rink, J.E. When should we becomes can we in curriculum. In: Carnes, M.; Stuek, P., eds. Proceedings of the 5th curriculum theory conference in physical education. Athens, GA: 1987 March.

10. Seefeldt, V. Developmental motor patterns: implications for elementary physical education. In: Nadeau, C.; Halliwell, W.; Newell, K.; Roberts, G., eds. Psychology of motor behavior and sport. Champaign, IL: Human Kinetics; 1980.

11. Siedentop, D.; Mand, C.; Taggert, A. Physical education: teaching strategies for grades 5-12. Palo Alto, CA: Mayfield; 1986.

Chapter 7

Teaching Fitness in Physical Education

Robert P. Pangrazi
Arizona State University

The focus of this chapter is to give teachers general guidelines for helping children develop positive attitudes toward fitness. How a teacher presents the fitness experience is as important as the actual fitness activities. Additionally, knowing how to motivate youngsters to participate in fitness experiences is requisite teacher behavior, and this chapter discusses a number of guidelines for creating positive fitness experiences.

A Brief Overview

Many schools have failed to provide a well-organized physical education program that teaches youngsters how to maintain health and vitality. A common belief among administrators and school boards is that physical education is a subject to be taught after all other subjects have received adequate support and coverage. Schools provide academic courses for children to live a productive life, and few people would question the importance of learning to read and write. However, these skills have little worth if one is near death or suffering from hypokinetic disease. There is no higher priority in life than health. Without it, all skills lack meaning and utility.

Childhood obesity is commonly regarded as the leading chronic pediatric disorder (6). A large number of children may be obese due to a lack of

exercise (3). Unfortunately, many obese children grow into obese adults; as children mature, the weight problem worsens (8). To improve fitness and conquer childhood obesity, children must develop active lifestyles at an early age. Children do not voluntarily engage in high-intensity activity when left to themselves. A study by Gilliam, MacConnie, Geenen, Pels, and Freedson (2) traced the intensity of voluntary activity patterns of 59 children by recording their heart rates. Results showed that youngsters seldom engaged in high-intensity activity that increased the heart rate into the training zone (160+ beats a minute). Exercising regularly and at proper intensity is a learned behavior.

Exercise programs for children should be designed to improve the self-confidence of children rather than to undermine it. The program should be tailored to the needs of each child (particularly in the case of obese youngsters) to assure the experience is a successful endeavor. The fitness program should be an enjoyable and positive social experience to assure that children develop a positive association with activity.

Focus on the Process of Fitness

Teachers and parents often talk only about *product* outcomes when they discuss fitness with children.

For example, teachers ask how fast students ran the mile, how many push-ups they performed, and how far they could stretch. Unfortunately, most youngsters would much rather talk about the *process* of participating in fitness activities. Children place great importance on being included in activity, being wanted by friends, and participating in "fun" activities (7). This "process versus product" conflict leads some children to believe that adults only value their performance when the product of fitness improves or increases. With excessive adult concern for the product of fitness, youngsters infer that fitness is an end product rather than an ongoing process. When children are forced to concentrate on the product of fitness, they seldom learn to understand the process.

Fitness is an ongoing process that involves learning to evaluate fitness levels, comparing types of activity, and designing personal fitness programs. Product orientation forces youngsters to focus on the intensity of their efforts and increases the odds that they will burn out and quit exercising. For example, when distance running against the clock, youngsters are expected to improve their time. Sooner or later, the point arrives when improvement no longer occurs. Regardless of training, improvement is limited by genetic factors. It can be discouraging (and nonreinforcing) to find it impossible to go any faster or jump any farther, and this lack of improvement may cause many people to quit.

When administering fitness programs, focus on the process of participation. If children participate in physical activity on a daily basis, the product of fitness will take care of itself. Praise children for physical participation rather than physical performance. Ask students how the game was, what they enjoyed, and who they visited—rather than how fast they ran or who won the contest.

Developing Positive Attitudes Toward Activity

Teachers can do a number of things to help students get "turned on" to activity. Fitness activity is seen as something good or bad, depending on one's experience. How fitness activities are taught influences how youngsters will feel about making fitness part of their lifestyles. The following strategies can help make activity a positive learning experience.

Individualize Exercise to Accommodate Various Stages of Physical Growth and Maturity

Students who are expected to participate in fitness activities and find themselves unable to perform certain exercises are not likely to develop positive attitudes about physical activity. Fitness experiences should be designed to let children determine their own work loads. Use time as the work load variable and ask children to do the best they can within a time limit. People dislike and fear experiences they perceive to be enforced from an external source. Voluntary long-term exercise is more probable when individuals are internally driven to do their best. Fitness experiences that allow children to control the intensity of their workouts offer better opportunity for the development of positive attitudes toward activity (4).

Expose Youngsters to a Wide Variety of Physical Fitness Routines and Exercises

Presenting a variety of fitness opportunities decreases monotony and increases the likelihood that all students will discover fitness activities that they like. Most youngsters are willing to accept activities they dislike if they know they'll get to do ones they enjoy sometime soon. A year-round routine of calisthenics and running laps forces children, regardless of ability and interest, to do the same activities all year. Avoiding potential boredom by systematically changing activities is a significant way to help students perceive fitness positively.

Give Youngsters a Basic Understanding of Physical Fitness

Knowing the values of physical fitness, how to apply the principles of exercise, and how fitness can become part of one's lifestyle can positively alter how students view physical activity. Bringing the class together at the end of a lesson to discuss the key fitness points presented promotes a clearer understanding of why fitness is important. To share cognitive information, teachers might establish a "muscle of the week," construct educational bulletin boards to illustrate fitness concepts, or send home handouts explaining principles of fitness development.

Give Students Meaningful Feedback About Their Performance

Feedback from a teacher contributes to the way children view fitness activities. Immediate, accurate, and specific feedback regarding performance encourages continued participation. Provided in a positive manner, this feedback can stimulate children to extend their participation habits outside the confines of the gym (7). Avoid falling into the trap of reinforcing only those students who perform well. All children need feedback and reinforcement even if they are incapable of performing at an elite level.

Meaningful feedback can help children understand that the fitness experience is a challenge—an experience they can conquer—rather than a threat (which appears impossible to accomplish). Goals must be established within the realm of challenge rather than the environment of threat, although they are viewed as one or the other depending on the perceptions of the student, not the instructor. It is important to listen carefully to participants rather than telling them to "do this for your own good!"

Teach Physical Skills *and* Fitness

Physical education programs should concentrate on skill development as well as fitness. Some states mandate fitness testing, which causes some teachers to worry about their students' failure to pass. Unfortunately, the skill development portion of PE is often sacrificed to increase the emphasis on teaching for fitness. The dual nature of physical education programs must continue by promoting both fitness *and* skill development. Skills are the tools that most adults use to attain fitness. The large majority of individuals maintain fitness through various skill-based activities, such as tennis, badminton, swimming, golf, basketball, aerobics, and bicycling. Children are more likely to participate as adults if they feel competent in an activity. School programs must graduate students with requisite entry skills in a variety of activities.

Role Model to Influence the Attitudes of Children Toward Physical Fitness

Appearance, attitude, and actions speak loudly about teachers and their values regarding fitness. Teachers who display physical vitality, take pride in being active, participate in fitness activities with children, and are physically fit will positively influence youngsters to maintain an active lifestyle. It is unreasonable to expect teachers to complete a fitness routine nine times a day and 5 days a week. However, teachers must exercise with a class periodically to assure students that they are willing to do what they ask others to do.

Motivating Children to Maintain Physical Fitness

Physical education programs should strongly motivate children to maintain fitness. Here are some suggestions for motivating positive fitness behavior.

1. Focus awards on the process of participation, rather than the product of fitness. Participation in exercise and physical activity are process goals, whereas fitness testing focuses on the product of fitness. When youngsters are involved in the process of fitness, the product takes care of itself. For example, fitness awards for scoring above the 85th percentile focus on product and motivate only a small minority of students. Results of the National School Population Fitness Survey (5) showed that only 0.1% of boys and 0.3% of girls could pass the six test items of the Youth Fitness Test (1). If only a few children are able to win an award, it discourages the others.

2. Set goals that are challenging yet attainable. When *all* children can achieve their goals through effort, this results in greater motivation and challenge. On the other hand, if youngsters find goals impossible to achieve, the system becomes discouraging and threatening. Develop a chart filled with goals that encourage participation and regular exercise.

3. Use bulletin boards in the gymnasium and classrooms to publicize items of interest about fitness. Rather than the typical posting of outstanding performances, list all youngsters who have participated. Bulletin boards are motivating devices when they attract the attention of all students.

4. Use visual aids such as films about fitness and related topics. For example, a number of films show people who have excelled despite physical handicaps.

5. Emphasize self-testing programs that teach children to evaluate their fitness levels. Children should have ongoing opportunities to assess their fitness, without concern for what others think. As

with adults, fitness is a personal matter with youngsters.

Figure 7.1 shows a self-testing card. Youngsters are told to find a friend and begin self-testing. This assures that students can test themselves with a friend of their choosing. The results are recorded, then cards are collected and distributed at a later time. Self-testing should be done two to three times during each school year so that students can evaluate their progress toward goals. Youngsters should not be required to share the results of their test unless they choose to do so.

6. Do not use fitness test results for grading purposes. This will certainly destroy any motivation youngsters have about participating in fitness activities. Children vary tremendously in terms of physical capability, and to grade them on their fitness scores is to penalize them for being born with a less productive body.

7. Involve parents in their children's fitness efforts. Cooperation at home can improve a youngster's level of motivation. Children are more likely to participate in fitness activities when their parents are supportive. Fitness homework that is sent home for weekend and vacation activity helps communicate to parents that regular activity is important. An effective technique is to develop a fitness calendar, listing activities to be performed on various days, and send a copy home to parents.

8. Feature a number of fitness routines and activities at physical education fitness exhibitions and school demonstrations for parents. Focus on all students participating in the program instead of using only elite performers. Another parent–student evening program to stimulate parental interest is a physical fitness activity night. Youngsters and their parents participate together in a number of fitness activities. After each one, teachers explain why these activities are included and what they contribute to the total fitness program.

Implementing Fitness Programs in the Elementary School

Fitness is part of the daily lesson and dedicated exclusively to the presentation of a wide variety of fitness activities (4). The following are suggestions to aid in the successful implementation of the fitness module:

1. Fitness instruction should begin with a 2- to 3-min warm-up period. Teach a number of methods for warming up (e.g., stretching, walking, slow jogging, and performing various exercises at a slower-than-usual pace). Youngsters should be offered the opportunity to prepare for strenuous activity in order to facilitate proper exercise habits.

2. The fitness portion of the daily lesson including warm-up should not extend beyond 10 to 15 min. Even though a higher level of fitness might be developed if more time were devoted to the area, emphasis must be placed on all phases of physical development. Physical education classes usually are 30 min long and are offered two to three times a week. It is necessary to compromise the length of the fitness session to assure that time is allowed for skill instruction.

3. Activities should be vigorous in nature, exercise all body parts, and cover the major components of fitness. Children are capable of strenuous work loads when they are properly designed for the age, fitness level, and ability of participants.

4. A variety of fitness routines comprising different aerobic activities and exercises for total body development are good alternatives to a year-long program of regimented calisthenics. An array of routines that appeal to the interest and fitness level of children should replace the traditional approach of doing one daily routine.

5. Conduct fitness routines during the first part of the lesson. Relegating fitness to the end of the lesson does little to enhance the image of exercise. Having the exercise phase of the lesson precede skill instruction reinforces the concept that you get fit to play sport; you do not play sport to get fit.

Teachers may ask whether to teach fitness if they only see a class once a week. The answer is yes; how else will youngsters learn to value fitness if it isn't part of school physical education lessons? Granted it is difficult to develop fitness levels on a once-a-week basis; however, attitudes can be developed that will last a lifetime.

6. Teachers should assume an active role during fitness instruction. Children respond positively to role modeling. A teacher who actively exercises with children, hustles to assist those youngsters having difficulty performing selected exercises, and is able to make exercise fun begins to instill in children the value of an active lifestyle.

7. Various forms of audio or visual assistance should be used to increase the child's level of motivation. Background music, colorful posters depicting exercises, a tambourine to provide rhythmical accompaniment for activity, and other instructional aids can make vigorous activity more enjoyable.

My Personal Fitness Record

Name_____ Age_____ School_____ Grade_____ Room_____

	Trial 1		Trial 2	
	Score	Acc	Score	Acc.
Body Composition				
Calf (arm) Skinfold				
Triceps (leg) Skinfold				
Total (arm + leg)				
Cardiovascular Endurance PACER				
Mile Run/Walk	:		:	
Abdominal Strength Curl-ups				
Upper Body Strength Push-ups				

The following items are pass-fail only.

Back Strength Trunk Lift				
Lower Back Flexibility Sit & Reach				
Upper Body Flexibility Shoulder Stretch				

Note: Acc. indicates that you have scored above the minimum criterion referenced health standard. This means that you possess the minimum fitness required for good health and minimal health risk. Even though you may have passed all the tests, you may not be active enough It is most important to be active for at least 30 minutes everyday.

You do not have to share your results. They are only meaningful to you and should help you determine whether you are active enough. See your teacher if you need ideas for increasing your activity level.

Figure 7.1   Example of a fitness self-testing card.

8. Determine work loads for children based on time rather than on a specified number of repetitions; this allows children to adjust their work load within personal limits. Having children perform as many sit-ups as possible within a time interval (in contrast to requiring that the entire class complete 30 sit-ups) will result in more children feeling successful.

9. If only 2 to 3 min are allowed for warm-up activity and 10 min for fitness, the importance of efficient use of time becomes obvious. Fitness activity should be continuous and demanding. Heart rates should be elevated into the target heart rate zone.

10. Class management skills should be effectively used to assure that the maximum amount of activity will occur in the allotted time. Students can lead the activity so that the teacher can move throughout the area and offer individualized instruction. During class there are a number of transitions from one activity to another. This is often time when children stand around. As an alternative, ask youngsters to move, and allow them to talk among themselves while doing so. This assures that moving will be associated with a positive reinforcer (being able to talk with a friend).

11. Fitness activities should *never* be assigned as punishment. Such a practice teaches students that, for example, push-ups and running are things you do when you misbehave. The opportunity to exercise should be a privilege as well as an enjoyable experience. Be an effective salesperson: Sell the joy of activity and the benefits of physical fitness to youngsters.

Summary

Fitness should be a positive experience and focus on success. Teachers can encourage student participation by demonstrating that they personally enjoy fitness activity. The opportunity for students to accomplish work loads by permitting adjustment with their capabilities assures a positive attitude. Little is gained if students are trained physically but develop a negative feeling about the experience. Move forward in small increments, and worry less about whether enough was accomplished and more about whether the experience was positive.

References

1. American Alliance for Health, Physical Education, Recreation and Dance. Youth fitness test manual. Reston, VA: Author; 1987.
2. Gilliam, T.B.; MacConnie, S.E.; Geenen, D.L.; Pels III, A.E.; Freedson, P.S. Exercise programs for children: a way to prevent heart disease? Phys. Sportsmed. 10(9):96-108; 1982.
3. Mayer, J. Obesity during childhood. In: Winick, M., ed. Childhood obesity. New York: Wiley; 1975:p. 73-80.
4. Pangrazi, R.P.; Dauer, V.P. Dynamic physical education for elementary school children. 10th ed. New York: Macmillan; 1992.
5. Reiff, G.G.; Dixon, W.R.; Jacoby, D.; Ye, X.Y.; Spain, C.G.; Hunsicker, P.A. The president's council on physical fitness and sports 1985 national school population fitness survey. Washington, DC: U.S. Department of Health and Human Services; 1987.
6. Ward, D.S.; Bar-Or, O. Role of the physician and physical education teacher in the treatment of obesity at school. Pediatrician 13:44-51; 1986.
7. Weiss, R.M. Self-esteem and achievement in children's sport and physical activity. In: Gould, D.; Weiss, M.R., eds. Advances in pediatric sport sciences. Vol. 2. Champaign, IL: Human Kinetics; 1987:p. 87-120.
8. Williams, M.H. Weight control through exercise and diet for children and young athletes. In: Stull, G.A.; Eckert, H.M., eds. Effects of physical activity on children. Champaign, IL: Human Kinetics; 1986:p. 88-113.

Chapter 8

Enhancing Fitness and Activity Motivation in Children

James R. Whitehead
University of North Dakota

In all areas of life, including the physical domain, some conceptual knowledge of motivation is crucial for understanding people's behavior. The study of motivation has progressed over the years, and theories have evolved that have expanded our understanding. In addition to explaining behavior, these theories can guide the choice of strategies to change it.

Unfortunately, there are differences between motivation theories, and thus it is advisable to have a good understanding before using them as a framework for writing practical guidelines. Even then, it is vital to evaluate their utility when applied to specific areas, such as physical fitness. This really can only be done by putting them to the test.

Organized in two parts, this chapter discusses an account of the development and content of pertinent motivation theory. This is supported by a review of studies that have tested theory credibility relevant to fitness through physical education. Second, and following from the theory, some guidelines for enhancing fitness and activity motivation are suggested for the practitioner.

You may want to read (and reread) the theory section from a critical perspective, draw your own conclusions, and devise your own practical methods. Other readers may trust the theory and find the practical guidelines stand alone. Ideally, readers will read all of this chapter and then will choose what is best for them.

Part One: Theoretical Background

The first part of this chapter considers motivation theories, especially about intrinsic motivation. Various studies on positive motivation in the classroom and in physical activity programs are next examined to see how intrinsic motivation might play out in practice.

Developments in Motivation Theory

Until relatively recently the major theories of motivation assumed that human behavior is determined by internal or external forces that are not amenable to conscious control. For example, Freudian, learning, and behavioral theorists cited (respectively) the unconscious mind, physiological drives, or environmental stimuli and reinforcements as the motivators of behavior. However, in the late 1950s it became obvious that data did not always fit the models. Some researchers noted the tendency of animals and humans toward curiosity, exploration, and excitement-seeking behaviors that could not be explained by existing theories!

These anomalies led to a significant addition to motivation theory. White (34) in a major psychological monograph proposed a theory of motivation that viewed humans as *intrinsically* active in efforts to master their environments. His proposal led to a wealth of research (9-11,13,20-23) which has shown enough consistency that the main tenets can be summarized and used as a guide for future research and practice.

These principles can be stated quite simply as follows: We are intrinsically motivated to master our environment, whether it be social, intellectual, or physical. When we feel that our mastery attempts are successful, we feel *competent* and experience feelings of intrinsic pleasure and a desire to further master the task at hand. We particularly experience intrinsic joy when we perceive *self-determination*—a feeling that our successes were produced by our own efforts and were initiated through our own choice.

Conversely, if we fail to attain mastery over an aspect of our environment then we feel incompetent, and this, in turn, is associated with feelings of pressure and tension and a disinterest in further mastery attempts. These negative feelings are also produced, or exacerbated, if we perceive external causation. That is, a feeling that the main reason for doing a task is extrinsic—such as for pay, rewards, or because of coercion. In short, self-determined success increases intrinsic motivation, but external controls and/or lack of success undermine it.

Inevitably, life is more complicated than the simplified statement of a psychological theory, and it should be noted that an individual's *perceptions* of competence and causality are the key to his or her motivational outcome. However, this apparent complication has a positive aspect for teachers, because it provides extra scope for planning strategies to achieve positive motivational outcomes for students.

For example, the perceived competence (and thus the intrinsic motivation) of relatively unfit children is theoretically enhanced if the focus is put on their personal improvement at a task, rather than how they compare to other kids. Similarly, the perception of self-determined choice should be promoted if kids are allowed to choose from a range of alternatives—even if those alternatives have already been decided upon by the teacher! However, because theories do not always translate successfully into practice, it is wise to review results of previous attempts at application. Some of these efforts are described later.

Sound Theory or Dogma: What Educational Research Shows

The ideal way to judge the relevance of a psychological theory to a particular area is to test it in practice and evaluate the results. Because few studies have directly analyzed fitness motivation enhancement, physical educators themselves must examine the results of related research and make a professional judgment of its success and relevance. Two aspects are of particular interest:

1. How well did students learn the material taught?
2. To what extent were positive motivational and affective outcomes produced by the experience?

There is abundant classroom research literature about student learning that shows the effectiveness of meticulously explaining how to learn as well as what to learn. This teaching procedure is known as *direct instruction* and consists of setting and explaining clear learning goals, sequencing assignments, explaining and illustrating subject materials, monitoring progress, and providing frequent opportunities for students to practice what they have learned (16,31). In simple terms, it is a strategy for setting, achieving, and providing feedback on the attainment of learning goals.

Unfortunately, the effectiveness of this strategy in physical education is not so clear. The method appears very effective for teaching physical skills, however, there is some concern that it may limit students' creativity, autonomy, and affective feelings toward the learning (19). This seems logical in light of intrinsic motivation theory because of the emphasis on external control implicit in the concept of direct instruction.

However, other classroom research indicates that promoting a useful reason for learning the material may be a means of producing positive motivation and affect as well as enhancing cognitive gains. For example, research has consistently shown that asking students to learn in order to teach the material to others (peer tutoring) produces positive attitudes toward the task—besides academic benefits (6,31). Benware and Deci (4) specifically tested the effects of this "active learning" method on intrinsic motivation. The study showed clear academic and motivational benefits for the students who had used this method compared to those who had merely "passively" learned the material in preparation for an exam. Again, these results fit the theory because increased personal involvement in the use of the material shifts the perception of learning causality from external to internal.

The importance of the role of the teacher in determining the "motivational atmosphere" of the classroom has been shown in other studies. Deci et al. (12,14) rated teachers on the extent to which they promoted autonomy as opposed to exerted control over their students. They found that as time went by, the children of the autonomy-oriented teachers became more intrinsically motivated and had higher self-esteem than the children taught by the control-oriented teachers.

However, as mentioned earlier, it seems to be the perception of control that counts. In another study of control in the classroom, Koestner, Ryan, Bernieri, and Holt (26) found that informing children of the good reasons for limits on their behavior still allowed them to feel self-determined in their learning within the defined limits. Teachers merely avoided the use of controlling phrases like "should," "must," and "have to." Rather, they acknowledged the temptation and fun inherent in breaching limits while asking children not to breach them nevertheless. Thus being informational—not controlling—seems to promote a perception of autonomy.

These studies apparently support the applicability of the intrinsic motivation theory to classroom education—but do they apply to fitness education? Although there are only a few relevant studies in the fitness education domain, they also add support. An evaluation of the "Know Your Body" curriculum that District of Columbia elementary and junior high schools use to teach health-related concepts found that effective teachers produced measurable improvements in their pupils' physiological and behavioral cardiovascular risk factors (30). Effective teaching was judged by rating instructors on a list of variables that included direct instruction methods, attempts at promoting student involvement, observable teacher and student enthusiasm, and positive role modeling. Unfortunately, no direct measures of student affective or motivational change were made. It can be logically argued, however, that their improvements reflected positive attitudes and that their enthusiasm (which correlated with learning) showed positive affect and motivation.

Similar results were noted in a study of a curriculum designed to reduce the cardiovascular risk factors of 10th graders in northern California high schools (25). As in the previous study, beneficial changes were observed in the students' risk factor profiles. Measurable improvements in knowledge were also demonstrated, but motivational and affective improvement can only be inferred as before from the positive physiological and behavioral changes.

However, direct measurement of attitude was made in two other studies. Research in Florida high schools showed that a compulsory personal fitness course designed to enhance cognitive, attitudinal, and fitness parameters was successful in meeting its objectives. Significant improvements were shown in all three areas (27). Another study, and perhaps one of the most convincing in the scant literature, was a long-term follow-up evaluation of a compulsory college fitness education program. Several years after graduating, students who had taken the class showed positive attitudinal, knowledge, and physical activity profiles, compared to students who had not taken the class (because they had transferred traditional PE credit from another university or had "tested out" of the course) (29).

In summary, it appears that the education research reviewed does support the application of intrinsic motivation theory to fitness education. Of course other evidence would be desirable, even from outside the school classroom or gymnasium. Fortunately, there are other relevant data available from research on the reasons children give for voluntarily participating in physical activity.

Research on Physical Activity Participation Motives

Before looking at actual research, it is worthwhile to restate the expectations predicted by intrinsic motivation theory. We should expect to find that participants (as compared to nonparticipants) experience feelings of competence, intrinsic pleasure, and self-determination from their physical activity involvement.

Unfortunately, there has been little research with children on participation motives in planned exercise or fitness situations. In contrast, there has been a wealth of study on sports participation; and because an important product of sports involvement is improved physical fitness, this research has an obvious relevance. The available research literature is too vast to review comprehensively here, so only main references will be cited. Interested readers who wish more detailed information are recommended to use those as a starting point for further study.

In terms of the experience of intrinsic pleasure, studies have indicated that "fun" is a primary reason given by young athletes for participating in sports (17,28). Wankel and Kreisel (32) examined the determinants of this generic enjoyment motive in detail, and they found that intrinsic aspects of sport activity (such as excitement, personal accomplishment, and skill improvement) were the most important to enjoyment. Social factors (such as being with friends) were of secondary importance, and extrinsic factors (such as winning, getting rewards, and pleasing others) were of least importance.

The primary importance of experiencing enjoyment along with personal improvement and skill mastery clearly indicates that the need to feel competent is a motivator. In contrast, the low ranking of the extrinsic factors suggests that external control undermines the perception of self-determination.

These points are given added emphasis by studies of reasons for dropout from children's sports. In a summary of research on the problem, Gould (18) cited several common reasons given by children. Affect- and competence-related reasons for quitting included interest in other activities, lack of success, little skill improvement, and lack of fun or a feeling of boredom. Reasons that could be seen as likely detractors from a perception of self-determination included overemphasis on competition, competitive stress, and dislike of the coach.

These common perceptions align clearly with intrinsic motivation theory. However, an interesting corollary is the question of what leads to them, particularly where it applies to the possible ways that children may perceive and assess their own ability or competence. Research literature indicates three principal ways that children make judgments of their success in trying to achieve competence.

Ames and Ames (3) have neatly summarized these competence-judging orientations as (a) *competitive*, (b) *cooperative*, and (c) *individualistic*. In the competitive orientation, children assess their competence by comparing their performance to that of their peers. In the cooperative orientation, social interdependence is salient and may lessen the focus on competitive ability while promoting social approval within a group. In an individualistic orientation, attention is focused on personal improvement or task mastery over time. Because an individualistic (and, to some extent, a cooperative) orientation primarily depends on personal effort for success, professionals strongly prefer and advocate it over the more ability-dependent competitive orientation.

This supports intrinsic motivation theory; when perceived competence grows out of personal improvement, the likelihood of perceiving success is maximized by self-determined effort. In other words, competence is under one's own control. In contrast, with a competitive orientation, whatever the level of personal effort, someone else can deflate a person's perception of ability by performing at a higher level. Therefore, these different orientations of events are of great importance to fitness teachers and leaders. Wankel and Sefton's (33) recent study on fun in youth sports appropriately sums up the main points:

> A positive fun experience in sport is dependent upon an organizational structure wherein skill development is emphasized, realistic challenges are provided, success is determined largely in terms of personal skill mastery, and there is not excessive emphasis on winning (1989, p. 364).

Part Two: Guidelines for Practice

As the first part of this chapter has shown, recent developments in motivational theories and subsequent studies indicate that students who become intrinsically motivated will be more likely to take personal pride in the process of becoming physically fit. The challenge, then, is how to help students internalize motivation and take on responsibility for their becoming more active. This part of the chapter first offers guidelines for putting theory into practice and then examines the possible motivational outcomes of fitness testing.

From Concepts to Practical Suggestions

Almost 10 years ago in the midst of attempting lifetime fitness concept teaching in a high school PE curriculum, an unforgettable event happened. I had already noticed that maintaining discipline was much easier with the addition to the traditional curriculum of both classroom fitness education lessons and individual and lifetime practical activities. However, it was a surprise nevertheless when one particularly troublesome student, who tried to disrupt my explanation of the importance of cardiovascular exercise, was told by fellow students, "Shut up—can't you see we're trying to listen to this!"

No formal explanation of the basic elements of intrinsic motivation theory had been available to me at that time, but I could recognize a surge in student interest when I saw one. My teaching had actually become more engaging than the antics of the class clown! Several years later, relating theory to practice is easier, now having had the benefit of reviewing and applying the research literature. Hopefully, my summary of intrinsic motivation guidelines reflects this in a practical way:

1. Help all children *feel competent* at physical activity, exercise, and fitness. To do this, try to structure teaching sequences and learning evaluations relative to individual task mastery. Remember that peer comparisons of ability may be highly counterproductive, particularly to those children who need our help the most—those most unfit.

2. Promote *perceptions of self-determination* and choice in fitness activity and programming. Remember that, like most adults, children feel coerced when told what activities they must do.

3. Be *informational* rather than controlling when giving necessary directions or feedback, take care to explain the good reasons for and meanings of instructions and rules.

4. Kids are intrinsically interested in what they think is *important* to them personally. Foster children's interest in activity by making them aware of its benefits. This can range from helping elementary kids equate sports with fun to teaching the social, appearance, and health benefits of exercise to high school students.

5. Enhance the intrinsic pleasures of physical activity by heightening *interest, fun, and excitement* in exercise-learning and fitness-promoting situations. Don't unnecessarily turn healthful exercise into competition, drudgery, or punishment. It should feel like play, not work!

These guidelines take for granted that paramount among our fitness education objectives are goals such as helping the inactive to become active, helping the unfit to improve, and helping those who are or become fit to maintain a desirable level. With these objectives in mind, and with the demand for evaluation of educational aims today, the flowchart in Figure 8.1 further illustrates the main points of the guidelines and possible motivational outcomes of establishing and teaching a fitness education curriculum.

Notice that it is the students' perceptions of the teacher's style, the relevance of the material, and the evaluation of their own competence that predict the motivational outcomes. The importance of these points is bound up with the issue of when programs should produce fitness—now or in the future. If we are prepared to accept that fitness education should enable students to maintain fitness for life, then the significance of intrinsic versus extrinsic motivation and the ways of promoting one or the other become more apparent.

Quite simply, if fitness is something we "do" to children then they will probably quit when they grow up or we relinquish control of their lives. A similar result may also occur if we make children feel incompetent. It is easy to do both by setting up "boot camp" and making kids run laps and do push-ups, while lowering their sense of competence by telling them that they are unfit compared to the norm.

In contrast, working *with* children to help them learn and understand the importance of activity and fitness and to help them appreciate that sports and exercise are interesting and exciting fosters their desire to continue in the future. This may happen particularly if they feel that they have a choice in or ownership of their personal activity programs and if they feel confident that they have a capacity for mastering fitness through their own efforts in the future. It goes without saying that achieving this state of "fitness independence" requires a good base of fitness knowledge and skills.

In fairness to teachers and other youth leaders, it is often tough to achieve the latter happy state of affairs because of the constraints and pressures that commonly affect their teaching (15). For example, administrators may want to see action from the children now, but they may not be willing to provide the money, resources, and facilities that help add interest, excitement, and choice to the curriculum. Teachers then are almost forced to become extrinsic motivators lest they themselves be perceived as ineffective.

Perhaps one way to counter that problem is to use the strength of the research presented here to argue the case for educationally sound improvements and to counter conflicting motivational dogma. With that in mind, Table 8.1 has been included as an aid for understanding the meanings and expressions of an intrinsic versus an extrinsic motivational orientation toward children's fitness programs. A final caution: Personal experience has shown that there is a persuasive tendency to lapse into the language of the extrinsic motivator. It's well worthwhile rehearsing the words and expressions that connote intrinsic motivation before attempting the argument!

Fitness Testing: A Suitable Case for Analysis

The final section of this chapter discusses fitness testing as a means of achieving the fitness-related

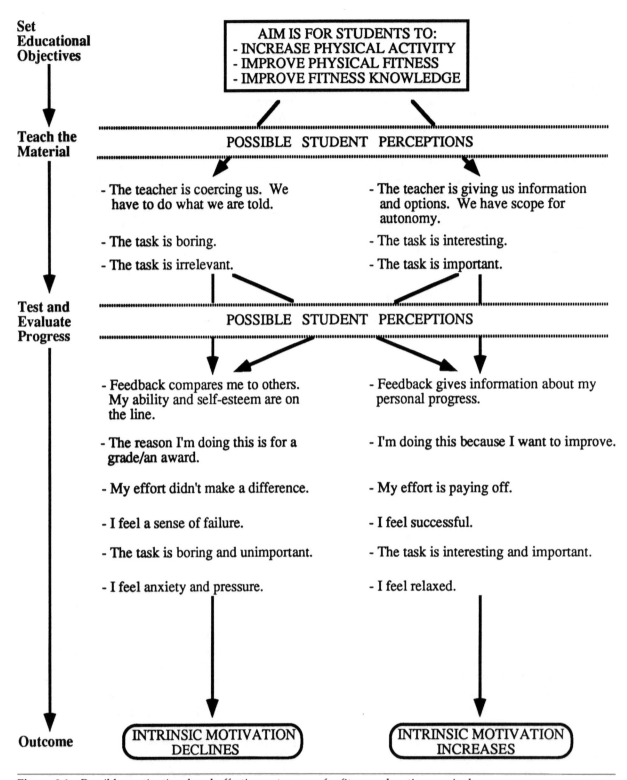

Set Educational Objectives

AIM IS FOR STUDENTS TO:
- INCREASE PHYSICAL ACTIVITY
- IMPROVE PHYSICAL FITNESS
- IMPROVE FITNESS KNOWLEDGE

Teach the Material

POSSIBLE   STUDENT   PERCEPTIONS

- The teacher is coercing us. We have to do what we are told.

- The task is boring.

- The task is irrelevant.

- The teacher is giving us information and options. We have scope for autonomy.

- The task is interesting.

- The task is important.

Test and Evaluate Progress

POSSIBLE   STUDENT   PERCEPTIONS

- Feedback compares me to others. My ability and self-esteem are on the line.

- The reason I'm doing this is for a grade/an award.

- My effort didn't make a difference.

- I feel a sense of failure.

- The task is boring and unimportant.

- I feel anxiety and pressure.

- Feedback gives information about my personal progress.

- I'm doing this because I want to improve.

- My effort is paying off.

- I feel successful.

- The task is interesting and important.

- I feel relaxed.

Outcome

INTRINSIC MOTIVATION DECLINES

INTRINSIC MOTIVATION INCREASES

Figure 8.1   Possible motivational and affective outcomes of a fitness education curriculum.

objectives of a physical education curriculum. This discussion particularly concerns the possible motivational outcomes of fitness tests and the award schemes that commonly accompany them.

As in the previous sections, the approach is based on evaluations using the intrinsic motivation theory: Does fitness testing increase children's perceived competence? Does it give them a perception

Table 8.1 Meanings and Expressions of Intrinsic Versus Extrinsic Motivation

Words that connote or promote feelings about motivation

Intrinsic	Extrinsic
Play	Work
Excitement	Tension
Fun	Pressure
Interest	Disinterest
Curiosity	Boredom
Importance	Irrelevance
Mastery	Incompetence
Success	Failure
Improvement	Deterioration
Choice	Coercion
Freedom	Constraint

Expressions of motivational mind-sets

Intrinsic	Extrinsic
"Let's help kids get fit."	"We must make kids fit."
"Let's help the kids motivate themselves."	"We have to motivate kids."
"Let's make exercise fun for kids."	"We must make the kids work harder."
"These are your exercise choices."	"You should/must do these exercises."
"This information will help you set goals and plan your exercise program."	"Your goal is to achieve X fitness level in Y weeks' time."
"These are the good reasons for taking part in an exercise program."	"You have to take part in this exercise program because I say so!"

of control? Does it highlight the importance of fitness? Are aspects of intrinsic motivation and pleasure—such as interest, excitement, and fun—a part of the experience of being tested? The first part of this analysis requires an examination of the reasons why fitness tests are used in the curriculum, because they could yield either or both positive and negative outcomes.

For example, if fitness tests are used to give personal relevance to fitness concepts, then they will have served an informational function and will most likely boost intrinsic motivation. Learning the concept of cardiovascular fitness by plotting heart rate responses to different work rates in a step test would be an example of this personalized learning approach. In contrast, if fitness tests are used for grade determination, or to identify winners of an award, then children are likely to perceive an extrinsic reason for doing them. In that case the tests would play a controlling function, and intrinsic motivation would likely decline (8).

The effect on children's perception of fitness competence is also largely dependent on how tests are administered and interpreted. In the past, norms and percentiles have been the most commonly used means of interpreting results. By definition, the use of norms means that children are ranked on ability against their peers. This almost forces children into a competitive orientation in judging their competence, and this has potentially serious motivational consequences for those who are relatively unfit. This concern has recently been supported by a study that clearly showed that receiving a low percentile ranking on a fitness test lowers children's intrinsic motivation (36).

Recently, there has been a move toward the use of criterion-referenced interpretation of fitness test results based on health, and minimal fitness standards associated with present and future health have been set (1,2,24). In theory this approach seems to avoid the competitive orientation of norm-based evaluation by emphasizing informational aspects and reducing peer comparisons; in practice, a note of caution is advised: An extrinsic motivation mind-set easily turns interpretation into evaluation by viewing health criterion scores as standards for passing or failing. Again, the potential danger of this, like norm-referenced interpretation, is that low-fit children may be made to feel incompetent, and, consequently, their intrinsic motivation may be reduced.

To avoid this trap, two suggestions are offered. First, carefully consider what is behind a focus on fitness testing. For example, when someone talks about fitness *testing* programs, they probably have in mind an extrinsic objective such as grading or awards, possibly at the expense of intrinsic motivation. However, when someone talks about fitness tests as part of fitness *education* programs, they are probably concerned about facilitating fitness learning and diagnosing fitness needs for exercise prescription and personal goal setting. In this case the potential for increasing intrinsic motivation is improved through the focus on information and individualized mastery. A second suggestion is to shift the primary emphasis of test interpretation from normative comparisons to explanation of the meaning of the score, its health implications, which is the concept of *interpretation zones* (35).

As an example, imagine that the three methods shown in Figure 8.2 are used to interpret a 12-min run score. The norm-referenced method would tell a child the percentage of his or her peers who are better or worse at the test. Use of the criterion-referenced method should tell a child the meaning of the score in terms of health risk but, in practice, is often interpreted in terms of passing or failing—perhaps because of the connotations of the term "criterion standard."

Because of this apparent confusion of meaning, the concept of interpretation zones is advocated here. It describes the probable intention of criterion-referencing. The interpretive focus should be on using the health implications of test scores to determine future fitness planning. Thus, in this example, an interpretation of a slow mile walk/run might include information about the difficulty of weight control when oxygen uptake is limited and the significance of coronary heart disease (CHD) risk at that level. At the other extreme, the cost–benefit ratio of potential health gain to injury risk would be a suitable topic for discussion with those who aspire to train to athletic performance levels of cardiovascular fitness.

The final aspect of fitness testing to consider is the use of awards. Ostensibly, awards are advocated as a means of motivating exercise behavior and fitness improvement. Unfortunately, there is mounting evidence that their use may do more harm than good, especially when they are linked to high percentile scores on a test. As well as producing an extrinsic focus on the reasons for actually doing fitness tests, it seems that most such awards are only "winnable" by children who already receive letters and medals for competitive athletics. This has led professionals to question whether or not this additional rewarding of the gifted is worth the potential motivational harm to other less fit children (7). It is worth noting in this respect that a recent evaluation of the percentile-based Canada Fitness Award scheme revealed that children tended to perceive those awards below the elite gold standard as virtual badges of demerit (5).

Other more recently constructed schemes have awards that are contingent on exercise behavior rather than high fitness levels. This approach is commendable for two reasons: The awards are available to all children on the basis of effort regardless of their initial fitness levels, and perceptions of self-determined individual mastery are facilitated by the personal effort involved.

In the final analysis, it seems that the role of awards should be viewed from the same perspective as the other aspects of fitness education discussed here. If awards are perceived as a recognition of self-determined mastery of exercise behavior and fitness achievement, then they may promote intrinsic motivation. If they are perceived as the major pay-off for fitness involvement (and it is worth pointing out that "award" and "reward"

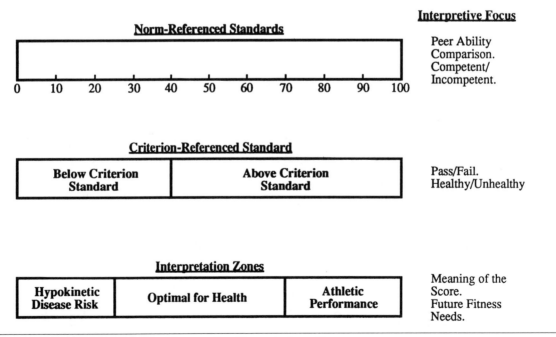

Figure 8.2   Three possible methods of interpreting fitness test results.

imply extrinsic motivation), then they may undermine intrinsic motivation.

Summary

If in theory and in practice intrinsic motivation is a key to making physical activity a lifelong habit, then working toward facilitating the internalization of student motivation and instilling in students a sense of accomplishment that comes from within is a proper goal for physical educators. Perhaps the best possible conclusion is to note that when intrinsic motivation for physical activity is present, awards, prizes, and payments become superfluous. The fun, thrills, excitement, and health benefits of sports, exercise, and physical activity in general are quite sufficient to keep us hooked for life. That happy state is a worthy goal to work toward cooperatively. However, let's not repeat decades-old mistakes. Let us form partnerships between schools, private organizations, and universities to plan model fitness education and enhancement programs for physical education. Above all, let's do it right this time by critically evaluating and improving as we go—otherwise we may simply replace old dogma with new. With those who are motivated it surely can be done.

References

1. American Alliance for Health, Physical Education, Recreation and Dance. Physical best: the AAHPERD guide to physical fitness education and assessment. Reston, VA: Author; 1989.
2. American Health and Fitness Foundation. Fit youth today: educating, conditioning, and testing students for health fitness. Austin, TX: American Health and Fitness Foundation; 1986.
3. Ames, C.; Ames, R. Goal structures and motivation. Elem. Sch. J. 85(1):39-52; 1984.
4. Benware, C.A.; Deci, E.L. Quality of learning with an active versus passive motivational set. Am. Educ. Res. J. 21(4):755-765; 1984.
5. Butler Research Associates. An evaluation of Canada fitness awards—interim report: phase 1. Report to the committee evaluating the Canada Fitness Award by Butler Research Associates; 1990 June.
6. Cohen, P.A.; Kulik, J.A.; Kulic, C.-L. Educational outcomes of tutoring: a meta-analysis of findings. Am. Educ. Res. J. 19(2):237-248; 1982.
7. Corbin, C.B.; Lovejoy, P.Y.; Steingard, P.; Emerson, R. Fitness awards: do they accomplish their intended objectives? Am. J. Health Prom. 4:345-351; 1990.
8. Corbin, C.B.; Whitehead, J.R.; Lovejoy, P.Y. Youth physical fitness awards. Quest 40:200-218; 1988.
9. Deci, E.L. Effects of externally mediated rewards on intrinsic motivation. J. Pers. Soc. Psychol. 18:105-115; 1971.
10. Deci, E.L. Intrinsic motivation. New York: Plenum Press; 1975.
11. Deci, E.L. The psychology of self-determination. Lexington, MA: Lexington Books; 1980.
12. Deci, E.L.; Nezlek, J.; Sheinman, L. Characteristics of the rewarder and intrinsic motivation of the rewardee. J. Pers. Soc. Psychol. 40:1-10; 1981.
13. Deci, E.L.; Ryan, R.M. Intrinsic motivation and self-determination in human behavior. New York: Plenum Press; 1985.
14. Deci, E.L.; Schwartz, A.J.; Sheinman, L.; Ryan, R.M. An instrument to assess adults' orientations toward control versus autonomy with children: reflections on intrinsic motivation and perceived competence. J. Educ. Psychol. 73:642-650; 1981.
15. Deci, E.L.; Spiegel, N.H.; Ryan, R.M.; Koestner, R.; Kauffman, M. Effects of performance standards on teaching styles: behavior of controlling teachers. J. Educ. Psychol. 6:852-859; 1982.
16. Doyle, W. Effective secondary classroom practices. In: Kyle, R.M.J., ed. Reaching for excellence: an effective schools sourcebook. Washington, DC: U.S. Government Printing Office; 1985.
17. Gill, D.L.; Gross, J.B.; Huddleston, S. Participation motivation in youth sports. Int. J. Sport Psychol. 14:1-14; 1983.
18. Gould, D. Understanding attrition in children's sport. In: Gould, D.; Weiss, M.R., eds. Advances in pediatric sport sciences. Vol. 2. Champaign, IL: Human Kinetics; 1987:p. 61-85.
19. Harrison, J.M. A review of the research on teacher effectiveness and its implications for current practice. Quest 39:36-55; 1987.
20. Harter, S. Effectance motivation reconsidered: toward a developmental model. Hum. Dev. 21:34-64; 1978.
21. Harter, S. A model of mastery motivation in children: individual differences and developmental change. In: Collins, W.A., ed. Aspects of the development of competence: the Minnesota symposium on child psychology. Vol. 14. Hillsdale, NJ: Erlbaum; 1981:p. 215-255.

22. Harter, S. Competence as a dimension of self-evaluation: toward a comprehensive model of self-worth. In: Leahy, R.L., ed. The development of the self. New York: Academic Press; 1985:p. 55-121.

23. Harter, S.; Connell, J.P. A model of children's achievement and related self-perceptions of competence, control, and motivational orientation. In: Nicholls, J., ed. The development of achievement-related cognitions and behaviors. Greenwich, CT: JAI Press; 1984:p. 219-250.

24. Institute for Aerobics Research. FitnessGram. Dallas, TX: Institute for Aerobics Research; 1987.

25. Killen, J.D.; Telch, M.J.; Robinson, T.N.; Maccoby, N.; Taylor, C.B.; Farquhar, J.W. Cardiovascular disease risk reduction for tenth graders. J. Am. Med. Assoc. 260:1728-1733; 1988.

26. Koestner, R.; Ryan, R.M.; Bernieri, F.; Holt, K. Setting limits on children's behavior: the differential effects of controlling vs. informational styles on intrinsic motivation and creativity. J. Pers. 52:233-248; 1984.

27. Rider, R.A.; Imwold, C.H.; Johnson, D. Effects of Florida's personal fitness course on cognitive, attitudinal, and physical fitness measures of secondary students: a pilot study. Percept. Mot. Skills 62:548-550; 1986.

28. Scanlan, T.K.; Lewthwaite, R. Social psychological aspects of competition for male youth sport participants: IV. Predictors of enjoyment. J. Sport Psychol. 8:25-35; 1986.

29. Slava, S.; Laurie, D.R.; Corbin, C.B. Long-term effects of a conceptual physical education program. Res. Q. Exerc. Sport 55:161-168; 1984.

30. Taggart, V.S.; Bush, P.J.; Zuckerman, A.E.; Theiss, P.K. A process evaluation of the District of Columbia "Know Your Body" project. J. Sch. Health 60(2):60-66; 1990.

31. U.S. Department of Education. What works: research about teaching and learning. Washington, DC: U.S. Department of Education; 1986.

32. Wankel, L.M.; Kreisel, P.S.J. Factors underlying enjoyment of youth sports: sport and age group comparisons. J. Sport Psychol. 7:51-64; 1985.

33. Wankel, L.M.; Sefton, J.M. A season-long investigation of fun in youth sports. J. Sport Exer. Psychol. 11:355-366; 1989.

34. White, R.W. Motivation reconsidered: the concept of competence. Psychol. Rev. 66:297-333; 1959.

35. Whitehead, J.R. Fitness assessment results— some concepts and analogies. JOPERD 60(6): 39-43; 1989.

36. Whitehead, J.R.; Corbin, C.B. Youth fitness testing: the effect of percentile-based evaluative feedback on intrinsic motivation. Res. Q. Exerc. Sport 62:225-231; 1991.

Chapter 9

Physical Fitness Education and Assessment: Addressing the Cognitive Domain

Clayre K. Petray
California State University, Long Beach

Physical fitness is an integral component of a quality physical education curriculum (1,2,3,22). The major goal of the fitness component of the physical education program is to provide students with the knowledge, attitudes, and skills that will allow them to develop healthy activity habits and will motivate them to continue appropriate activity in pursuit of physical fitness throughout life. To accomplish this goal, the cognitive, affective, and motor domains of learning must be addressed (6). In particular, it is essential for students to acquire the necessary knowledge to establish and maintain an active, healthy lifestyle (7,11,24,30).

The federal government's Department of Health and Human Services underscores the significance of the cognitive (or knowledge-based) domain in its document *Healthy People 2000* (36). For example, two objectives in the priority area of physical activity and fitness have the premise that knowledge about fitness is necessary for students to achieve optimal health (see Table 9.1).

Unfortunately, physical education programs that incorporate fitness knowledge throughout the curriculum are virtually nonexistent in the schools. Few physical education curricula include cognitive objectives that focus on enhancing students' appreciation of the role and value of exercise on physical fitness and health (3). Where health-related fitness concepts are taught, teachers rarely

utilize a preplanned, sequential approach (12). The cognitive domain can no longer be overlooked; cognitive teachings related to physical fitness are not only integral to the development of a physically educated person, they are critical to the health of our nation.

Table 9.1 *Healthy People 2000* **Objectives and the Cognitive Domain**

1.3 Increase to at least 30% the proportion of people aged 6 and older who engage regularly, preferably daily, in light to moderate physical activity for at least 30 minutes per day.

1.4 Increase . . . to at least 75% the proportion of children and adolescents aged 6 through 17 who engage in vigorous physical activity that promotes the development and maintenance of cardiorespiratory fitness 3 or more days per week for 20 or more minutes per occasion.

In the cognitive domain: Students must understand how to calculate their maximum heart rate for age and understand that light to moderate physical activity is performed at less than 60% of maximum heart rate for age, and that vigorous physical activity uses large muscle groups at 60% or more of maximum heart rate for age.

This chapter provides a structured approach for incorporating health-related fitness concepts into the physical education program at all grade levels. The comprehensive education plan included in *Physical Best: The Instructor's Guide to Physical Fitness Education and Assessment* (20) (see Figure 9.1) is utilized as a framework for incorporating fitness concepts into the program. Although this educational plan is included in the Physical Best program, this approach can be adapted for use with any of the fitness programs currently in existence. Although the focus of this chapter is on the cognitive domain, it should be noted that all three learning domains are interrelated and essential; one domain should not be sacrificed for another.

A Plan for Teaching Fitness Concepts

The Physical Best Comprehensive Educational Plan consists of nine phases that comprise a continuous cycle (20). Starting with Establishing Values and continuing through Evaluation, the cognitive domain should be addressed during each phase. Implications for the cognitive domain and specific examples of health-related physical fitness concepts that may be taught during each phase follow.

Establishing Values

The initial phase of the plan involves the identification of values upon which a program will be based. Corbin and Fox (7) have identified values that underlie the physical fitness component of the physical education program. Each of these values and its implication for the cognitive domain is shown in Table 9.2.

Establishing Objectives

Cognitive objectives for physical fitness are developed based upon the values. Corbin (5) has developed a taxonomy of objectives for health-related fitness. This taxonomy, described as the "Stairway to Lifetime Fitness," (see chapter 5 in this book) focuses on the importance of higher order objectives such as establishing personal exercise patterns, self-evaluation, and problem solving. Specific cognitive objectives covering the knowledge outlined in Table 9.3 must be developed at each grade level to enable students to climb the stairway and achieve the ultimate goal of physical fitness instruction, which is to educate and motivate students to establish and maintain a healthy lifestyle.

Preinstruction Physical Fitness Testing

Fitness testing conducted prior to the implementation of fitness activities should serve primarily as a

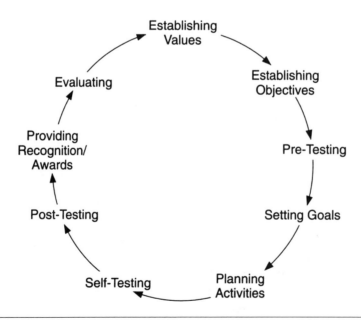

Figure 9.1 Physical Best comprehensive education plan.
Reprinted from *Physical Best Instructor's Guide* with permission of the American Alliance for Health, Physical Education, Recreation and Dance, 1900 Association Dr., Reston, VA 22091.

Table 9.2   Implications of Health-Related Physical Fitness Values for the Cognitive Domain

Value	Implication
1. Physical fitness is for a lifetime.	Students need to understand the difference between skill-related and health-related physical fitness and lifetime health.
2. Physical fitness is for everybody.	Students need to understand that fitness is not just for athletes; all people should lead active, healthy lifestyles. Every person can enjoy exercise and can achieve fitness for a healthy, active life.
3. Each person is responsible for her or his own fitness.	Students need to understand how to incorporate physical fitness into their own lives. They need the knowledge that will allow them to set up their own fitness program and to make wise fitness choices throughout their lives.

Table 9.3   Fitness Knowledge to Be Addressed in Grade-Level Objectives

1. *Why* exercise is important
2. *How* to develop and maintain health-related physical fitness
3. *What* one's personal exercise and fitness needs are

cognitive learning experience (6,13,15,19,24,31,38). Prior to and during this phase fitness concepts are taught, which may stimulate the desire for self-improvement and may help students in setting personal goals and planning individualized exercise programs. Concepts appropriate for inclusion in preinstruction testing experiences are identified in Table 9.4. Teaching these concepts during the pretesting phase establishes a comfortable atmosphere in which individual fitness levels, not peer comparisons, are the focus.

Setting Personal Fitness Goals With Students

Goal-setting experiences provide an opportune time to teach concepts, which ultimately lead to

Table 9.4   Fitness Concepts Taught During the Preinstruction Testing

1. Health-related physical fitness is a personal issue. Students are not compared to each other; individual progress is emphasized.
2. Fitness scores are confidential. Scores are used to help each student set personal fitness goals and measure his or her individual progress.
3. There are four major health-related physical fitness components: aerobic endurance, body composition, flexibility, and muscular strength and endurance.
4. Each fitness component is specifically related to lifetime health.
5. Each fitness test measures one of the health-related physical fitness components.
6. The criterion-referenced standards represent an estimate of minimal health standards. The standards differ depending on the gender and age of each student.
7. Interpretation of test scores is sometimes difficult. Each student's personal progress is what counts.

Table 9.5   Fitness Concepts Taught During the Goal-Setting Phase

1. Self-improvement is the focus: Goals are individual and confidential.
2. The student participates in the goal-setting process.
3. Goals are specific.
4. No more than one or two goals are set at one time.
5. Goals should not be difficult to achieve; they challenge, yet are within reach.
6. Opportunities to measure individual progress at various intervals will be provided.
7. Goals can extend beyond the scope of the health fitness standards to include participation in activity outside the school setting, improvement or maintenance of test scores, and the attainment of healthy standards, knowledge, and attitudes.

giving students responsibility for their own fitness (26). Table 9.5 identifies fitness concepts that students need to understand and be able to apply for positive, successful goal-setting experiences. When students begin to understand and apply these concepts, they become more aware of their own fitness levels and capabilities.

Planning and Implementation of Activities

The Planning and Implementation phase is the most extensive phase of the educational plan. Fitness concepts that should be included in this phase are presented in Table 9.6; the complexity of the information depends upon grade level and prior fitness experiences of the students.

When implementing health-related physical fitness activities, the teaching of physical fitness concepts should be planned as a continuum throughout the year. A daily, weekly, or monthly plan may be developed to ensure a sequential progression of fitness concepts. The Fitness for Life (9) program includes a weekly schedule for teaching fitness concepts to middle, junior high, and high school students; this schedule is organized in progression so that each concept or series of related concepts builds upon the previous concepts. Petray, Leeds, Blazer, and McSwegin (32) provide a plan for teaching fitness concepts to high school students that emphasizes a different major category of fitness each month. A preplanned approach ensures that concepts are introduced and reinforced sequentially.

Three methods may be utilized to provide a comprehensive approach for incorporating fitness concepts into the Planning and Implementation phase.

Table 9.6 Fitness Concepts Taught
During the Planning and Implementation Phase

1. Why physical fitness is important and its relationship to lifetime health.
2. The four components of health-related physical fitness.
3. How physical fitness is developed: the FITT guidelines (Frequency, Intensity, Time, and Type of exercise) and principles of exercise (overload, specificity, and progression) for each fitness component.
4. Safe and dangerous exercises.
5. Simple anatomy and physiology: skeletal system, muscular system, circulatory system, respiratory system, digestive system, and nervous system.
6. Nutrition as it relates to exercise (e.g., the relationship of exercise to energy expenditure).
7. Benefits of physical fitness.
8. How to evaluate personal fitness.
9. How to plan and carry out a personal exercise program.
10. Activity can be fun!

These methods, aimed at providing students with the understanding necessary to establish and maintain healthy lifestyles, are

a) to teach fitness concepts within the framework of the physical education class,
b) to integrate fitness concepts into other subjects in the school curriculum, and
c) to educate parents and the community about the value of regular activity.

Teaching Fitness Concepts Within the Framework of the Physical Education Class

A variety of strategies can be utilized to introduce and reinforce fitness concepts in the physical education class. Three recommended strategies are to

a) teach fitness concepts during activity,
b) conduct classroom lessons on fitness concepts, and
c) assign homework related to fitness concepts.

Teaching Fitness Concepts During Activity. Fitness concepts can be introduced and reinforced while students are active. This approach is most effective when the fitness concepts relate directly to the activities in which the students are involved. Concepts are brief and simple and are interspersed appropriately throughout the lesson. It should take no longer than 10 to 20 sec to explain a concept; complex concepts that take over 20 sec to explain are more difficult for students to learn and will result in decreased activity time for students. One major conceptual theme should be presented each day because students may be confused if numerous, unrelated concepts are presented during one class period.

Numerous strategies have been developed to teach fitness concepts during activity. For example, Kern (16) utilizes a jogging course that models the circulatory system; the students, acting as the blood, travel through the heart, arteries, and veins. Petray and Blazer (30) teach elementary school students about the changes in heart rate during activity. Prior to, during, and following vigorous physical activity, students feel their hearts beat and signal their pulse rate by opening and closing their fists. Leeds (32) teaches high school students the concept of recovery heart rate at the conclusion of an aerobic workout.

Conducting Classroom Lessons on Fitness Topics. Physical educators can reinforce and expand upon concepts taught during activity through a lecture and laboratory format in a classroom setting. The classroom is an appropriate environment for the following: self-evaluation work sheets, activity work sheets, the planning of personal fitness programs, discussions on fitness topics, and written quizzes and tests. Classroom lessons actively involve students in the learning process. A lecture and laboratory approach to teaching concepts that maximizes student participation has been developed by Corbin and Lindsey (8,9). It is recommended that teachers who see students 4 to 5 days per week schedule classroom lessons on a regular basis. Teachers who see students 1 to 3 days per week may utilize a classroom setting to teach fitness concepts in circumstances where inclement weather or other conditions restrict vigorous activity.

Assigning Homework Related to Fitness Concepts. Homework assignments related to fitness concepts involve implementing outside the school setting fitness concepts that have been taught during the physical education class. A variety of homework assignments aimed at motivating students to make physical fitness part of their lifestyle have been developed; these assignments may be oral, written, or physical. For example, Kopperud (17) implemented a take-home exercise program in which the student is given an exercise sheet to bring home; with assistance from parents or guardians, the student performs the activities listed on the sheet. Virgilio and Berenson (37) instituted the Superfit Exercise Log Book in which each student records the following information on a daily basis:

- Minutes of exercise
- Time of day
- Weather conditions
- Fitness activities
- Comments

Parent involvement in homework assignments is encouraged. The purpose of physical education homework assignments is to motivate students to incorporate fitness into their lives on a regular basis outside the school setting.

Supplemental materials may be used to instill fitness concepts in the physical education class. Elementary teachers may use educational materials such as the *Feelin' Good Series* (18). Secondary teachers may also use Feelin' Good as well as physical education textbooks such as *Fitness for Life* (9), *Moving for Life* (14), *Personal Fitness: Looking Good/Feeling Good* (39), and *Personal Fitness and You* (35).

Visual aids, such as pictures, posters, drawings, charts, task cards, transparencies, books, magazines, and newspaper articles may be used to enhance students' grasp of conceptual information (24,33). A physical education library may be established and computer software may be utilized. Individual learning centers may be set up so students can work independently with minimal teacher involvement (12).

Integrating Concepts Into Other Subjects in the School Curriculum

A multidisciplinary approach, in which the physical educator works with other faculty and staff in the school to coordinate the teaching of health-related physical fitness and to establish physical fitness as a schoolwide concern, may also be employed to teach physical fitness concepts. Many opportunities exist within the school setting for collaboration in teaching physical fitness concepts. School nurses, health educators, and other school personnel may join with physical educators in a team approach to fitness assessment (23,25,27,28).

A multidisciplinary approach can be implemented in a variety of ways. For example, on the elementary school level, the physical educator can collaborate with the classroom teacher to implement a Physical Education Notebook (34). When students return to the classroom after completing physical education class with the physical educator, the classroom teacher devotes part of a language arts lesson to writing in the Physical Education Notebooks. The notebooks, designed by the physical educator, include questions such as, What was your favorite activity today? What did you improve in today? What is the bone or muscle of the week, where is it located, and what type of action does it perform? and What is the fitness fact of the week? On the high school level, teachers of subjects such as health education, home economics, biology, and general science may provide discussions of the health benefits of exercise (25). A well-coordinated, schoolwide approach to teaching health-related physical fitness concepts will maximize the effectiveness of the physical educator in imparting fitness concepts to students within the school setting.

Educating Parents and the Community About the Value of Regular Activity

Physical fitness is not an objective that can be accomplished entirely in the school setting. If students are to make physical activity a part of their lifestyles, physical educators must educate the parents and community (6,11,20,36). The fitness concepts taught in physical education, as well as in other curricular areas, should be conveyed to parents. Parental involvement should be a part of students' homework assignments.

Numerous strategies have been developed for educating parents and community about the whats, whys, and hows of health-related physical fitness. Activities such as newsletters, family fitness contracts, parent nights, health fairs, fun runs, field days, and parent-volunteer programs have been used to educate parents and the community (4,29,30,37). Educating parents and community not only increases the effectiveness of the physical education program, it also serves as an excellent opportunity to publicize and promote the program.

Well-defined, intentional learning experiences related to physical fitness should occur both in and out of the physical education class. Although the teaching of physical fitness concepts begins in the physical education class, the physical educator will be most effective if the teaching of fitness concepts is coordinated schoolwide and if parents and community are educated.

Self-Testing

Physical fitness self-testing experiences provide students with the opportunity to learn how to measure and evaluate their personal fitness levels, both in and out of school (11,13,28). People who know how to evaluate their own fitness can determine their own fitness and exercise needs. During the self-evaluation phase of the program, students need to understand and apply the concepts listed in Table 9.7. Self-testing experiences that include

Table 9.7   Fitness Concepts Taught During the Self-Testing Phase

1. How to self-test each fitness component.
2. How to interpret criterion-referenced standards.
3. How to reevaluate and modify personal goals when appropriate.
4. Individual progress is what counts.
5. Grades should not be based on fitness scores; the self-testing process is more important than the product of test scores.
6. Dependence to independence—students learn that taking responsibility for their own fitness is important.

these concepts provide students with the knowledge necessary to ultimately take responsibility for their own fitness.

Postinstruction Testing

Physical fitness assessment held at the conclusion of the school year is used as a tool to facilitate the educational process; during this phase students are given the knowledge necessary to make intelligent decisions about their future health and fitness (11,13,38). During postinstruction testing experiences students need to understand and apply the concepts depicted in Table 9.8. Again, the *process* of evaluation is more important than the product of test scores.

Providing Recognition and Awards

The process of providing recognition for fitness goal achievement should be used as a learning experience that encourages lifetime activity rather than performance of arbitrary standards (10,20). Students need to understand the concepts presented in Table 9.9 to ensure that this phase is a positive learning experience. The concepts focus on the use of awards to recognize achievement; the *accomplishment*, not the award, is emphasized.

Evaluation

The Evaluation phase of the comprehensive plan functions as a process that allows teachers to determine whether or not objectives are being met in the cognitive domain, as well as in the affective and motor domains. Work sheets, questionnaires, exercise diaries, and written tests may be used to evaluate students' knowledge, understanding, and application of fitness concepts (8,9,21). This information is used to evaluate the effectiveness of the

Table 9.8   Fitness Concepts Taught During the Postinstruction Testing Phase

1. The emphasis is on individual progress—on the entire process of pretesting, goal setting, fitness activities, self-evaluation, and posttesting.
2. Testing at the conclusion of the program may be used to provide students with information concerning goal achievement.

Table 9.9   Fitness Concepts Taught During the Recognition Phase

1. The process of setting a goal, measuring progress, and reevaluating is to be emphasized.
2. If a goal is not attained, students should not give up. Goals can be reevaluated and modified if appropriate. Students can continue to work on a goal until it is achieved.
3. The process of setting fitness goals is similar to setting goals in life. Not all goals are achieved.
4. The focus is on the process of setting and attempting to achieve one's fitness goal rather than on the award.
5. The purpose of the awards is to recognize achievement of fitness goals. The award is not the focus of the goal-setting process.
6. Awards may be related to the fitness process or performance (17).
   A. Process
      1. Participating in regular exercise outside of the physical education class
   B. Performance
      1. Criterion: students understand rationale for criterion
      2. Goals for maintenance or improvement of fitness

program and can serve as a guide for making changes in the program.

Once the evaluation phase has been completed, the educational cycle continues. Values are reexamined; objectives are modified and changed when necessary. The educational cycle is continuous; it involves constant reevaluation and modification to meet the needs of students.

Conclusion

Physical fitness concepts aimed at teaching students to lead active lifestyles and to be wise fitness consumers should be part of each student's learning experience in physical education. Students should be taught the facts about exercise, how to evaluate their own fitness, and how to plan their own exercise programs. Students need to understand that physical fitness is an ongoing, lifetime process. Ultimately, the students are given the responsibility for their own fitness. Teachers help them along the way by using a comprehensive plan that establishes values and objectives, provides preinstruction fitness testing, helps students

set personal goals, carefully implements activities designed to help students achieve those goals, encourages self-testing and postinstruction testing, gives awards to recognize the students' achievements in the *process* of physical fitness, and provides for evaluation of the program. The physical education program can provide students with learning experiences that will enable them to achieve and maintain optimal personal fitness for life!

Acknowledgments

The author wishes to thank Margaret Leeds, Beverly Hills High School, Beverly Hills Unified School District, Beverly Hills, California, and Leslie Skow, Lincoln Elementary School, Newport/Mesa Unified School District, Costa Mesa, California for their assistance with the early revisions of this chapter.

References

1. American Academy of Pediatrics. Physical fitness and the schools. Pediatrics 80(3):449-450; 1987.
2. American Academy of Physical Education. The American academy of physical education newsletter. 8(1):6; 1987.
3. American College of Sports Medicine. ACSM opinion statement on physical fitness of children and youth. Med. Sci. Sports Exerc. 20(4): 422-423; 1988.
4. Bushnell, R. Witness fitness. Paper presented at the AAHPERD annual convention. Boston, MA; 1988 April.
5. Corbin, C.B. The fitness curriculum: climbing the stairway to lifetime fitness. In: Pate, R.R.; Hohn, R.C., ed. Fitness through physical education. Champaign, IL: Human Kinetics; 1994.
6. Corbin, C.B. Physical fitness in the K-12 curriculum: some defensible solutions to perennial problems. JOPERD 58(7):49-54; 1987.
7. Corbin, C.B.; Fox, K.R. Fitness for a lifetime. Br. J. Phys. Educ. 16:44-46; 1985.
8. Corbin, C.B.; Lindsey, R. Concepts of physical fitness with laboratories. Dubuque, IA: Brown; 1990.
9. Corbin, C.B.; Lindsey, R. Fitness for life. Glenview, IL: Scott, Foresman; 1990.

10. Corbin, C.B.; Whitehead, J.R.; Lovejoy, P.Y. Youth physical fitness awards. Quest 40(3): 200-218; 1988.
11. Espiritu, J.K. Quality physical education programs—cognitive emphases. JOPERD 58(6): 38-40; 1987.
12. Espiritu, J.K.; Loushrey, T. The learning center approach to teaching in physical education. Phys. Educ. 43(3):112-128; 1985.
13. Fox, K.R.; Biddle, S.J.H. The use of fitness tests—educational and psychological considerations. JOPERD 59(2):47-53; 1988.
14. Hennessy, B.; Monti, W.; Spindt, G. Moving for life. Dubuque, IA: Kendall/Hunt; 1991.
15. Jenkins, D.; Staub, J. Student fitness—the physical educator's role. JOPERD 56(2):31-32; 1985.
16. Kern, K.A. Teaching circulation in elementary P.E. classes—a circulatory systems model. JOPERD 58(1):62-63; 1987.
17. Kopperud, K. An emphasis on physical fitness—elementary physical education. JOPERD 57(7):18-22; 1986.
18. Kuntzleman, C. Feelin' good series. Reston, VA: AAHPERD; 1991.
19. McSwegin, P.J. Assessing physical fitness. JOPERD 60(6):33; 1989.
20. McSwegin, P.J.; Pemberton, C.; Petray, C.; Going, S. Physical best: the AAHPERD guide to physical fitness education and assessment. Reston, VA: AAHPERD; 1988.
21. Melville, S. Teaching and evaluating cognitive skills in elementary physical education. JOPERD 56(2):26-28; 1985.
22. National Association of Sport and Physical Education. COPEC position statement: physical fitness and physical education. Reston, VA: AAHPERD; 1986.
23. Parker, M.; Pemberton, C. Elementary classroom teachers—untapped resources for fitness assessment. JOPERD 60(6):61-63; 1989.
24. Pate, R. Teaching physical fitness concepts in public schools. In: Cundiff, D., ed. Implementation of health fitness exercise programs. Reston, VA: AAHPERD; 1985:p. 70-72.
25. Pate, R.; Corbin, C.; Simons-Morton, B.; Ross, J. Physical education and its role in school health promotion. J. Sch. Health 57(10):445-450; 1987.
26. Pemberton, C.; McSwegin, P.J. Fitting in fitness: goal setting and motivation. JOPERD 60(1):39-41; 1989.
27. Petray, C. Classroom teachers as partners: teaching health-related physical fitness. JOPERD 60(7):64-66; 1989.
28. Petray, C. Organizing physical fitness assessment for grades kindergarten through two: strategies for the elementary physical education specialist. JOPERD 60(6):57-60; 1989.
29. Petray, C. Physical Best: PR tool for the elementary physical educator. JOPERD 62(8):23-26; 1990.
30. Petray, C.; Blazer, S. Health-related physical fitness: concepts and activities for elementary school children. Edina, MN: Burgess; 1991.
31. Petray, C.; Blazer, S.; Lavay, B.; Leeds, M. Fitting in fitness: designing the fitness testing environment. JOPERD 60(1):35-38; 1989.
32. Petray, C.; Leeds, M.; Blazer, S.; McSwegin, P.J. Fitting in fitness: programming for physical fitness. JOPERD 60(1):42-45; 1989.
33. Sander, A.M.; Burton, E.C. Learning aids—enhancing fitness knowledge in elementary physical education. JOPERD 60(1):56-59; 1989.
34. Skow, L. Teaching strategies: cognitive concepts in physical education. Presented at the annual conference of the California Association of Health, Physical Education, Recreation and Dance. Long Beach, CA; 1990 March.
35. Stokes, R.; Moore, C. Personal fitness and you. Winston-Salem, NC: Hunter Publications; 1987.
36. U.S. Department of Health and Human Services Public Health Service. Healthy people 2000: national health promotion and disease prevention objectives. 1991. Available from: U.S. Government Printing Office. Washington, DC: (DHHS Pub. No. [PHS] 91-50213).
37. Virgilio, S.J.; Berenson, G.S. Super kids–superfit: a comprehensive fitness intervention model for elementary schools. JOPERD 59(8): 19-25; 1988.
38. Whitehead, J.R. Fitness assessment results—some concepts and analogies. JOPERD 60(6): 39-43; 1989.
39. Williams, C.; Harageones, E.; Johnson, D.; Smith, C. Personal fitness: looking good, feeling good. Dubuque, IA: Kendall/Hunt; 1988.

Chapter 10

Exercise for Children With Special Needs

Dianne S. Ward
University of South Carolina, Columbia

Children are by nature active, energetic people. Even without parental encouragement most children are busy learning and moving about the world around them. Infants explore their immediate environment with their hands and slowly gain voluntary control over their muscles. Shortly thereafter, infants learn to turn over, pull up to a standing position, and begin to interact physically with their world.

This chapter will focus on those children who, because of some cognitive or physical impairment, have experienced restricted physical activity contributing to an often reduced level of physical fitness. In the recent past, impaired children have frequently been discriminated against when programs of physical activity have been implemented. Increased emphasis on providing the child having special needs with opportunities similar to the nonimpaired has resulted in a greater emphasis on fitness programming for the impaired.

Principles and guidelines established for the development and implementation of fitness programs for the nonimpaired are also appropriate for children with unique needs (29). The material covered in this chapter will be presented in a *noncategorical* manner. Thus, no specific impairments will be discussed, but rather general guidelines are presented. In addition, a section of this chapter will deal with the low-fit and the overweight child.

Fitness and the Impaired Child

Physical fitness is composed of two types: *health-related* and *performance-related*. The purpose of health-related physical fitness is twofold: prevention of disease that could alter the quality of life, and rehabilitation of conditions that are currently affecting the quality of one's life. Performance-related physical fitness focuses on the acquisition of motor skills for better participation in sports and recreational activities. Although both of these aspects of physical fitness are worthy endeavors, this chapter will focus only on health-related physical fitness, because there are obvious rehabilitative benefits available for special children—which are beyond the scope of this chapter. For more information on performance-related physical fitness, the reader is referred to other sources (e.g., 11,29).

Children with impairments often exhibit low levels of physical activity, termed *hypoactivity* (2,26). A number of pediatric conditions have been linked with reduced physical activity. Bar-Or (2) divides these impairments into two categories: those in which hypoactivity is inherent and directly related to the impairment, and those that result in children having lower levels of physical activity incidental to the impairment itself. The first group of conditions creates physical limitations resulting in reduced physical activity; the second group results in restricted physical activity not caused directly by the impairment but imposed by external factors.

Impairments that affect the physical ability of children can reduce their participation in two ways: by a decreased health status, imposed by the condition itself, and by reduced physical activity that can result in additional health problems (2). For example, the child with arthritis faces pain caused by joint inflammation on a daily basis; the child with cystic fibrosis continually endures reduced respiratory function. A secondary impact of these conditions, which directly results from reduced physical activity, is increased risk of heart disease, potential for developing obesity, and susceptibility to other lifestyle-related conditions, such as hypertension, insulin-independent diabetes mellitus, and osteoporosis. These secondary conditions can be more debilitating than the original cause of the inactivity. Table 10.1 provides examples of childhood impairments that limit physical activity of children either by a physical or an incidental restriction.

Children with impairments tend to be less physically active than nonimpaired children (5). Reasons for this hypoactivity are numerous and often interrelated, including

- neuromuscular or structural impairments that limit efficient motor skill performance,
- cardiovascular impairments that limit endurance,

Table 10.1   Childhood Impairments Resulting in Hypoactivity

Direct physical restrictions of physical activity
  Juvenile arthritis
  Cerebral palsy
  Cyanotic heart disease
  Cystic fibrosis (severe)
  Scoliosis
Indirect restrictions of physical activity
  Bronchial asthma
  Cystic fibrosis (mild/moderate)
  Juvenile diabetes
  Juvenile hypertension
  Noncyanotic heart disease
  Obesity

Note. From *Pediatric Sports Medicine for the Practitioner* (p. 68) by O. Bar-Or, 1983, New York: Springer-Verlag. Copyright 1983 by Springer-Verlag. Adapted by permission.

- specific physical limitations that restrict movement,
- overprotective parents who restrict the child's involvement in normal play experiences, and
- lack of opportunities for strenuous physical activity.

High levels of physical fitness are necessary for many children with impairments to perform functional activities that nonimpaired children consider routine (6). To the physically handicapped child, getting dressed represents a major energy expenditure. The child walking with an above-knee prosthesis requires adequate cardiovascular efficiency to manage the increased energy demand of locomotion.

It has been assumed that impaired children, because of their physically exhausting daily routines, have high levels of physical fitness. However, this often is not true, because of the restricted level of activity and sedentary lifestyle. This reduced activity begins a spiral of reduced fitness that ultimately results in a decreased functional ability. For example, the young child who can self-ambulate with the aid of an assistant device often will be restricted to a wheelchair soon after adolescence. This reduced mobility is a direct result of a reduced level of fitness and a lowering of aerobic capacity associated with increased age (1).

Restriction of physical activity early in life reinforces a sedentary lifestyle later and often results in further limitations. It is critical to provide children with special needs numerous opportunities to successfully participate in physical activities to help obtain and maintain lifelong high levels of physical fitness.

Like nonimpaired children, children with special needs experience similar benefits from regular physical activity. In addition, exercise can facilitate rehabilitation and reduce the limitations of an impairment, thereby improving functional ability. Participation in regular physical activity has a number of benefits for children and youth, and these are summarized in Table 10.2.

The Impaired Child and Physical Education

A primary objective of the physical education program is to assist students in beginning and maintaining a regular pattern of physical activity. It is thought that from this regular physical activity

Table 10.2 Benefits of Regular Physical Activity for Children With Special Needs

General benefits	Specific benefits
1. Increased muscle mass and movement efficiency	1. Increased ambulatory ability
2. Better heart and lung efficiency	2. Improved range of motion in restricted joints
3. Greater endurance	3. Decreased incidence of contractures
4. Lower levels of body fat	4. Increased stamina for daily living
5. Increased flexibility	5. Change in calorie balance
6. Social opportunities	6. Improved lung function

students will limit unnecessary health problems and improve their functional ability.

For some time children with disabilities usually were excluded from PE by either medical or parental request. Some disabled children were excluded from the physical education program by the instructor who assumed the child could not effectively participate in the regular program; no alternative or special physical education was available. The implementation of Public Law 94-142 makes provision of appropriate PE for all students mandatory. Most professional physical educators and school administrators endorse the inclusion of children with impairments in the physical education program and continually seek ways of incorporating these children into the regular or an adapted program.

Even for nonimpaired children physical education programs have not been completely successful in improving physical fitness (4,28). Reasons for this poor showing are numerous, but one may be the generally high level of physical conditioning naturally existing in healthy children, leaving little room for improvements in performance. Children with impairments, however, due to poor entry levels of physical fitness, should be able to demonstrate significant strides in the development of physical fitness through the school physical education program—even more so than the nonimpaired.

Program Design

The development of physical fitness programs for children with impairments should have a primary purpose of improved functional capacity and increased habitual physical activity. Functional capacity is improved by appropriately designed and implemented *exercise prescriptions*; and increased physical activity in students is facilitated by *modifications* in the classroom learning environment.

Exercise Prescriptions

Training programs for impaired children should have characteristics similar to those for nonimpaired students. Prior to the development of a training program, however, teachers must execute three preliminary steps:

1. Assessment
2. Goal setting
3. Individualization of training

Table 10.3 illustrates how these processes should occur. Following these preliminary planning activities, the exercise prescription should be developed.

The components of health-related physical fitness include cardiovascular fitness, muscular fitness (strength, endurance, and flexibility), and body composition. The manner in which exercise is prescribed is specific to each of these components of fitness.

Cardiovascular Fitness. Cardiovascular training is appropriate for most children regardless of

Table 10.3 Planning Steps Prior to Exercise Training

1. Assessment
   - Execute appropriate health-related physical fitness tests, modified when necessary to meet the needs of the child.
   - Retest at certain intervals to monitor progress and reassess exercise prescription.
   - Record results in student folder.
   - Recognize achievement, no matter how small.
2. Goal setting
   - Go over the physical fitness test results.
   - Set goals for training in collaboration with students.
   - After each retesting, reevaluate student goals.
3. Individualized training
   - Develop individual prescriptions for each student based on fitness assessment and disability.
   - Allow for different paces among the children.
   - Use a variety of teaching techniques (e.g., station teaching, circuit training, and interval training).

condition. Students with cardiovascular impairments (e.g., children with Down's syndrome) should have specific prescriptions for exercise developed in conjunction with their physicians. Children who are ambulatory can use typical aerobic training techniques: fast walking, jogging, swimming, and so on. Nonambulatory students will be required to increase their metabolic demand using arm work, such as arm ergometry and wheeling (wheelchair mobility), or seated aerobics. Novel routines, developed for use with music, that employ continuous arm movement and the use of small dumbbells can be incorporated into the exercise program.

Muscular Fitness. Muscular training—endurance, strength, and flexibility—are important components of physical fitness. Many impaired students need additional muscular training to support ambulation, to counteract disease-related decrements, or to improve range of motion affected by impairment and inactivity. Specific activities such as resistance weight training can be used effectively to increase muscle strength and endurance even in young children (35). Flexibility is critical for many impaired students, particularly those susceptible to muscular contractures (e.g., children with cerebral palsy). Furthermore, impaired children are just as interested in improved body image as are the nonimpaired.

Body Composition. Excess body fat commonly seen in children with impairments is due to their lower potential for mobility and their correspondingly reduced physical activity. Impairments like spina bifida, juvenile hypertension, and chairbound cerebral palsy may result in excess body fat from reduced physical activity. The obese but otherwise healthy child has the need to alter body composition for fitness as well as for social reasons. In many cases, increased physical activity alone may not be adequate. It is suggested that some type of dietary education be incorporated with exercise for these children. Altering energy balance by increasing physical activity, however, is an excellent start.

An appropriate exercise prescription must include the principles for developing a training program: mode, dosage, and progression. The *mode* is the type of activity selected and should reflect the outcomes desired. If children with neuromuscular impairments need to develop muscular strength, they should be involved in progressive resistance activities (weight training). Overweight children who need to increase energy expenditure and cardiovascular endurance should have exercise prescriptions that include aerobic activities like walking or interval dancing.

The *dosage* of the exercise prescription is comprised of the frequency, duration, and intensity of the activity. Frequency and duration depend on the current level of conditioning of the child as well as the time available during class. Regular frequency (2-3 bouts a week) and reasonable duration (15-30 min) are necessary for increasing fitness. However, modifications in these guidelines may have to be considered when providing activities for the impaired child. Interval training has been used successfully with impaired children as a way to individualize the dosage of an exercise prescription (27). Intensity refers to the level of difficulty required. Although much has been written on the importance of establishing the minimum level of intensity (75%-85% of maximal heart rate or HRmax), controlling precise intensity with these children may, by necessity, be less feasible.

Progression in a prescription requires that the exercise begin gradually and be periodically monitored. For some conditions (e.g., cardiovascular impairments or asthma) the intensity of the physical activity must be carefully monitored. Children often have difficulty self-monitoring heart rate by palpation and may require excessive amounts of time for heart rate checks. The use of a self-rating scale such as the Borg RPE (ratings of perceived exertion) scale (7) has demonstrated promise for intensity control (3).

Examples of how principles of prescription modification may be applied with specific disorders are presented in Cases 10.1 and 10.2.

Modifications of the Learning Environment

Increasing the physical activity level for children with impairments requires fostering an enjoyable learning atmosphere with reasonable expectations for students. Franklin (14) gives a number of guidelines that may assist the physical educator in the development of fitness programs. Several important ones should be highlighted when working with children with special needs.

1. Use moderate-intensity exercise prescriptions.
2. Emphasize variety and fun.
3. Use behavior change strategies.
4. Chart individual progress.
5. Reinforce achievements.
6. Include modified recreational games for conditioning.

CASE STUDY #1

Billy, a 9-year-old boy with mild-to-moderate asthma, is enrolled in a regular physical education class that meets three times per week. As part of the fitness unit the teacher has designed an individualized program.

Assessment

Fitness test	Achievement	% rank
1-mile run[a]	n/a	n/a
Sit-and-reach	25 cm	60th
Sit-ups	29 in 60 sec	40th
Push-ups[b]	10 modified	n/a
Body composition	10 mm (2 sites)	90th

Goal Setting

Short-Term
1. To increase exercise stamina
2. To increase arm and shoulder-girdle strength
3. To improve abdominal strength and endurance

Long-Term
1. To decrease frequency of asthmatic events
2. To increase student's participation in movement-related experiences within the classroom and at home
3. To decrease the fear associated with exercise

Prescription Modification

Cardiovascular

Intensity: HR 160-180 bpm; RPE 12-14
Duration: Intervals of 6-8 min each
Frequency: 3 × week (class), 1 × week (home)

Muscular strength and endurance

Sit-ups: 30 sec trials, 3 × week
Weights: Dumbbell work, 3 × week: biceps, triceps, and deltoids

Comments

Exercise has been identified as a primary initiator of an asthmatic event, although participation in exercise programs is thought to improve the functioning of the asthmatic child (21). Exercise-induced asthmatic attacks usually *follow* exercise and can result in the child's reluctance to participate in future activity. It has been found that gradual increases in the intensity and duration of submaximal levels of exercise will not induce bronchospasm. Activities should be less than 8 min in duration, although the intensity can be up to 85% of maximal predicted heart rate (2). Cold air and airborne irritants (such as grass clippings) can increase the sensitivity of the asthmatic child. With physician approval, most children with asthma are able to participate in regular physical education class.

---

[a]Care must be taken when testing the cardiovascular fitness of children with asthma. Many currently used assessment techniques require an intensity and duration of activity that places the child at risk. It is suggested that the instructor rely on a subjective assessment of this measure or some submaximal (below 85% predicted HR) technique.

[b]No child-based norms available.

CASE STUDY #2

Sarah is a 12-year-old student with spina bifida who is enrolled in an adapted physical education class. She has been restricted to her wheelchair for several years. Her physical condition is well controlled, and the family physician encourages increased physical activity.

Assessment

Fitness test	Achievement	% rank
Arm cranking test[a]	50 RPM, 4 min	n/a
Dumbbell lift	Bicep curls, deltoid lifts, and overhead lifts (5 × 2 lb)	15th
Body composition	40 mm (sum of 2 sites)	15th

Goal Setting

Short-Term

1. To improve arm-cranking time to 10 continuous min
2. To increase the number of dumbbell lifts by 50%
3. To decrease skinfold thickness by 2 mm

Long-Term

1. To increase participation in regular physical activity when not in school
2. To increase knowledge about weight control

Prescription Modification

Cardiovascular

Intensity: HR 130-150 bpm; RPE 12-14

Duration: Intermittent arm cranking; 2 min bouts, increasing to 3 min each, with 1 min rest between; 15-20 min total

Frequency: 5 × week (class)

Muscular strength and endurance

Arm and shoulder-girdle activity using small dumbbell weights (2-5 lb)

Comments

Children with spina bifida often are ambulatory (with crutches or braces), but many use wheelchairs. In either case, arm and shoulder-girdle strength and endurance are extremely important. Consultation with the school district's physical therapist can provide pertinent information about which muscles to target. Use of a weight-training program (specific number of sets and repetitions) or a musical dumbbell program (like aerobic dance using small-weight routine performed to music) can be very effective. Obesity in chair-bound children often results in youth with excess body fat. Some type of weight-control intervention may be useful.

---

[a]Arm cranking can be executed on a modified arm ergometer constructed from a bicycle crank mounted on an adjustable table. Many school districts have woodshop classes that are able to create adapted equipment.

---

7. Establish a regular workout schedule.
8. Test fitness periodically to assess the program.
9. Use music during training.
10. Use group exercise opportunities.

Guidelines 1 through 5 will now be considered more fully.

Using Moderate-Intensity Prescription. Developing exercise prescriptions requires selection of the proper dosage of exercise. Frequency and duration are easily quantifiable. The conventional standard of 3 days a week, 20 min a day is typically employed in the development of physical fitness. Intensity, however, is more difficult to prescribe.

Research has demonstrated that children and adults alike respond better to a level of intensity that they perceive is not too difficult for them. If an educator uses the standard 75% to 85% HRmax for training the impaired, early drop-out or noncompliance may result (12,13). Also, it is well known that injury results from exercise that is too difficult for the performer.

Emphasizing Fun and Variety. Fitness programs for all young people should emphasize fun and variety. Class activities should have gamelike qualities. Unlike adult fitness programs that employ discipline and individual motivation, children enjoy physical activity because of its playlike atmosphere. Teachers should take games and modify them for purposes of conditioning (see 19). Aerobic games can be developed from typical elementary activities such as "Musical Hoops"—a game that requires students to move between hoops placed on the floor until the music stops. The addition of music to exercise training always improves classroom atmosphere, particularly music that children themselves recommend.

Using Behavior Change Strategies. Adherence to exercise programs is influenced by the social context in which exercise is carried out. Few studies have investigated the school as a social support network for behavior change. Other social support sources such as family, friends, and the work site have been observed and found to be powerful mechanisms for assisting in behavior change. School programs could use approaches taken from the workplace or community. One such example is Bell Telephone, which formed exercise groups with its employees and reinforced attendance at weight-control group meetings (9).

Poor adherence to an exercise program is a predictable consequence of the lack of prompt rewards. Exercise for the novice also has several immediate, negative consequences, such as discomfort, soreness, and awkwardness. The positive benefits such as weight loss, improved health, and feeling better are less immediate. More immediate awards such as stickers, certificates, and class recognitions can be designed to maximize adherence (10,22).

Charting Progress and Rewarding Achievement. Children usually need only opportunities, not motivational techniques, to be physically active. This may not be the case with the low-active or low-fit youngster. As children approach adolescence, however, even healthy youth begin to demonstrate a decline in activity level. Therefore, both

physical condition and age can contribute to the decline in physical activity level observed with impaired youth. Rowland (26) lists a number of suggestions for motivating children and adolescents to exercise (see Table 10.4) and suggests that if children can be motivated to exercise during class, eventually they will participate in physical activity at will—apart from the request of someone else.

Changing behavior requires constant attention to progress, achievement, and recognition. Children who have special exercise needs require the same techniques as others when attempting to alter physical fitness levels and habitual physical activity. Setting short-term goals works best for children. Following some type of assessment, exercise goals should be set in collaboration with the students themselves. This works better than teachers setting goals for students.

After the goal is set, some type of progress charting system should be used. This could be a poster or a bulletin board or individual progress sheets where the teacher or the student records daily achievements. Recognizing progress also is necessary. Certificates of achievement can be made by the teacher using clip art or magazine cut-outs arranged on a form and photocopied for the students (see Figure 10.1). It matters little whether the award says "Most Steady Walker" or "Physical Fitness Weekly Award." Children enjoy and benefit from regular recognition of their progress.

Organizational Considerations

The most difficult problem facing the physical educator in aiding the exercise-impaired youth is the

Table 10.4 Factors in Motivating Children to Exercise

Positive	Negative
Fun	Discomfort
Success	Failure
Peer support	Embarrassment
Family involvement	Competition
Variety	Boredom
Supportive leaders	Injuries
Freedom	Regimentation

Note. From *Exercise and Children's Health* (p. 267) by T.W. Rowland, 1990, Champaign, IL: Human Kinetics. Copyright 1990 by Thomas W. Rowland. Adapted by permission.

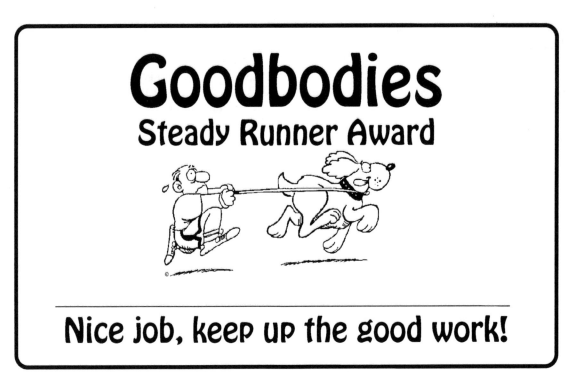

Figure 10.1   Example of award certificate used for motivation and reinforcement in an ongoing weight-control program for children—The Goodbodies Program. (Reprinted from reference 17.)

problem of heterogeneity in the classroom. Within a group of healthy children there are normally wide ranges of physical abilities. When impaired children are included within the regular PE class, the range of abilities widens significantly, thus placing demands on the teacher beyond the scope of normal instructional planning. There are instances when the impaired child cannot be provided an opportunity to succeed during a regular physical education class, and there are other times when the child can easily be integrated into the regular class. Many factors contribute to the success of mainstreaming the impaired child into the regular PE environment, including the ability level of the child and the willingness of the instructor to individualize instruction.

Consideration must be given first to which environment will benefit the child most. Whenever possible, the exercise-impaired child should be instructed within the regular class. Provision of special or adapted physical education should be restricted to those children who because of their impairment cannot successfully participate in the regular class. A third option, not typically viewed as part of the physical education teacher's primary duties, is the multidisciplinary program or after-school program. Just as there are after-school opportunities for the child who excels in sport, special

programs after school designed to remediate the low fit may work well. In some instances the physical education teacher may work with the guidance counselor, the school nurse, district dietician, or a local pediatrician to provide a special in-school program designed specifically for a special needs group. This type of program has worked well for obesity intervention (8,31,34). Table 10.5 describes possible program structures.

Efforts to individualize exercise training require thorough planning. Accommodating the child with special needs is no different than planning for individual differences. When low-fit students are present within a regular physical education class, the teacher should plan for activities and exercise prescriptions that allow all students to improve physical functioning at an individual rate. Use of station teaching, circuit training, drill sheets, or task cards can aid in personalizing the program. Sherrill (27) details the idea of using interval training with individuals or small groups. Students are given Interval Training Prescriptions (ITP) that list the specific activities and number of repetitions required. This technique can work well when a class contains many levels of physical conditioning.

Special PE classes work best for many students with special fitness needs. However, physical fitness education and training must be included as

Table 10.5 Program Structures for Children With Special Needs

Program structure	Description
In class	Children of all ability levels are integrated into the regular physical education program.
Special class	Children with special needs are provided a separate class.
In-school program	Program provided within the school day by a group of school professionals.
After-school program	Program provided by the physical education teacher or a group of school professionals immediately after school.

part of these classes. The inclusion of physical fitness education into the special physical education curriculum is crucial to these students' quality of life and sense of well-being.

The Low-Fit and Overweight Child

Estimates of the prevalence of obesity among childhood populations range from a low of 10% to as high as 25% (15). Obesity is considered the leading nutritional disorder in developed countries (20). As previously discussed in this chapter, a child with an impairment often exhibits lower levels of fitness due to reduced physical activity. Commonly this decreased activity also results in a child who exhibits difficulty controlling weight.

Childhood obesity is a problem that continues to plague American youngsters, and indications are that the levels of body fat in children are increasing. A study by Gortmaker (18) and recent evidence obtained in the National Youth Fitness surveys (24,25) confirm that American children are getting fatter. It is unclear whether this phenomenon is caused by increased calorie consumption, choice of calories, low energy expenditure, or some genetic factor. It is clear, however, that obesity affects physical activity and physical fitness.

Obese children usually score low on the cardiovascular component of physical fitness tests. Older

children and adolescents find PE classes troublesome and often exclude themselves from participation by "sitting out" or not dressing. In some cases antisocial behavior toward the teacher or classmates results. Younger children who have weight problems still want to participate but are often ridiculed by their classmates during times when their physical differences are more apparent.

The physical education teacher can be an important influence in the attitude toward physical activity that the overweight or obese youth develops. When an individual carries excess body weight as adipose tissue, this weight contributes nothing to the energy production process, but adds a considerable burden. Obese children may complain about the difficulty of an activity. Erroneously, teachers may feel that these objections are part of the problem, that this child is simply lazy.

Studies comparing exercise perception between overweight and nonoverweight adolescents found that obese youth rate exercise similarly to normal-weight youth (32) and that, in fact, during weight-bearing activities (walking or running) overweight children worked harder at a given exercise prescription than required (30). It is important that overweight children feel support rather than disapproval from the physical education teacher.

Experts are in agreement as to the benefits of increased physical activity and physical fitness for overweight youth—improved functional capacity, greater social acceptance, and regular caloric expenditure, all of which can contribute to weight loss. However, there is no general consensus on accommodating these children within the physical education program.

Selecting a training regime for the overweight child requires some adaptation of the exercise prescription. The modes of exercise should be primarily aerobic but can take any form. Activities such as walking, interval jogging, aerobic dance (either continuous or interval), or aerobic games work well with children. Teachers should resist prescribing adult-like activities for children. Self-motivation to exercise does not exist in these children and an element of fun must be included.

Duration of exercise depends on the child's current level of functioning, and frequency depends on the time limitations of the physical education class. Progression of a prescription will depend on the initial fitness level of the child, the time available for training, and the child's own motivation. Getting the child to *like* being active is more important than fulfilling an exercise guideline.

The most important adaptation to the exercise prescription is the modification of the intensity component. Due to their low fitness status and general inexperience with exercise, a low level of intensity (50%-60% HRmax, HR 120-150 bpm) works better with these children. Because heart rate is sometimes difficult for children to palpate, ratings of perceived exertion (RPE) using some type of scale has been suggested (3,30). Instead of giving children a range of HR beats, children are given a range of numbers representing a level of exertion. The Borg scale (7) has been used successfully for prescribing exercise to overweight children (30), although adjustments are suggested for weight-bearing activities (33). Stick figures accompanying the RPE numbers have also been used (23). (See Figure 10.2 for a copy of the Borg scale and Table 10.6 for prescription suggestions.)

Changing habits requires that, in addition to developing fitness and having fun within the physical education class, teachers should attempt to

6	**No exertion at all**
7	
	Extremely light
8	
9	**Very light**
10	
11	**Light**
12	
13	**Somewhat hard**
14	
15	**Hard (heavy)**
16	
17	**Very hard**
18	
19	**Extremely hard**
20	**Maximal exertion**

Figure 10.2 The Borg scale.
Note. From "Psychophysical bases of perceived exertion" by G. Borg, 1982, *Medicine and Science in Sports and Exercise,* **14,** pp. 377-387. Copyright 1982 by ACSM. Reprinted by permission.

Table 10.6   Use of the Borg Scale for Exercise Prescription With Overweight Children

---

Basic Assumptions

The child has adequate cognitive ability to understand the scale.
* Children age 9 years and above may be able to use the scale effectively. Younger ones may be able to use the scale with careful training.

Teacher will take time to instruct students on what the scale means and how to use it.
* Children need instruction on using the scale, but the extent of need will depend on age and experience.

Prescribing Intensity

Children rate exercise at levels slightly lower than do adults.
* ACSM guidelines indicate that RPE 11 to 16 is approximately equivalent to 50% to 75% max. When prescribing intensity using RPE, use an RPE between 10 and 15.

Overweight children tend to run at speeds faster than required when using RPE to control intensity.
* If jogging or running is the mode of exercise, use a slightly lower RPE prescription.

---

develop exercise *habits* in overweight and obese youth. This is more difficult than the in-class instruction but overall may be more important to include. One way to develop exercise habits is to use an activity contract. An activity is assigned for the weekend (or days without physical education class) using the exercise prescription as homework, extra credit, or simply as enrichment. Parents are asked to validate the activities to develop accountability. Figure 10.3 shows examples of activity contracts from an ongoing weight-control program (see 17, The Goodbodies Program).

The school can be an important agent for change in the overweight or obese child. (For a thorough review of the role of the school in the treatment of obesity, see 31). It should be noted that the most important roles the school physical education program can play are primary obesity prevention for all children and early intervention for children with moderate degrees of overweight or obesity. The school setting, however, may not be adequate for treating the severely obese child who needs intensive, long-term diet and exercise therapy (16).

At-Home Activity Contract

THE GOODBODIES PROGRAM

Name:_____

Time period: From: ___/___/_____   To: ___/___/_____

Cardiovascular

Activity: Walking, bike riding, jogging, or skating

Time: <u>15 continuous minutes</u>

No. of repetitions: _____once_____

Muscle Fitness

Body helpers: Sit-ups and push-ups

Time: _____1 min each_____

No. of repetitions: _____2 each_____

Recreational

Activity: Select an activity of your choice

Time: _____30 min_____

No. of repetitions: _____once_____

Activity selected: _____

I,_____, agree to engage in the above activities under the conditions specified and will record information accurately and honestly.

Student's signature: _____ Date: _____

Parent's signature: _____ Date: _____

Figure 10.3 Example of an activity contract to be used by physical education instructors to increase physical activity adherence. The Goodbodies Program (reference 17) is an ongoing weight-control program for children.

Summary

Physical activity is an integral component in the life of a child. Children learn about themselves and their environment when they are active. Physical impairments can rob children of a fundamental need—the need to be physically active. Physical education programs can assist children who show decreased levels of physical activity by providing opportunities to improve physical fitness. The health-related components of physical fitness (cardiovascular fitness, muscular fitness, flexibility, and body composition) should be emphasized in order to improve the child's exercise capacity.

Assessment, goal setting, and individualization of training should be completed for each child based on the impairment. The learning environment must be modified to encourage ongoing participation. Children with special fitness needs may be accommodated within the regular PE program, but in many cases, specially adapted physical education programs are necessary. Making physical activity a habit is the ultimate goal of the physical education program. This goal is even more important when the child is limited by a health condition.

Acknowledgments

Special thanks are given to Dr. Bruce McClenaghan for his careful review and suggestions for this chapter.

References

1. Anderson, D.A.; Levine, A.A.; Gellert, H. Loss of ambulatory ability in patients with old anterior poliomyelitis. Lancet 2:1061-1063; 1972.
2. Bar-Or, O. Pediatric sport medicine for the practitioner: from physiologic principles to clinical applications. New York: Springer-Verlag; 1983.
3. Bar-Or, O.; Ward, D.S. Ratings of perceived exertion in children. In: Bar-Or, O., ed. Advances in pediatric sport sciences. Vol. 3. Champaign, IL: Human Kinetics; 1989: p. 151-168.
4. Bar-Or, O.; Zwiren, L. Physiological effects of increased frequency of physical education classes and of endurance conditioning on 4- to 10-year-old girls and boys. In: Bar-Or, O., ed. Pediatric work physiology. Natanya, Israel: Wingate Institute; 1971:p. 183-198.
5. Blair, S. Physical activity leads to fitness and pays off. Phys. Sportsmed. 13:153-157; 1985.
6. Blair, S.; Pate, R.R.; McClenaghan, B. Current approaches to physical fitness education. In: Kratockwill, T.R., ed. Advances in school psychology. Vol. 2. Hillsdale, NJ: Erlbaum; 1982: p. 315-361.
7. Borg, G. Physical work and effort. Oxford: Pergamon, 1977.
8. Brownell, K.D.; Kaye, F.S. A school-based behavior modification, nutrition education, and physical activity program for obese children. Am. J. Clin. Nutr. 35:277-283; 1982.
9. Brownell, K.D.; Stunkard, A.J. Physical activity in the development and control of obesity. In: Stunkard, A.J., ed. Obesity. Philadelphia: Saunders; 1980:p. 300-324.
10. Brownell, K.D.; Stunkard, A.J. Behavioral treatment of obesity in children. Am. J. Dis. Child. 35:277-283; 1982.
11. Corbin, C.; Lindsey, R. Fitness for life. Glenview, IL: Scott, Foresman; 1985.
12. Dishman, R.; Dunn, A.L. Exercise adherence in children and youth: implication for adulthood. In: Dishman, R.K., ed. Exercise adherence: its impact on public health. Champaign, IL: Human Kinetics; 1988:p. 155-202.
13. Epstein, L.H.; Koeske, R.; Wing, R. Adherence to exercise in obese children. J. Cardiac Rehabil. 4:185-195; 1984.
14. Franklin, B.A. Program compliance. In: Storlie, J.; Jordan, H.A., eds. Behavioral management of obesity. New York: Spectrum Publications; 1984:p. 115-128.
15. Forbes, G.B. Prevalence of obesity. In: Bray, G., ed. Obesity in perspective. Vol. 2. Washington, DC: U.S. Government Printing Office; 1975: p. 75-78.
16. Foster, G.D.; Wadden, T.A.; Brownell, K.A. Peer-led program for the treatment and prevention of obesity in the schools. J. Consul. Clin. Psychol. 53:538-540; 1985.
17. The goodbodies program. Unpublished document by Dianne Ward. University of South Carolina.
18. Gortmaker, S.L.; Dietz, W.H.; Sobol, A.M.; Wehler, C.A. Increasing pediatric obesity in the United States. Am. J. Dis. Child. 141:535-540; 1987.
19. Graham, G.; Holt-Hale, S.; Parker, M. Children moving: a teacher's guide to developing a successful physical education program. 2nd ed. Palo Alto, CA: Mayfield; 1987.

20. Mayer, J. Overweight: causes, cost and control. Englewood Cliffs, NJ: Prentice Hall; 1968.
21. McClenaghan, B.; Balog, L. Exercise and the asthmatic child. S.C. J. Health, Phys. Ed., Rec. Dance 15:11-13; 1982.
22. McClenaghan, B.; Ward, D.S. Health and physical education. In: Maher, C.A.; Forman, S.G., eds. A behavioral approach to education of children and youth. Hillsdale, NJ: Erlbaum; 1987:p. 131-151.
23. Nystad, W.; Oseid, S.; Mellbye, E.B. Physical education for asthmatic children: the relationship between changes in heart rate, perceived exertion, and motivation for participation. In: Oseid, S.; Carlsen, K.-H., eds. Children and exercise XIII. Champaign, IL: Human Kinetics; 1989:p. 369-377.
24. Ross, J.G.; Gilbert, G.G. The national children and youth fitness study: a summary of findings. JOPERD 56:45-50; 1985.
25. Ross, J.G.; Pate, R.R. The national children and youth fitness study II: a summary of findings. JOPERD 58:51-56; 1987.
26. Rowland, T.W. Exercise and children's health. Champaign, IL: Human Kinetics; 1990.
27. Sherrill, C. Adapted physical education and recreation. Dubuque, IA: Brown; 1986.
28. Shephard, R.J.; Lavallee, H.; Jéquier, J.-C.; Rajic, M.; LaBarre, R. Influence of added activity classes upon the working capacity of Quebec schoolchildren. In: Lavallee, H.; Shephard, R.J., eds. Frontiers of activity and child health. Quebec: Pelican; 1977:p. 237-245.
29. Short, F. Physical fitness. In: Winnick, J., ed. Adapted physical education and sport. Champaign, IL: Human Kinetics; 1990:p. 301-314.
30. Ward, D.S.; Bar-Or, O. Use of the Borg scale in exercise prescription for overweight youth. Can. J. Sport Sci. 15:120-125; 1990.
31. Ward, D.S.; Bar-Or, O. Role of the physician and physical education teacher in the treatment of obesity at school. Pediatrician 13:44-51; 1986.
32. Ward, D.S.; Bar-Or, O.; Blimkie, C.R.J. Rating of perceived exertion in obese adolescents. Med. Sci. Sports Exerc. 18:s72; 1986.
33. Ward, D.S.; Jackman, J.; Galiano, F. Exercise intensity reproduction: children vs. adults. Pediatr. Exerc. Sci. 7:24-30; 1991.
34. Ward, D.S.; McClenaghan, B.A. Special programs for special people: ideas for extending the physical education program. Phys. Educ. 37:63-68; 1980.
35. Weltman, A. Weight training in prepubertal children: physiologic benefit and potential damage. In: Bar-Or, O., ed. Advances in pediatric sports sciences. Vol. 3. Champaign, IL: Human Kinetics; 1989:p. 101-129.

Chapter 11

Fitness Programming and the Low-Fit Child

Patricia J. McSwegin
University of Missouri, Kansas City

Not all children are physically fit. Fortunately, even low-fit children can benefit from a well-planned and carefully executed physical education program. This chapter focuses on designing physical education programs that are effective in helping low-fit children overcome their fitness problems. This chapter presents a definition of the term *low-fit children*, reviews the reasons for being concerned about low fitness, outlines a systematic way to organize an effective fitness education program, and offers suggestions for modifying activity for various fitness conditions.

Who Are the Low-Fit Children?

The major surveys on youth fitness (2, 3, 4, 5) reveal two common findings. First, many children and youths are fairly fit, especially in the areas that support sport participation (i.e., speed, agility, power, etc.). Second, a sizeable percentage of children and youths (perhaps 30%) rate low in two key aspects of fitness related to health: namely, body composition and aerobic endurance. The surveys, which assessed youth activity habits and fitness patterns as well as fitness per se, reveal students have an alarming lack of knowledge about fitness, lack skill in solving fitness problems, and do not understand the need for an active lifestyle. These data indicate that many of the children who

score well currently on fitness tests might be at risk of diminished fitness status later in life because they do not know how to sustain fitness. Nor are they aware of the implications of remaining or becoming sedentary.

Simply administering fitness tests and then identifying as low-fit the number of children who scored below some standard on each test is inaccurate and inappropriate. Because lifelong fitness requires lifelong habits and because habits developed early in life influence adult behavior, there is a need to approach fitness education from cognitive and affective perspectives as well as psychomotor perspectives. The cognitive abilities needed to recognize, to understand, and to implement appropriate fitness behaviors are important elements in the process of developing appropriate fitness habits for life. For example, a youngster blessed with good heredity might test well on body composition throughout childhood, even though he eats poorly and avoids exercising whenever possible. His fitness test scores would classify him as "fit," but his lack of understanding about weight-control principles and his poor habits put him at risk. Is he fit? A skinfold test would indicate yes; a knowledge test or physical activity attitude test might indicate no.

Habitual physical activity level is another factor to consider in determining fitness status. Recent findings on weight-control studies with adults conclude that regular exercise is a key element of a successful weight reduction program. A study from the Centers for Disease Control (1) showed that even a minimal addition of physical activity in sedentary individuals may significantly and positively reduce risk of coronary heart disease (CHD). Thus, willingness to regularly engage in any physical activity is an important factor in fitness.

Unfortunately, there are not a lot of data on the cognitive and affective aspects of fitness, especially those related to children. But, reports on the increasing number of hours that children spend watching television or sitting at a computer suggest that even children with good fitness test scores might have fitness problems. National Children and Youth Fitness Study (NCYFS) data (4, 5) reflect this in revealing that few parents are providing encouragement for their children to engage in moderate to vigorous activity three to four times per week. In fact, socialization pressures such as peer interest in sedentary activities (computer games and television), poor parental role models, and discouragement from sport participation limit the physical activity patterns of children.

If fitness test scores alone are used to define fitness levels, we might conclude that a majority of children are fit, especially if the items test sport-related fitness components. But, if determination of fitness level takes a broader view, which includes adequate knowledge about fitness and a positive attitude toward physical activity, then vast numbers of children appear in danger of being "low fit."

Why Be Concerned About Low Fitness Levels in Children?

Not all children have the potential to be great athletes—despite years of diligent practice to throw far, run fast, or jump high! Fortunately, having a high level of athletic skill is not a requirement for living a happy, healthy life. Basic fitness, however, is an important component of well-being, and the ability to achieve basic fitness is within the potential of all but the most severely disabled child.

As described in previous chapters, basic fitness refers to having sufficient levels of fitness components that underlie various facets of health, especially cardiovascular health, joint and muscle function, and body composition. High levels of these components provide abundant energy, endurance, strength, and freedom of joint movement to carry

out daily activities and still enjoy leisure-time activities. Low-fit children are not only denied those benefits, they become caught in a vicious cycle: Their low energy, poor flexibility, minimal strength, and limited endurance discourage them from being active. The more sedentary they become, the worse their fitness becomes, prompting them to avoid activity even more! This situation also affects the social interactions of these children as they are left out of the sport and play experiences of their peers. Worst yet, in attempting to participate, they experience failure, which further alienates them from physical activity.

Low-fit, sedentary children suffer from both the physical and social consequences of their condition. In addition, they suffer from lack of attention to their particular needs. Teachers and parents often excuse the over- or underweight child from activity that might be challenging. The child with low energy levels is not expected to run for the ball or hustle. Children with poor flexibility are often cautioned against stretching too hard. All of these practices discourage low-fit children from doing the activities they most need encouragement to do. However, that encouragement needs to be founded upon sound pedagogical, psychological, and physiological principles.

Planning an Effective Fitness Program

The keys to effective fitness programming are the same for all children: The teacher must plan carefully, observe regularly, and adjust appropriately; the children must be motivated to take part appropriately and must be given opportunities for stimulation in all learning domains. An effective fitness plan starts with review of the program's basic philosophy and asks if the program is focused on all children or on a select group only (i.e., elite children or special children)? Then student needs must be determined both through testing and through observation, the results of which should be used to help students establish goals and objectives.

Establish first the individual goals and program objectives, then plan and implement the program. The program design should include checkpoints that indicate how well each student is progressing toward goals and how well the program is providing them with the activities, knowledge, skills, and motivation necessary to achieve their goals. Such checkpoints might include self-testing by the children, systematic observation of specific behaviors, informal checklists of attitudes, participation, or other pertinent behavior, and simple conversation with the children about what they are doing at home, what they like to do, how they feel, and so on. More formal and systematic assessment of progress toward goals should be done at the end of each unit of activity and the end of the school year.

Effectiveness of the program should be evaluated, both in regard to the children's attainment of their personal goals and to the overall success of the program, including its various units. Throughout the program, and definitely at the end, children should be recognized for their successes and encouraged to continue striving for goals not met. The program should be revised, reinforced, and recognized when and where appropriate, keeping in mind that the process is integrated. Testing should be related to goal setting, goal setting should guide program planning, and program evaluation should provide information for revision. Figure 11.1 demonstrates the steps necessary to planning and implementing an effective fitness program.

Programming for Low-Fit Children

How does programming for low-fit children differ from programming for average or high-fit children? The answer to this question is: not much . . . and a lot! The systematic plan outlined in Figure

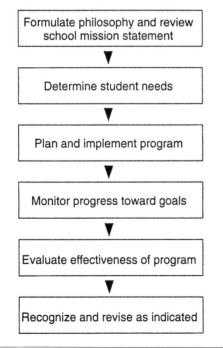

Figure 11.1   Components of effective planning for fitness.

11.1 should be used as a guide for all children low- to high-fit. Children themselves must take part in goal setting, remembering that all need realistic opportunities to reach their goals, cognitive, affective, and psychomotor stimulation, and encouragement to develop and maintain good fitness behaviors. The fitness plan for the low-fit child, incorporating cognitive, affective, and psychomotor elements, parallels a program for high-fit children although it differs in a few significant ways. Table 11.1 lists key points to consider in planning fitness activities for the low-fit child.

The planning process begins by recognizing that some children are low in fitness. Then the low-fit children must be identified, their specific fitness problems must be delineated, and a plan for dealing with those factors interfering with or limiting the fitness of each child must be made. It is crucial that teachers first rule out disease, health disorders, and hereditary problems as a cause of the fitness problem before undertaking the suggestions in Table 11.1.

The most limiting aspect of poor fitness is being overweight and/or overfat. An overweight child is one whose body weight is at least 20% more than expected on height-weight charts; an overfat child is one who, regardless of weight, has excess body fat (i.e., has too much fat in comparison to nonfat tissue like muscle). It is possible for a child to be at normal weight and still be overfat, or, due to extraordinary amounts of muscle, to be overweight without being overfat. As used in this chapter, overweight will refer to the condition in which a child has excess weight not accounted for by extra muscle.

Both overweight and overfat children are disadvantaged by having to move nonfunctional excess weight (in the form of fat). Children with either condition can benefit from resistance activities that will increase their muscular strength. In addition, both need plenty of aerobic activity, even though problems of excess body weight and fat are particularly great in endurance activities and in all activities requiring movement of one's own body.

Excess body weight can interfere with flexibility, agility, and mechanics of motion and contributes to poor perceptions of body image, potentially undermining self-esteem. Unless modifications are made for activity in these children or for their expected performance, they will usually fail. This failure is magnified when the physical education teacher promotes an environment where children are continually compared to other children.

Table 11.1 Points to Consider in Planning Activity for Low-Fit Children

Fitness problem	Possible cause	Suggested action
Fatigue	Low aerobic endurance	Regular aerobic activity
	Poor muscle endurance	Repeat contractions of specific muscles
	Unbalanced diet	Eat from all basic food groups including plenty of complex carbohydrate
	Insufficient strength	Resistance activities for specific muscles
	Dehydration	Drink sufficient water
Weakness	Insufficient strength	Resistance activities
	Low muscle endurance	Repeat contractions
Muscle tightness	Lack of flexibility	Stretching of key muscles
		Proper warm-up and cool-down
Overweight/overfat	Sedentary living	Become regularly active
	Low muscle mass	Resistance activity
	Overeating	Eat in moderation
Inactive	Unaware of importance	Develop awareness
	Poor role models	Identify good models
	Poor motivation	Provide encouragement and success opportunities

Note. In addition to the psychomotor suggestions listed above, it is important to provide cognitive learning opportunities that prepare the child to make objective decisions and to lend support to affective behaviors that lead to establishment of appropriate habits.

Overweight children should be allowed to work at their own rate, get assistance in moving their weight, and engage in activities that do not require lifting of their full body weight. For example, they can do modified pull-ups with feet resting on the floor, they can do wall push-ups, and they can have a partner assist on sit-ups. They can assist themselves in whatever way they discover helpful to complete the task, allowing them to work at their own speed. These children can benefit greatly from play on jungle gyms and other outdoor play equipment requiring them to hang, climb, and crawl while only partially supporting their weight. Such activities permit overweight children to participate successfully with their peers while gradually developing strength. When doing aerobic activities (large muscle, rhythmical actions), which are critical to weight loss, it is essential that overweight children be allowed to move at their own pace.

Overfat children who are not overweight should focus on resistance activities that will increase their muscular strength but not cause them to lose weight. Because they tend to be weaker and fatigue easily, they need opportunities to start at low resistance levels and progress slowly. Children who are both overfat and overweight should have a balance of resistance and aerobic activities.

Modification of intensity level is an important adaptation to make for low-fit children. They must be allowed to participate at levels of exertion that are manageable but still reflect effort comparable to what high-fit children exert. Both low- and high-fit children need to understand that fitness benefits result from effort that is relative to an individual's capability, not from effort compared to some absolute standard. For example, expecting all children to run a mile in 11:00 min is not reasonable unless they already have fairly good aerobic endurance. For high-fit children, an 11-min goal would require only moderate effort (i.e., 60%-70% of maximum effort), whereas a low-fit child might not achieve that time even with 100% effort!

Shortening distances of continuous runs or walks, alternating types of activity (e.g., run—walk—skip—gallop—jog), using intermittent bouts of activity with varying intensity (walk-rest, jog-rest, walk-rest, etc.), and allowing opportunity to set personal endurance goals can aid low-fit children in identifying and striving for a realistic endurance goal. Circuits and station drills are good opportunities for children to work at individual levels of effort without feeling embarrassed. The focus at each point in the circuit or at each activity station is on continuing the exercise for a specified time period—not on how many repetitions can be completed. This allows the lowest fit child to exercise along with the highest fit child and still achieve a realistic personal goal.

Some children are low in fitness because they have inadequate levels of muscular strength. Their lack of muscular strength may negatively influence the performance of many motor skills, such as striking a ball with a bat, shooting a basket, throwing for distance, jumping, or moving with speed. If a child has insufficient strength to meet minimal performance standards, then activities for this child should be modified to focus effort on accuracy and form rather than on distance and speed until strength is improved. Light bats, lower baskets, lighter and smaller balls, and shorter distances to targets can help the child with low strength have successful movement experiences while developing correct motor skill form.

It is not always easy to distinguish strength problems from body weight or fatness problems. A child who can match peers in throwing a softball for distance, lifting a barbell, or pushing a cage ball probably has sufficient muscular strength and can participate comfortably with peers. But if that same child has trouble completing whole-body movements (skipping, jumping, rope climbing, running through cones, working out on gymnastics equipment, etc.), then make activity modifications like those for overweight children.

Children who have both body-weight and strength problems are particularly disadvantaged because their ability to move (either for fitness or motor skill development) is severely limited. Their first need is to move, beginning at low intensity with frequent rest periods and without focus on performance goals. Then they need increasingly more challenging activity that is longer in duration, higher in intensity, and greater in complexity but with each step only slightly more challenging than what they can already handle. They need opportunities to grow in both understanding of movement and fitness principles and in responsibility for helping themselves solve their fitness problems. Finally, they need encouragement to be active and eat properly at school and at home.

In addition to their obvious physical limitations, low-fit children often exhibit a diminished sense of self-worth, lack of confidence, and poor attitude toward participation in any physical activity. It is easy to ignore the fact that some children quietly slip to the back of the balance-beam line never having taken a turn, or that some children always get excused from "gym" when it is time to run a mile or try a new activity. Low-fit children need to be encouraged to take part, to understand that

they can enhance their fitness and motor skills, and to have successful, fun experiences.

They need to understand that school alone cannot solve their problems but that they must take action at home as well, particularly in regard to dietary habits. For example, a 20-min PE class twice weekly cannot provide sufficient activity to make significant changes in the body composition of an overweight or overfat child. But discussion of dietary guidelines, understanding of exercise principles related to weight control, and encouragement to make small, positive changes in eating and exercising habits can provide the overweight or overfat child with the skills, knowledge, and motivation to move toward a healthful level of body composition. Fitness and nutrition fact sheets on the bulletin board or short comments about such facts at the start of each class period open opportunities for the low-fit child to successfully take part in class (e.g., by answering questions or bringing in articles, etc.) while adding to everyone's knowledge base.

Articulating physical education activities, knowledge, and skills with other subjects serves to reinforce and often expand what can be accomplished in class time alone and further teaches that physical activity is not just something done in the isolation of PE class. Such integration might be of particular value to the child who is reluctant to participate or who lacks knowledge about the benefits and principles of exercising and nutrition. The classroom fitness, activity, and nutrition corner is a good way to add support to physical education subject matter. (See chapter 16 for a description of the North Dakota fitness corner.) The low-fit child can more easily and quickly succeed in fitness corner activities than he or she can succeed in improving fitness per se. Such success might keep the low-fit child committed to the long process of changing exercise and dietary habits.

Many current events lend support to physical education subject matter: professional sports, Olympic events, recreational programs, diet fads, and so on. The low-fit child is on equal ground with the high-fit child when cognitive and affective goals are established. Such goals are not just substitutes for "real" fitness goals; knowledge and attitudes are legitimate goals themselves. A teacher can regularly lead students through exercises in such a way that students do improve their fitness, but such a program would lack the important elements that prepare children to make wise fitness decisions for life. For example, even if PE class time is sufficient to significantly alter fitness directly (i.e., 1 hr per day, five times per week), there should be cognitive and affective experiences that teach young people the whys, whats, and hows of exercise and nutrition, that teach children to analyze their own fitness status, and that challenge children to design and implement their own fitness plan.

Once general activities have been matched to the fitness problem (e.g., stretching for poor flexibility), then select specific activities that will be attractive to the low-fit child. Often those activities can be the same as those planned for all of the other students, but with modification. Table 11.2 lists factors that signal a possible need for activity modification.

Table 11.2 Characteristics of Activity That Signal Need for Modification for Low-Fit Children

Activity factor	Need	Modification
Bear body weight	Less weight to handle	Self-assistance Partner assistance Change action angle
Endurance or set number of reps	Decreased time per work bout Decreased number of reps	Intermittent work Work within own time frame Flexible goals
Use of an implement	Changes that allow control of implement	Use shorter, lighter, or different type
Speed	Slower pace	Match partners Flexible goals Self-paced
Power	Reduced strength or speed	Decreased intensity Self-paced
Quick changes of direction	Decreased speed	Self-paced Flexible goals

Summary

Low-fit children should be identified and then helped to deal with the limitations imposed by their specific fitness problems. As often as possible, the low-fit child should be included in peer activities, but with modifications that increase the likelihood of successful participation. The characteristics of certain activities suggest room for modification, including activities that require strength, speed, and movement of the entire body weight. The underlying causes of low fitness levels include inadequate knowledge, poor fitness skills, and poor attitudes as well as the obvious ill-effects of overweight, minimal strength, lack of endurance, and muscle tightness. In addition to the physical risks and limitations imposed by low fitness status, low-fit children also may suffer from psychological and social consequences of their condition. A major responsibility for the teacher of low-fit children is to implement a systematic plan that offers both emotional support and sound physiological guidance. Such a plan holds the potential for helping even low-fit children to develop skills, knowledge, and attitudes leading to a more active lifestyle.

References

1. Casperson, C.J.; Christenson, G.M.; Pollard, R.A. Status of the 1990 physical fitness and exercise objectives—evidence from NHIS 1985. Public Health Reports 101:587-592; 1986.
2. Chrysler-AAU physical fitness program. In: Updyke, W., ed., Physical fitness trends in American youth 1980-1989. Bloomington: Indiana University, 1989.
3. President's Council on Physical Fitness and Sports. A review of physical activity research. Washington, DC: U.S. Government Printing Office, 1989.
4. Ross, J.G.; Gilbert, G.G. The national children and youth fitness study: a summary of findings. JOPERD 56(1):45-50; 1985.
5. Ross, J.G.; Pate, R.R. The national children and youth fitness study II: a summary of findings. JOPERD 58(9):51-56; 1987.
6. Williams, M.H. Nutrition for fitness and sport. 3rd ed. Dubuque, IA: Brown; 1992.

Chapter 12

Fitness Testing: Current Approaches and Purposes in Physical Education

Russell R. Pate
University of South Carolina, Columbia

Physical fitness testing has a long history in American physical education programs. The recent history of this process has been controversial and dynamic; the past decade has been dominated by debate and change. Unfortunately, some of the debate has been rancorous and much of the change has been slow and painful. Nonetheless, I believe the debate has been productive, stimulating thinking and action toward much improved fitness evaluation. The current programs for youth fitness testing, however imperfect, are vastly improved over past programs.

Despite improved fitness testing, the debates have had at least one negative side effect. Many practitioners have been confused by the apparently conflicting viewpoints espoused by various organization and professional leaders, all of whom seem credible and authoritative. This discord has left many teachers and administrators uncertain as to which testing program is best for them. I hope this chapter will assist readers in making decisions about the proper role of fitness testing in a physical education program and in becoming familiar with various fitness testing options available in the current market. The specific purposes of this chapter are to describe the current "state-of-the-art" physical fitness testing protocols and to make recommendations concerning how fitness tests are used in school physical education programs.

Current Physical Fitness Test Batteries

Between the mid-1950s and 1980 there was one dominant physical fitness test battery in the United States, the AAHPER Youth Fitness Test (1). It was aggressively promoted by both the American Alliance for Health, Physical Education, Recreation and Dance and the President's Council on Physical Fitness and Sports. Although this testing protocol underwent several revisions, throughout its lifespan it was appropriately labeled a test of "motor fitness," due to its measurement of a rather heterogeneous array of physical fitness components. As shown in Table 12.1, the final version of the Youth Fitness Test includes seven items that measure fitness components ranging from speed and anaerobic power to cardiorespiratory endurance.

Beginning in the mid-1970s the motor fitness approach to youth fitness testing came under attack for its failure to focus on the health-related aspects of fitness and for its inclusion of test items that measured traits specific to athletic performance rather than fitness as it relates to normal, day-to-day life. By the late 1980s AAHPERD had ceased promotion of the Youth Fitness Test, and other fitness testing programs were developed to fill the void. The remainder of this section is dedicated to describing the fitness testing programs

Table 12.1   AAHPER Youth Fitness Test, 1976 Version

Test items	Fitness component
600-yd run-walk or mile run-walk	Cardiorespiratory endurance
Pull-ups (boys)	Muscular strength and endurance
Flexed arm hang (girls)	Muscular strength and endurance
Sit-ups	Muscular strength and endurance
50-yd dash	Speed
Standing broad jump	Anaerobic power
Shuttle run	Agility, speed

Table 12.2   AAHPERD Physical Best

Test items
  1-mile walk/run
  Sum of triceps and calf skinfolds
  Sit-and-reach
  Modified sit-ups (1 min)
  Pull-ups
Other features
  Criterion-referenced standards
  Two-tiered award scheme
  Activity award
  Computerized feedback system
Organizational contact
  American Alliance for Health, Physical Education, Recreation and Dance
  1900 Association Drive
  Reston, Virginia 22091

Table 12.3   FitnessGram

Test items
  1-mile run/walk *or* multistage 20-m shuttle run
  Sum of triceps and calf skinfolds *or* body mass index
  Curl-up
  Trunk lift
  Push-up, modified pull-up, pull-up, *or* flexed arm hang
  Back-saver sit-and-reach *or* shoulder stretch
Other features
  Criterion-referenced standards
  Activity behavior recognition
  Performance recognition
  Computerized feedback system
  Curricular materials
Organizational contact
  Cooper Institute for Aerobics Research
  12330 Preston Road
  Dallas, Texas 75230

that are currently being promoted on a national scale in the United States. After briefly describing the several testing programs, an analysis follows showing the common threads that run through them.

AAHPERD Physical Best

AAHPERD has replaced the Youth Fitness Test with a health-related physical fitness testing program entitled *Physical Best: A Physical Fitness and Education Assessment Program* (2). The key feature in the Physical Best program is a five-item battery that includes tests of cardiorespiratory endurance, body composition, flexibility, abdominal muscle strength and endurance, and upper-body muscle strength and endurance. The specific test items are listed in Table 12.2 as well as other features of the Physical Best program. Among these are curricular materials and a two-tiered award system based on attainment of performance standards that are linked to health criteria (i.e., criterion-referenced standards). The program also provides a computer software package for generation of individual student report cards.

FitnessGram

FitnessGram is a health-related physical fitness testing program that centers around a computerized system for processing, interpreting, and providing test result feedback (4). The test protocol itself includes items that measure five components

of fitness: aerobic capacity, body composition, abdominal muscle strength and endurance, upper-body muscle strength and endurance, and trunk extension strength and endurance. Flexibility is an optional component. Four of the required components also offer optional test items, and several are innovative. For example, the multistage, 20-m shuttle run is included as an optional aerobic capacity test; a paced curl-up test is used to measure abdominal muscle strength and endurance. As shown in Table 12.3, other features of FitnessGram are criterion-referenced standards, behavioral as well as performance recognition systems, and curricular materials.

President's Challenge

The President's Challenge is a physical fitness test battery that can be used to qualify youngsters for the Presidential Fitness Award (9). The battery includes five test items and these are listed in Table 12.4. In contrast to Physical Best and FitnessGram, the President's Challenge test does not evaluate body composition but does measure speed and agility via the shuttle-run test. This program uses norm-reference standards that serve as the basis for a three-tiered award system. The Presidential Physical Fitness Award is reserved for youngsters scoring at the 85th percentile or better on all test items. The National Physical Fitness Award is earned by students scoring at the 50th percentile or better on all test items. Others receive a Participant Physical Fitness Award.

YMCA Youth Fitness Test

The YMCA Youth Fitness Test is similar to FitnessGram and Physical Best in that five health-related fitness components are measured and criterion-referenced standards are provided (6). Two of five test items distinguish this battery (see Table 12.5). The protocol for the curl-up test calls for a limited range of motion at the hip and no anchoring of the feet. Also, a modified pull-up test is used to evaluate upper-body muscular strength. The latter test item makes use of a low bar, and the youngster's feet are in contact with the floor. This procedure, sometimes referred to as the Vermont pull-up, was used in the National Children and Youth Fitness Study II (8). Also included with the YMCA Youth Fitness Test package is a set of lesson plans that can be used to incorporate the test into a physical education curriculum.

Chrysler Fund/AAU Test

The Chrysler Fund/AAU test protocol shares some characteristics with each of the aforementioned test batteries (3). Like all those previously mentioned, the Chrysler Fund/AAU test includes distance run, bent-knee sit-up, and sit-and-reach test items. Like the President's Challenge test, this test requires either the pull-up (boys) or flexed arm hang (girls) test items. Also,

Table 12.4   President's Challenge

Test items
   1-mile run/walk
   Pull-ups or flexed arm hang
   V-sit-and-reach or sit-and-reach
   Curl-ups (1 min)
   Shuttle run
Other features
   Norm-referenced standards
   Presidential Physical Fitness Award (85th percentile)
   National Physical Fitness Award (50th percentile)
   Participant Physical Fitness Award
   School Demonstration Center Program
   State Champion Program
Organizational contact
   President's Council on Physical Fitness and Sports
   Washington, DC 20001

Table 12.5   YMCA Youth Fitness Test

Test items
   1-mile run
   Sum of triceps and calf skinfolds
   Curl-ups (40 maximum)
   Sit-and-reach
   Modified pull-ups
Other features
   Criterion-referenced standards
   Fitness program lesson plans
Organizational contact
   YMCA Program Store
   P.O. Box 5076
   Champaign, Illinois 61825-5076

as shown in Table 12.6 (page 122), several optional "skill component" test items, many of them carry-overs from the old AAHPER Youth Fitness Test (e.g., the 50-yd sprint and standing long jump) are included. No measure of body composition is provided. Award certificates linked to a two-tiered set of standards are made available. Also, instructional materials and a data management software package can be obtained.

Common Threads and Recent Trends in Fitness Testing

A review of the descriptions above and the material in Tables 12.2 through 12.6 may lead to the

Table 12.6 Chrysler Fund-AAU Physical Fitness Test

Test items
  Required
    Endurance run (1/4 mile to 1 mile, depending on
      age)
    Bent-knee sit-ups (1 min)
    Sit-and-reach test
    Pull-ups (boys)
    Flexed arm hang (girls)
  Optional events
    Standing long jump
    Isometric push-up
    Modified push-up (girls)
    Isometric leg squat
    Shuttle run
    Sprints (50 yd-100 yd, depending on age)
  Other features
    Promotional materials
    Newsletter for instructors
    Three-tiered, norm-referenced award scheme
    Computer software
    Curricular materials
  Organizational contact
    Chrysler Fund/AAU Physical Fitness Program
    Poplars Building
    Bloomington, Indiana 47405

conclusion that the current major fitness test batteries are much more alike than they are different. Because all the testing programs described have been either developed or revised within the last 5 years, collectively these tests reflect the contemporary thinking about appropriate approaches to fitness measurement in youngsters. Several important trends are evident.

Emphasis on Health-Related Fitness

Whereas there are some differences across the five testing programs, clearly all emphasize evaluation of the health-related fitness components. This represents a major change from the situation 10 to 20 years ago, reflecting a heightened appreciation for the role that exercise and fitness can play in promoting health and preventing disease.

Criterion-Referenced Standards

Several of the major testing programs have developed criterion-referenced standards for interpret-

ing test results and test levels of performance associated with good health (5). These standards, which currently vary considerably between programs, are used as the basis for award systems. The trend toward inclusion of criterion-referenced standards in fitness testing programs probably reflects two concerns. First, there has been dissatisfaction with the traditional norm-referenced approach to interpretation of test performance, because this approach tends to emphasize competition and elite performance. Second, there is a desire to communicate to youngsters that there is a level of fitness (probably below that needed to be a successful athlete) that is satisfactory for health maintenance. At present, establishing criterion-referenced standards for physical fitness is an imperfect process but one that is attractive from a theoretical standpoint.

Feedback Systems

To facilitate the process of communicating fitness test results to students and their parents, several computerized systems have automated the production of fitness report cards. These systems, which are currently offered with the FitnessGram and Physical Best programs, provide a graphic presentation of the youngster's performance on each test item and indicate how each performance rates relative to a criterion-referenced standard. These feedback systems have been developed to overcome an often-cited criticism of school-based fitness testing programs, that test results are not presented to students or parents in a meaningful way. Understandably a student's enthusiasm for the testing process could be blunted if neither students nor their parents are informed of the meaning of the test results. Also, as personal computers have become more readily available in the schools, these computerized feedback systems have made it easier for the teacher to manage fitness test data on large numbers of students.

Curricular Plans and Instructional Materials

Other innovations evident in several current fitness testing programs are curricular guidelines and instructional materials. The purpose of these resource materials is to assist the teacher in building the testing process into the physical education curriculum in a meaningful and pedagogically sound fashion. In the past, fitness tests, too often administered "in a vacuum," have failed to link the testing process to the rest of the physical education curriculum. However, administration of a fitness test can be an opportunity to promote valuable cognitive and affective learning. The inclusion of curricular materials with testing guidelines indicates an effort to meaningfully incorporate fitness tests into physical education programs.

Physical Activity Assessment

Over the years great attention has been given to refinement of the methods for measurement of physical fitness, and much energy has been invested in promoting the use of fitness tests in PE programs. However, only in recent years has much attention been given to measurement of physical activity behavior in children, which in my opinion will become an important component of physical education programs in the future. Currently, both the FitnessGram and Physical Best programs include program components that encourage students to become more active and provide awards that encourage this. Although these aspects of fitness testing programs are not highly developed at this point, it does seem appropriate to shift some of the emphasis toward activity assessment and away from fitness measurement.

Purposes of Fitness Testing

In my view the most critical step in any physical fitness testing program is one that the teacher should take long before any child completes a single test item: that is, determining the goal of the overall physical education program. Fitness testing should be undertaken only if it makes an important contribution to attainment of the program goals. It is this author's opinion that the goal of physical education should be to promote adoption of a physically active lifestyle, thereby promoting maintenance of good health and fitness throughout life. Fitness tests can and should be used to help attain this goal.

After establishing the overall goal of the physical education program, specify objectives for the fitness testing process. This too is a critical, preliminary component of the testing program. Tests should be used with specific instructional outcomes in mind—*not* just because they are a traditional component of PE. Following is a discussion

of several objectives that can be attained with fitness testing, not all of which will be appropriate for all physical education programs.

Promotion of Cognitive Learning

One of the most readily attainable objectives of fitness testing is promotion of cognitive learning. The fitness test provides an ideal opportunity for students to learn about the meaning of health-related physical fitness and its components. However, such learning will occur only if effective instructional techniques are planned and implemented with the test. Helpful guidelines on how this can be accomplished are provided in chapter 9 of this book.

Promotion of Affective Learning

From a psychological perspective, participation in a fitness test can be either a very positive or negative experience. Conducting a fitness test in a way that demeans or embarrasses the student can extinguish intrinsic motivation to be active and fit (7). On the other hand, conducted in an environment that rewards participation and effort, a fitness test can enhance a student's interest in fitness and an appreciation of its importance. A key ingredient is test success. Students are more likely to find fitness tests a positive experience if they succeed. Therefore, it is critical to carefully establish the criteria for success.

Motivation for Improved Fitness

Many educators assume that participating in a fitness test will motivate youngsters to work toward improved fitness. I believe this is possible only if the testing process is carefully and properly designed. "Failure" on a fitness test can be deflating to children. The motivational outcome of test participation depends on how the testing process is presented initially to the student, how the results are interpreted, and what types of learning activities follow the test (see chapter 9 for a discussion of how the testing process can be properly integrated into a physical education curriculum).

Identification of Children in Need of Improvement

A rationale often cited for administration of fitness tests is that low-fit youngsters should be identified using objective procedures. An assumption perhaps implicit in this reasoning is that an appropriate intervention program will be available for youngsters with fitness deficiencies. In my view only when this assumption is borne out is this objective appropriate. Few physical education programs, however, have the resources (or commitment) to deliver special intervention programs for low-fit youngsters. (This most unfortunate situation is addressed in chapters 10 and 11.) In the ideal setting, fitness tests would be used as the basis for referral of low-fit youngsters to programs specially designed to meet their needs. Even in conditions that are far less than ideal, reasonable and appropriate follow-up to the testing process is essential. Otherwise, the utility of the testing process would be questionable.

Identification of Children With Athletic Potential

Fitness tests, because they provide objective measures of physical performance, can be used to identify youngsters who rank at the high end of the performance spectrum on the fitness components measured. An "elite" performance on a specific test item or set of items may indicate that a youngster has the potential to excel in an athletic activity that requires a high level of fitness in the corresponding fitness component. For example, a youngster who performs well on the mile-run test may have the potential to excel in athletic activities that require high levels of cardiorespiratory endurance (e.g., cross-country running, swimming, or wrestling). However, applying this objective is complicated.

First, contemporary fitness testing procedures do not usually focus on those fitness components, such as speed, anaerobic power, and agility, that are important in many of the most popular athletic activities. Second, performance in most athletic activities depends on a complex mix of factors including specific motor skill performance, motivation, and experience as well as fitness; of course, fitness tests do not measure most of these factors. So, I believe fitness test results can provide some information that is useful in guiding youngsters into appropriate athletic activities. But the benefits in this area are probably quite limited, and this objective alone would not constitute a strong rationale for fitness test administration.

Program Evaluation

In many school districts administration of physical fitness tests is mandated, often as part of an overall effort to evaluate the effectiveness of the physical education program. Although program evaluation is important, I do not recommend use of fitness tests for this purpose. Many factors affect the fitness levels of children, and it is unrealistic to expect a high correlation between the quality of the physical education program and the performances of children on fitness tests. Also, there is a risk that teachers would feel pressure to produce short-term gains in fitness at the expense of other program goals such as developing positive attitudes toward physical activity. It is preferable to focus relevant program evaluation activities on documentation showing that an appropriate fitness test was administered and that the results were used in meaningful ways.

Recommended Approaches to Fitness Testing

As noted in the opening paragraphs of this chapter, physical fitness tests have held a prominent place in physical education programs for many years. Despite this long history there is very little scientific evidence to guide us in deciding how to best incorporate fitness tests into PE. Most of the research on fitness testing has dealt with identification of valid test items. Very little research has been directed toward understanding how youngsters respond to fitness tests and how tests can best be used to attain important educational objectives. Because there is so little scientific information on which to base recommendations, the ideas that follow are only sensible conclusions. Many of the recommended procedures have been used by some teachers and, based on anecdotal reports, appear to be reasonable and consistent with the philosophy upon which this book is based.

Test Preparation

Performance of a physical fitness test, with its requirement of peak effort, can be an activity that is both physically and psychologically stressful for youngsters. In addition, lower stress and greater enjoyment is evident if the individual is familiar with the testing procedures and experiences success in the testing process. Accordingly, it is essential that youngsters be well prepared before taking a physical fitness test. This preparation should involve actual exercise training as well as familiarity with the test items. Fitness tests do not lend themselves to the "pop quiz" approach. Too often fitness tests are scheduled at the very beginning of the school year or at other times that preclude careful preparation of youngsters for the testing process. Therefore, it is not surprising that many adults have only negative recollections of their participation in fitness tests.

Single-Test Administration

In many physical education programs, physical fitness tests are administered at the beginning of the school year and again at the end of the year. On the surface this scheme may make sense, because we hope to observe improved physical fitness as a result of the intervening program. However, for several reasons, this pattern may not be useful. First, fitness tests are time consuming, and the time required for two may not be warranted. Second, the time requirement may cause the teacher to force each of the two tests into the shortest possible time block, and this may preclude using the test as an opportunity for cognitive and affective learning. Third, the second test makes sense only if the intervening program can be expected to produce change; often this is unlikely. In some situations a second test in a given school year may be appropriate and useful, but only with specific and predetermined educational objectives. Again, fitness testing should be seen as a means of meeting a valuable educational end, not as an end in itself.

Append Cognitive and Affective Learning Activities to the Testing Process

As noted, fitness testing can be used as an activity that promotes attainment of learning in the cognitive and affective domains. However, these desirable outcomes are likely to result only if specific learning activities are built into the testing process. Accomplishing this may be facilitated by thoroughly integrating the test into the curriculum and by spreading it across a period of several weeks. For example, the mile-run test could be administered as part of an instructional unit dealing with cardiorespiratory fitness and the ways in which it can be developed and maintained. Too often fitness tests have been administered in a curricular vacuum, that is, with nothing to link them to meaningful educational outcomes. This problem can be

overcome by treating fitness tests as tools in facilitating cognitive and affective learning.

Communicate and Interpret Test Results in a Meaningful Way

Administration of a physical fitness test is worth the time and effort involved only if results are meaningful to the students. Careful plans should be laid for communication of test results to students and, ideally, their parents. The appropriate and useful techniques for feedback of test results vary greatly in terms of formality, time requirement, and expense. Using a "low-tech" example, the teacher might simply discuss with a class of fourth graders what it means to be able to run a mile without stopping to walk. Such a discussion should help students understand the meaning of their test performance, should positively reinforce those who were able to run the whole mile, and (if handled sensitively) should help those who did not run the whole mile to understand why they were unable to meet that standard and how they might do better next time. At the "high-tech" end of the continuum are the computer-generated individual report card systems now available in the FitnessGram (4) and Physical Best (2) programs. In any case, the feedback procedures should be planned carefully and designed to promote attainment of important affective and cognitive learning objectives.

Apply Criterion-Referenced Standards

As previously discussed, several of the available fitness testing programs include guidelines for interpretation of test performances that use criterion-referenced standards rather than the more traditional norm-referenced standards. Although we are currently limited in our ability to establish fitness test standards on the basis of anticipated future health benefits, it is my view that the benefits of using criterion-referenced standards outweigh the associated problems and limitations.

Criterion-referenced fitness test standards that are established on the basis of the relationship between exercise and health tend to reflect levels that are attainable by the vast majority of youngsters (5). Therefore, participation in the test is likely to be a successful experience for youngsters and should help to build what has been called *exercise self-efficacy*, that is, a sense of personal mastery of exercise participation and fitness. Too often in the past fitness tests have been a failure experience for most children, because norm-referenced standards, set at an arbitrary and high level, have been used in interpreting test results.

Other benefits of using criterion-referenced fitness test standards are their reinforcement of the fitness–health link and their emphasis that one can be fit without being an elite athlete. These benefits occur most effectively, of course, when teachers take the time to discuss with students the origins of the standards and their relationship to health maintenance.

Plan and Implement Intervention Programs for Low-Fit Youngsters

A fitness testing program will inevitably identify some youngsters who fail to meet reasonable health fitness standards. It is, in my view, fundamentally corrupt to administer a fitness test, identify those who need remediation, and then do nothing to help them. Of course, some schools are limited in their ability to provide the individual (or small-group) programming that would be desirable in many cases. Despite this limitation, I still consider it essential that youngsters who manifest fitness deficiencies be provided some sort of intervention program. This might be limited to suggestions for home exercise, referral to a community-based youth fitness program, or communication with parents concerning recommended activities. Understandably, teachers cannot and should not bear all the responsibility for remediating fitness deficiencies, however, it seems essential to implement any feasible intervention in a given setting.

Design and Apply Award Systems Carefully

Tangible awards (e.g., patches, certificates, etc.) have become a common component of fitness testing programs. Typically these awards have been given to youngsters who attain some predetermined level of performance (norm- or criterion-referenced standards). Presumably these awards have been provided for the purpose of motivating youngsters to attain desirable levels of test performance. But, therein lies a potential problem. As discussed by Whitehead in chapter 8 of this volume, extrinsic rewards are motivating to a particular youngster only if the established standard is seen as attainable. Hence there is a need to set goals that are realistic for each student.

Furthermore, there is a risk that *intrinsic motivation* to attain a desirable fitness level can, in the long term, be extinguished by provision of tangible awards that are later unavailable (as almost certainly will be the case when the youngster leaves school).

Clearly there is a need to plan award schemes in a very careful manner. I believe that inexpensive, tangible awards, although not essential, can play a useful role in an overall plan that is designed to encourage activity and fitness. However, in my view, such awards should be used sparingly, should be provided primarily for attaining activity objectives (not arbitrary fitness standards), should be attainable by most youngsters, and should complement a well-designed set of intangible rewards. Overall, it is essential that we keep our focus on the big goal—enhancement of long-term physical activity behavior. Any award scheme should be evaluated first and foremost on the basis of its likely impact on this goal.

Evaluate Both Activity Behavior and Fitness

Physical fitness is a multidimensional trait determined by genetic, behavioral, and environmental factors. Consequently it is entirely possible for some youngsters to perform reasonably well on a fitness test while being rather sedentary. However, because low activity will ultimately lead to low fitness and increased disease risk, over time activity behavior will be more important than fitness during childhood. This suggests monitoring physical activity behavior during childhood, and as already mentioned, some of the current fitness testing programs include components that focus on activity promotion. I recommend that physical activity habits and overall activity level be assessed as part of a fitness measurement program. Such an approach provides information on both the product (fitness) and the process (physical activity) that leads to fitness.

Use Self-Testing Activities

One of the major deterrents to the use of fitness tests in physical education programs is the perception held by many teachers that tests must be administered in a highly controlled manner. Such control is sometimes seen as requiring more time and personnel than are available. There is no question that the validity and reliability of a fitness test item depends on the specific manner in which the test is administered. Therefore, if the test results are to be used for research purposes, great care must be taken to standardize testing procedures. However, if a test is being used primarily for pedagogical purposes, that is, to promote cognitive and affective learning, then standardization of testing procedures becomes much less important.

Youngsters at all ages are capable of administering fitness tests to themselves and their peers. This approach, although obviously sacrificing much in terms of standardization, has many benefits. First, responsibility is placed with the youngsters so that they learn how to administer the test. Second, there is no need for extra personnel or excessive amounts of time. Third, with self- and partner testing, performance can remain "confidential"—no one but the student and partner needs to know how the student performed. And fourth, the entire process is student-centered rather than teacher-centered. For more information on student self- and partner-testing of physical fitness, refer to the work of Ratliffe and Ratliffe (10).

Summary

Physical fitness testing, a common component of school physical education programs for over 30 years, has been a focus of controversy for the past decade. Fitness testing methods have changed dramatically, most of them now emphasizing components of health-related fitness that are important across the lifespan. Fitness tests have been used for various purposes, not all of which are realistic or pedagogically sound. However, if properly incorporated into a physical education curriculum, fitness tests can contribute to cognitive and affective learning. Concerns about the impact of fitness tests on attitudes toward physical activity and fitness have forced a reexamination of the role of fitness tests in PE. The future is likely to bring increased emphasis on measurement of physical activity behavior in children and youth. As this trend develops, use of physical fitness tests may be more limited. This change in emphasis will hopefully promote an appreciation for the important contribution that health-related physical fitness can make to the quality of life.

References

1. American Alliance for Health, Physical Education, and Recreation. AAHPER youth fitness test manual. Washington, DC: AAHPER; 1976.
2. American Alliance for Health, Physical Education, Recreation and Dance. Physical best: a physical fitness education and assessment program. Reston, VA: AAHPERD; 1988.
3. Chrysler Fund-Amateur Athletic Union. Chrysler Fund-AAU physical fitness program. Bloomington, IN: Chrysler Fund-AAU; 1991.
4. Cooper Institute for Aerobics Research. FitnessGram test administration manual. Dallas, TX: Cooper Institute for Aerobics Research; 1992.
5. Cureton, K.J.; Warren, G.L. Criterion-referenced standards for youth health-related fitness tests: a tutorial. Res. Q. Exerc. Sport 61:7-19; 1990.
6. Franks, B. YMCA youth fitness test manual. Champaign, IL: YMCA of the USA; 1989.
7. Hopple, C.J. Children's perceptions of physical tests. Teach. Elem. Phys. Educ. 3(2):10-11; 1992.
8. Pate, R.R.; Ross, J.G.; Baumgartner, T.A.; Sparks, R.E. The modified pull-up. JOPERD 58(9):71-73; 1987.
9. President's Council on Physical Fitness and Sports. The president's challenge physical fitness program packet. Washington, DC: President's Council on Physical Fitness and Sports; 1992.
10. Ratliffe, T.; Ratliffe, L. Partner self-test: encouraging on-task practice and accountability. Teach. Elem. Phys. Educ. 2(4):14; 1991.

Chapter 13

Physical Fitness and Activity Standards for Youth

Kirk J. Cureton
University of Georgia

The development of physical fitness and physical activity standards for youth (children and adolescents) is relatively new. Until recently, the question of how much fitness and activity is needed by youth had not been directly addressed. However, information establishing the importance of adequate fitness and physical activity for health (8,10,13,17) and the belief that early intervention is important for establishing an active lifestyle (13,20,28) have brought these questions to the forefront. Despite the lack of scientific information needed to establish definitive, valid standards, many health and fitness experts have become convinced that at least tentative criterion-referenced standards are needed (6).

Failure to identify the minimum levels of physical activity and fitness required by youth has contributed to conflicting views about the level of fitness and activity of U.S. youth (6). One view, the predominate one conveyed to the public, is that youth engage in too little physical activity and have low levels of fitness. It has been based primarily on the lack of improvement in test scores on national youth fitness surveys conducted between 1965 and 1985 and arbitrary judgments about what levels of fitness should be (23). An alternate view is that children and adolescents are naturally physically activity and fit and, in fact, are the most active and fit segments of the U.S. population. This view has been based on epidemiologic studies comparing levels of physical activity and fitness of youth with levels in adults associated with reduced risk of coronary heart disease or all-cause mortality, or with recently developed criterion-referenced standards for the youth health-related fitness tests (6,28). Which of these views is correct? No answer is possible without a definition of the minimum criterion levels of physical fitness and activity required by youth. Hence, the need for standards.

Youth Fitness Standards

Criterion-referenced standards identifying desirable levels of fitness have not been developed and utilized until recently. Part of the reason is that normative standards such as percentiles have been used almost exclusively for interpretation of youth fitness test results (3,22-25). Normative standards make possible the comparison of a child's score with that of a reference group, such as a national probability sample of children of the same age and gender, but they do not directly indicate a level of physical fitness that is desirable. With the development of health-related physical fitness tests in the late 1970s and early 1980s (3,5,19), physical fitness and measurement specialists pointed out that there were at least two limitations to the use of normative standards for the interpretation of health-related physical fitness tests. First, normative standards are based on the level of physical fitness in a reference group, which may or may not possess a desired level of fitness. And second, the level of fitness required for promotion of health and well-being is not identified by normative standards. Instead, it was suggested that criterion-referenced standards should be developed that would specify the minimal level of fitness required for maintenance of health and performance of daily tasks.

The first youth health-related fitness criterion-referenced standards were developed in 1978 as part of the South Carolina Physical Fitness Test (19). These standards consisted of scores for field tests that represented levels of cardiorespiratory endurance, body composition, low-back and hamstring flexibility, and abdominal strength and endurance thought to be necessary for good health in children and youth. They were established by a panel of physical fitness experts based on professional judgment, available scientific information, and normative data for children in South Carolina. Since that time, four national youth health-related physical fitness tests have developed criterion-referenced standards: the Fit Youth Today Program (30), FitnessGram (14), Physical Best (4), and the YMCA Youth Fitness Test (12). The criterion-referenced standards have taken the place of normative standards in each test.

Criterion-referenced standards have a number of advantages in the assessment of health-related physical fitness (9). First, they are absolute standards that specify the minimum levels of fitness thought to be required to promote health (minimize disease risk) and perform daily tasks. Because the standards should be based on empirical scientific data and expert opinion, in theory they should be independent of the proportion of the population who can meet the standards. In practice, normative data have been used to establish some of the existing standards, and therefore the standards are to some extent a function of the fitness level of the population of U.S. youth. Normative standards, such as the 50th or the 85th percentile, are based entirely on the distribution of scores in a reference group and do not necessarily represent a desirable level of fitness.

A second advantage of criterion-referenced standards is that they provide immediate diagnostic feedback about whether or not performance is adequate. Passing the standard means that you have the minimum level of fitness required for health promotion and performance of daily tasks, whereas failing to pass the standard means you need additional physical activity or diet designed

to improve your fitness. Normative standards do not directly address the question of whether or not a level of fitness or physical activity is adequate. Finally, criterion-referenced standards do not imply that "more is better." They are designed to categorize individuals into groups that either meet or exceed the minimum standard and those who do not. The degree to which a score is above or below the standard is not emphasized. In contrast, normative standards imply that high-percentile scores are "better," but with a health-based criterion this may be inappropriate.

There are also several disadvantages of criterion-referenced standards. First, they may be established arbitrarily. The extent to which this was done with standards for youth fitness tests is largely unknown. Except for the FitnessGram mile run/walk standard (9), the exact procedure used for establishing the standards has not been revealed. Although there is always some judgment used in establishing "cut-off" scores, it is important that the standards have a reasoned and scientific basis. Second, significant consequences may result if field test standards misclassify the level of fitness as assessed by a criterion measure. For example, a child may not meet the standard for the mile run/walk, despite having the desired level of cardiorespiratory fitness as judged by a laboratory test of maximal oxygen uptake. The negative outcome could discourage the child from further participation in vigorous physical activity if the child felt the goal was unattainable or not worth the effort needed to attain it. The proportion of children classified correctly on a criterion measure by a standard is a measure of its validity. To date, comprehensive studies of the validity of youth fitness criterion-referenced standards and the effects of misclassifications have not been published. A third disadvantage of criterion-referenced standards is that because they represent desired minimum levels of fitness, they do not provide incentive to achieve high levels of fitness. Safrit (26) has suggested that including normative standards (which provide incentive for high-level achievement) in addition to criterion-referenced standards in youth fitness test manuals would help overcome this limitation.

A major problem with the current youth fitness criterion-referenced standards is that standards developed for the same items on different youth fitness tests are not the same. Table 13.1 illustrates these differences. Included for reference also are the 85th-percentile standards used for the Presidential Physical Fitness Award by the President's

Table 13.1   FitnessGram and Physical Best Criterion-Referenced Standards and 85th-Percentile Standards for the President's Challenge Presidential Physical Fitness Award

Test item	FitnessGram			Physical Best			Presidential Award		
	8 yrs	12 yrs	16 yrs	8 yrs	12 yrs	16 yrs	8 yrs	12 yrs	16 yrs
					Boys				
Mile run/walk (min:sec)	13:00	10:00	8:30	10:00	9:00	7:30	8:48	7:11	6:08
% fat*	25	25	25	20	20	20	—	—	—
Pull-ups (number)	1	1	1	1	2	5	5	7	11
Sit-and-reach (in.)**	1	1	1	2	2	2	3	4	6
Sit-ups (number)	25	35	40	26	38	44	40	50	56
					Girls				
Mile run/walk (min:sec)	14:00	12:00	10:30	11:30	11:00	10:30	10:02	8:23	8:23
% fat*	32	32	32	30	30	30	—	—	—
Pull-ups (number)	1	1	1	1	1	1	2	2	1
Sit-and-reach (in.)**	1	1	1	2	2	2	3	7	9
Sit-ups (number)	25	30	35	26	33	35	38	45	45

*For Physical Best standards, sum of two skinfolds was converted to percent fat using the nomogram of Lohman (14). Only the highest value of the acceptable range is given.

**For FitnessGram and Physical Best standards, values were adjusted to reflect a deviation from a zero reference at the bottom of the feet.

Challenge test (published by the President's Council on Physical Fitness and Sports), which have functioned like criterion-referenced standards in the past. The biggest discrepancies can be seen in the mile run/walk test of cardiorespiratory fitness. For example, the AAHPERD Physical Best and FitnessGram standards for boys and girls under age 10 years differ by 2 to 3 min. The FitnessGram standards for children of this age correspond to the 20th to 35th percentile on national norms, whereas the AAHPERD Physical Best standards correspond approximately to the 50th percentile. Clearly, the standards represent quite different levels of fitness. Smaller differences also exist for the body composition, pull-up, sit-up, and sit-and-reach items. Both sets of standards represent very low levels of performance compared with standards for the Presidential Award.

The discrepancies in the standards established by different groups raise questions about the basis of the standards and their validity. As mentioned, none of the organizations that developed criterion-referenced standards has described in detail how the standards were developed. The general approaches used for setting the standards are known,

however (see Table 13.2 for an illustration). Three types of information were used as the basis for these standards: empirical, judgmental, and normative. The basis of the FitnessGram mile run/walk standards has been described in detail (9). Empirical data linking maximal oxygen uptake (laboratory criterion measure of cardiorespiratory fitness) to cardiovascular disease risk and all-cause mortality in adults were used, in part, to identify

Table 13.2   Approach Used for Setting FitnessGram Criterion-Referenced Standards

Test	Approach
Mile run/walk	Empirical, normative, judgmental
Skinfold measures, BMI	Empirical, normative, judgmental
Sit-and-reach	Normative, judgmental
Sit-ups	Normative, judgmental
Pull-ups	Normative, judgmental

criterion levels of maximal oxygen uptake considered consistent with good health and performance of daily tasks. Judgment was made by a panel of experts who took into account normative data on maximal oxygen uptake. Except for the study of Blair et al. (7) (which was not available at the time the standards were developed) these data did not identify a precise cut-off value above which disease risk is increased. Selected were values of 42 ml/kg × minutes for boys of all ages and 35 to 40 ml/kg × minutes for girls, depending on age. Mile run/walk times estimated to correspond to these values were then calculated.

The body composition standards were based on empirical data relating skinfold thickness measures and the body mass index (weight/height²) to estimates of total body fatness in children of different ages (15,29). The criterion levels of body fatness were set at values considered to represent the lower limit of obesity, 25% fat for boys and 32% fat for girls of all ages. These levels were based in part on normative data for percent fat and roughly correspond to the body mass index values above which disease risk is increased in adults (18). For the field test items assessing neuromuscular function, there were no objective criterion measures that had been empirically related to disease risk on which performance standards could be based. Therefore, the standards for these items were based on normative data and expert judgment as to what represented an adequate level of function.

The approach used in setting standards for the other youth fitness tests was probably like that used for the FitnessGram standards, although the judgment as to exactly what the standards should be obviously varied. Therefore, because most of the standards for FitnessGram and for the other youth fitness tests are based on judgment and normative data, they can be accused of arbitrariness. Additional empirical data are needed to establish more definitive standards.

Which set of criterion-referenced standards is most valid? At the present time, no data are available to answer this question precisely. To directly validate the standards, longitudinal data comparing disease rates or mortality of adults who scored above and below the standards as children would be needed. It will be many years, if ever, before this type of data is available. A limited number of studies have been published evaluating the validity of the field test standards for classifying laboratory criteria of fitness or for classifying physical activity. Cureton and Warren (9) evaluated the validity of the FitnessGram and AAHPERD Physical Best mile run/walk criterion-referenced standards in terms of accuracy in classifying maximal aerobic power (criterion measure of cardiorespiratory fitness) in 578 children 7 to 14 years old. They found both sets of standards reasonably valid; the proportion of children classified correctly averaged 0.85 for the FitnessGram standards and 0.61 for the Physical Best standards. Data were not available for analysis from children of other ages.

Looney and Plowman (16) validated the FitnessGram standards against measures of physical activity. Using the data from the National Children and Youth Fitness Studies (NCYFS) I and II (national probability sample of 8,800 children ages 8 to 18 years), they compared the percentage of youth passing the FitnessGram standards in those classified as "active" or "inactive" by a questionnaire of physical habits. The differences between active and inactive children in the percentage passing four of five items were relatively small: 28.1% versus 29.6% for boys and 34.2% versus 29.1% for girls. These findings indicate that the FitnessGram standards do not accurately differentiate activity level of children, although only relatively crude measures of activity level were used in these studies.

Research to date gives practitioners little direction about whether the criterion-referenced standards of the FitnessGram, Physical Best, and YMCA should be used. Each set of standards was developed by health and fitness experts; no one set is known to be definitely better than the others. The sets of standards differ in form and difficulty, however. The FitnessGram and Physical Best provide a single standard for each test item that classifies scores as above or below the minimal level considered consistent with good health. In general, the standards for Physical Best are more difficult than those for FitnessGram. The Physical Best standards correspond to approximately the 50th percentile on national norms, which means that approximately 50% of children will not pass the tests. The FitnessGram standards correspond to approximately the 20th to 35th percentile, meaning that only 20% to 35% of children typically will not pass.

The YMCA standards classify scores into three categories: "needs work," "borderline," and "good." For the mile run/walk and sit-up tests, the "good" standard is approximately the same as FitnessGram, whereas the standards separating the "needs work" from "borderline" categories are less stringent than the FitnessGram. For the body composition item, the YMCA standards separating the "needs work" from "borderline" categories are similar to those of FitnessGram. The more stringent standards of the Physical Best are based on the philosophy that scores of children need to be high enough to buffer the degeneration that typically occurs with middle age (4,11). The other test programs have not adjusted their standards for these possible changes, and the importance of this adjustment is unknown and controversial (9). Practitioners should consider the differences in the level of the standards when adopting a test and set of standards.

Another factor to consider in deciding which test and accompanying standards to use is what specific field test items make up the test. Although all of the test batteries assess the same health-related fitness components, some of the field tests for assessing these components differ. For example, to assess upper-body strength and endurance the Physical Best uses a regular pull-up, whereas the FitnessGram provides the option of a regular pull-up or flexed arm hang and the YMCA utilizes a modified pull-up. Many youth cannot do one regular pull-up, so there will be many zero scores on this Physical Best test item. The modified pull-up requires construction of an apparatus on which to perform the test. The YMCA test utilizes a bent-knee curl-up without feet supported to assess abdominal strength and endurance, whereas the FitnessGram and Physical Best utilize a bent-knee sit-up with feet supported. Based on personal or practical considerations, one set of test items may be preferable.

Finally, the other support materials (computer software, reports, awards, and curriculum materials) that accompany a test or the technical assistance provided may be a basis for selecting one test and set of standards over another. Because of the differences in the test items and the level of the standards, one test and the standards that accompany it should be selected and utilized consistently.

Lack of consensus on youth fitness criterion-referenced standards has made it difficult to provide a definitive answer to the question of what proportion of the U.S. population is fit. Several studies have applied the FitnessGram criterion-referenced standards to large data bases in an attempt to address this question. Blair et al. (6) applied the FitnessGram standards to an opportunistic population of 37,454 children and youth age 6 to 17 years whose schools elected to participate in the FitnessGram program and who made the data available for use in research. The percentage of boys and girls, respectively, passing the different test items were 1-mile run, 69% and 63%; body composition, 83% and 84%; sit-and-reach, 96% and

89%; sit-ups, 74% and 67%; and upper-body strength and endurance, 58% and 40%. In addition, they compared the percentages of the boys and girls passing four of five items in the FitnessGram sample with the corresponding percentages passing the same standards from the NCYFS I, a nationally representative sample of children age 10 to 18 years. The percentages of boys who passed four of five items were 54.5% for FitnessGram and 63% for NCYFS I. The corresponding percentages for girls were 45.4% and 42.8%. Looney and Plowman (16) reported passing rates of children and youth in the NCYFS I and II on the FitnessGram criterion-referenced standards. The percentages of boys and girls, respectively, passing the different items were mile run/walk, 77% and 60%; percent body fat, 89% and 91%; sit-ups, 65% and 57%; sit-and-reach, 90% and 97%; and pull-ups, 73% and 32%. Seventy-two percent of boys and 48% of girls passed four of five test items. These data suggest that although a large number of children are unfit, a majority appear to have adequate fitness for health maintenance and performance of daily tasks—if the FitnessGram standards have validity.

Physical Activity Standards

In the past, level of physical fitness has often been considered synonymous with level of physical activity, and because it was simpler, emphasis was placed primarily on the assessment of youth physical fitness. However, the relationships among physical activity, physical fitness, and health are complex (8), and data on adults have suggested that physical fitness and physical activity may have independent effects on health status (7). Data on children have shown that measures of physical activity and physical fitness are poorly correlated (21). Therefore, Blair et al. (6) and others have suggested that separate standards for physical fitness and physical activity for children are needed.

A number of individuals and organizations have recommended levels of physical activity for youth (1,2,13,20,28), most of which have been based on guidelines established for developing cardiorespiratory fitness in adults. All the guidelines recommend that children participate in moderate-to-vigorous (50%-80% functional capacity) dynamic activities involving large muscle groups, 3 to 7 days a week, 20 to 30 min a day. These recommendations are probably appropriate for increasing levels of cardiorespiratory fitness in children but may be too stringent as minimum standards for promoting health and increasing the likelihood of participation in appropriate physical activity as adults. There are considerable data showing that an increase in cardiorespiratory fitness is not a prerequisite for acquiring health benefits (13). There is also a growing consensus that physical activity programs for youth should emphasize development of positive attitudes, knowledge, and behavioral patterns that will carry over to adulthood (13,28).

Blair et al. (6) have proposed that physical activity involving an energy expenditure of approximately 12 kilojoules per kilogram body weight per day (kJ/kg/day), a level associated with diverse health benefits and reduced mortality in adults, could be used as a criterion-referenced physical activity standard for children. This amount of energy expenditure is modest; it represents about 100 kcal per day in a 34-kg (100-lb) boy or girl. Regardless of age, gender, and weight, it represents about 20 to 40 min moderate-intensity daily physical activity. High-intensity activity is not needed to meet this standard; in other respects it is similar to other previous recommendations. This is the only recommendation that is based on health criteria and is probably the standard with the most justification. Applying this standard to students tested in the NCYFS I, whose physical activity was assessed by interview, Blair et al. (6) found that 88% of 956 girls and 94% of 1,307 boys met this activity standard. These data suggest that the physical activity level of a relatively high percentage of boys and girls in this country is adequate for maintenance of health.

Practical Recommendations

Based on the information presented herein, the following are recommendations concerning the use of physical fitness and activity standards:

1. Separate criterion-referenced standards should be used for physical fitness and physical activity. Youth should be encouraged to meet both sets of standards.

2. The recommendations of Blair et al. (6) for physical activity involving at least 12 kJ/kg/day of energy expenditure, or 20 to 40 min of moderate daily physical activity, should be utilized as a minimum criterion-referenced standard for physical activity needed to promote health in children and youth until new information suggests otherwise.

3. The health-related physical fitness criterion-referenced standards developed for the Fitness-Gram, AAHPERD Physical Best, or YMCA Physical Fitness tests should be used to evaluate whether or not students possess the minimum level of fitness required to promote health and perform daily tasks. Appropriate additional, remedial physical activity or diet designed to improve fitness should be prescribed for those not meeting the standards. At the present time, it is not known which set of standards is most valid. Therefore, until a consensus is reached, the test and standards that seem most appropriate should be selected and utilized consistently.

4. Physical activity behavior and criterion-referenced health-related fitness standards, rather than normative standards, should be used as the basis for health-related fitness awards.

5. As refinements occur and more information becomes available on the relation of physical activity and fitness to health, revisions in the criterion-referenced fitness and physical activity standards should be expected.

6. Normative standards may be useful in describing physical activity or health-related fitness levels of an individual or group relative to others. However, they should not be used in place of criterion-referenced standards for interpretation of individual test results because they do not indicate desired levels of physical activity or fitness, they do not provide diagnostic feedback about whether fitness and activity levels are adequate, and they imply that "more is better," which leads unjustly to rewarding only the most physically gifted.

Summary

In recent years, criterion-referenced physical fitness and activity standards for youth have been developed that provide estimates of the minimal levels consistent with good health and performance of daily tasks. These criterion-referenced standards have replaced normative standards as the principal means for evaluating and interpreting individual fitness and activity levels in youth. They provide objective benchmarks for interpreting national surveys of youth fitness and activity. These standards are tentative, and additional research is needed to validate them against health outcomes. Because several different youth fitness tests and sets of standards currently exist, teachers and other health and fitness professionals must select from among those available. Consensus on a single set of fitness and activity criterion-referenced standards is needed.

References

1. American Academy of Pediatrics. Physical fitness and the schools. Pediatrics 80:449-450; 1987.
2. American College of Sports Medicine. Opinion statement on physical fitness in children and youth. Med. Sci. Sports Exerc. 20:422-423; 1988.
3. American Alliance for Health, Physical Education, Recreation and Dance. Health-related physical fitness test manual. Reston, VA: AAHPERD; 1980.
4. American Alliance for Health, Physical Education, Recreation and Dance. Physical best. Reston, VA: AAHPERD; 1988.
5. Blair, S.N.; Falls, H.B.; Pate, R.R. A new physical fitness test. Phys. Sportsmed. 11:87-91; 1983.
6. Blair, S.N.; Clark, D.G.; Cureton, K.J.; Powell, K.E. Exercise and fitness in childhood: implications for a lifetime of health. In: Gisolfi, C.V.; Lamb, D.R., eds. Perspectives in exercise science and sports medicine: youth, exercise and sport. Indianapolis, IN: Benchmark Press; 1989:p. 401-422.
7. Blair, S.N.; Kohl, H.W.; Paffenbarger, R.S.; Clarke, D.G.; Cooper, K.H.; Gibbons, L.W. Physical fitness and all-cause mortality: a prospective study of healthy men. J. Am. Med. Assoc. 262:2395-2401; 1990.
8. Bouchard, C.; Shephard, R.J.; Stephens, T.; Sutton, J.R.; McPherson, B.D., eds. Exercise, fitness and health: a consensus of current knowledge. Champaign, IL: Human Kinetics; 1990.
9. Cureton, K.J.; Warren, G.W. Criterion-referenced standards for youth health-related fitness tests: a tutorial. Res. Q. Exerc. Sport 61:7-19; 1990.
10. Department of Health and Human Services. Promoting health/preventing disease: objectives for the nation. 1980:p. 155-161. Available from: U.S. Government Printing Office: Washington, DC.
11. Dotson, C. Health fitness standards: aerobic endurance. JOPERD 59:26-31; 1988.
12. Franks, D.B. YMCA youth fitness test manual. Champaign, IL: Human Kinetics; 1989.
13. Haskell, W.L.; Montoye, H.J.; Orenstein, D. Physical activity and exercise to achieve health-related physical fitness components. Public Health Rep. 100:202-212; 1985.
14. Institute for Aerobics Research. FitnessGram user's manual. Dallas, TX: Author; 1987.
15. Lohman, T.G. Assessment of body composition in children. Pediatr. Exerc. Sci. 1:19-30; 1989.
16. Looney, M.A.; Plowman, S.A. Passing rates of American children and youth on the Fitness-Gram criterion-referenced physical fitness standards. Res. Q. Exerc. Sport 61:215-223; 1990.
17. Malina, R.M. Growth, exercise, fitness and later outcomes. In: Bouchard, C. et al., eds. Exercise, fitness and health: a consensus of current knowledge. Champaign, IL: Human Kinetics; 1990:p. 637-653.
18. National Institutes of Health consensus development conference statement. Vol. 5, No. 9. Washington, DC: U.S. Government Printing Office; 1985.
19. Pate, R.R., ed. South Carolina physical fitness test manual test procedures and norms. 2nd ed. Columbia: South Carolina Association for Health, Physical Education, Recreation and Dance; 1983.
20. Pate, R.R.; Blair, S.N. Exercise and the prevention of atherosclerosis: pediatric implications. In: Strong, W., ed. Pediatric aspects of atherosclerosis. New York: Grune & Stratton; 1978: p. 251-286.
21. Pate, R.R.; Dowda, M.; Ross, J.G. Associations between physical activity and physical fitness in American children. Am. J. Dis. Child. 144: 1123-1129; 1990.
22. Presidential physical fitness award program: instructor's guide. Washington, DC: President's Council on Physical Fitness and Sports; 1987.
23. Reiff, G.G.; Dixon, W.R.; Jacoby, D.; Ye, G.X.; Spain, G.G.; Hunsicker, P.A. The president's council on physical fitness and sports national school population fitness survey. Ann Arbor: University of Michigan; 1986.
24. Ross, J.G.; Dotson, C.O.; Gilbert, G.G.; Katz, S.J. New standards for physical fitness measurement. JOPERD 56(1):62-66; 1985.
25. Ross, J.G.; Pate, R.R.; Delphy, L.A.; Gold, R.S.; Svilar, M. NCYFS II: new health-related fitness norms. JOPERD 58(10):66-70; 1987.
26. Safrit, M.J. The validity and reliability of fitness tests for children. Pediatr. Exerc. Sci. 2:9-28; 1990.

27. Simons-Morton, B.G.; O'Hara, N.M.; Simons-Morton, D.G.; Parcel, G.S. Children and fitness: a public health perspective. Res. Q. Exerc. Sport 58:295-302; 1987.

28. Simons-Morton, B.G.; Parcel, G.S.; O'Hara, N.M.; Blair, S.N.; Pate, R.R. Health-related physical fitness in childhood: status and recommendations. Annu. Rev. Public Health 9: 403-425; 1988.

29. Slaughter, M.H.; Lohman, T.G.; Boileau, R.A.; Horswill, C.A.; Stillman, R.J.; Van Loan, M.D.; Bemden, D.A. Skinfold equations for estimation of body fatness in children and youth. Hum. Biol. 60:709-723; 1988.

30. Squires, W.G.; Smith, E. Fit youth today program manual. Austin, TX: American Health and Fitness Foundation; 1986.

Chapter 14

Implementing Health-Related Physical Education

Bruce G. Simons-Morton
The National Institute of Child Health and Human Development

The benefits of physical activity and physical fitness have been long suspected, but documented only recently. It now appears that regular participation over the course of a lifetime in moderate physical activity (the type that increases cardiorespiratory fitness) is protective against all-cause mortality and cardiovascular disease (CVD) (1). Indeed, participation in regular physical activity is as important in preventing CVD as being a nonsmoker or eating a low-fat diet (19). In addition, physical activity is thought to improve sleep, increase capacity to perform daily functions, improve mental health, and help in maintaining weight (34).

Childhood physical activity provides immediate health benefits. Children who are physically active are less likely than inactive children to be obese (3), and higher levels of fitness during childhood are associated with generally lower blood pressure and lipids (12). Most experts agree that regular physical activity is important for growth and development (11), that it improves body composition (10), and that it may improve academic performance, moderate the effects of stress, and advance social development (23,24). The primary value of physical activity during childhood, however, is its impact on knowledge, attitudes, skills, and habits that may carry over into adulthood (2,22,29,31). Increasing the amount of appropriate physical activities, those likely to be continued into adulthood (21), is a national health objective (35).

Inclusion of physical education in the public school curriculum is perhaps one of the nation's greatest commitments to the health of American youth. During most of the 20th century, however, athletic skill and team sports have dominated the curriculum and instructional focus of PE, whereas health-related fitness has become a secondary objective. Sadly, most community programs also emphasize youth sports rather than health-related fitness. Hence, with some exception, both school and community programs have tended to service the small proportion of relatively more athletic children to the disadvantage of the vast majority of less athletic children whose need for organized physical activity probably is greater.

School physical education provides the ideal context for promoting health-related physical activity among children and youth because the magnitude and breadth of exposure can be sufficient to increase knowledge, affect attitudes, improve skills, and provide a substantial dose of physical activity (17,22,32). Nevertheless, school physical education is at a critical juncture in time. Funding for public education is more precarious and uncertain than ever. In many states, concerns about the preparation of American workers for the high-technology positions of the future have led to back-to-the-basics legislation for school curricula, providing little support for electives such as PE, music, and art. Physical education must compete for its place in the curriculum with computer labs, foreign language, field trips, and the arts. In many districts the number of physical education specialists has diminished in recent years. Perennial problems, such as the dominance of athletics over secondary PE and the uncomfortable curriculum integration of health and physical education, continue unresolved. Importantly, as evidence mounts showing that many school physical education programs do little to promote children's fitness (15,31,33), the profession finds that it may have squandered some of the public support upon which it has always relied.

Sadly, the apparent decline in the status of physical education in American schools comes just at the time when the benefits of physical activity are becoming known and concerns about children's fitness and inactivity are greater than ever before. The need to develop, implement, and diffuse quality, health-related physical education (HRPE) is now urgent.

This chapter describes HRPE, presents a case study involving the implementation of one elementary school HRPE program, and discusses the conditions required for the broad diffusion of HRPE among American schools.

Health-Related Physical Education as an Innovation

Despite a basis in the early history of the profession and evidence of its existence today in a few model programs, HRPE (also described elsewhere, see 2,4,26) is uncommon enough today to be considered an innovation. Further promotion of the innovation of HRPE requires that we define its special characteristics, identify its relative advantages over the approaches that dominate current practice, and establish the requirements for its implementation and diffusion.

The Nature of Health-Related Physical Education

The purpose of HRPE is to improve fitness, promote health, and prevent future disease in a population by increasing the amount of lifetime physical activity its individuals obtain. Stated differently, the goal is to increase the proportion of the population that maintains an adequate level of physical activity throughout their lives. The goals of HRPE

therefore are to assure that students obtain a substantial measure of physical activity during physical education classes and to encourage students to obtain physical activity outside school and throughout life. Increasing the amount of physical activity children obtain is largely a matter of developing activity- and fitness-oriented curricula and improving teaching effectiveness and efficacy. Increasing physical activity outside the classroom is largely a matter of making physical education classes highly enjoyable, increasing average motor skill development, and emphasizing lifetime activities during PE that can be engaged in easily outside structured programs.

Physical education cannot by itself be expected to reduce the prevalence of sedentary behavior among the population. Also required are increased availability and improved quality of public areas and facilities, expanded community programs, and changes in adult norms with respect to physical activity (28). Nevertheless, PE is a critical element in the process because it alone has the opportunity to educate the nation's youth in a systematic manner, thereby increasing the population's knowledge, improving attitudes and skills, and providing a substantial dose of correct practice.

Characteristics of the Innovation

HRPE is based on the principles of fitness development that specify the frequency, duration, type, and intensity of physical activity. In HRPE, these fitness principles are applied to the group rather than the individual. These principles can be applied in a variety of curricula emphasizing lifetime health and fitness.

Frequency

Although physical education accounts for less than half the physical activity children and youth obtain (21), it is the only source for many young children (27). Daily HRPE for all students in every semester of every grade is desirable (13), and 3 days a week is the minimum that is consistent with the goals of HRPE.

Duration

Both the actual time available for each class and the amount of time children are active during the class are important. It is very challenging to organize a class with less than 30 min of effective instructional time. Regardless of the length of the class, at least 40% of class time should be devoted to activity, that is, the median amount of activity students receive, averaged across the classes of each curriculum unit or grading period.

Type of Activity

A variety of physical activities and variations on each activity should be included in HRPE curricula (6,25). Physical activities that require gross motor movement and that can be engaged in easily outside of class and later in life should be emphasized. So-called lifetime or appropriate activities should dominate the curriculum, because they have limited requirements for equipment, facilities, and partners and therefore are likely to be continued during adulthood. Fitness units should be included, but all instructional units should emphasize fitness. Seasonal activities such as team sports, individual sports, games, and dance should be prominent and organized to foster maximum participation.

The seemingly endless professional debate between those who favor an emphasis on motor skills and those who favor an emphasis on health and fitness seems misdirected. Improvements in motor skills such as rope jumping, ball tossing, or running are important objectives of physical education because skill increases enjoyment and interest in further participation and allows children to maintain continuity of activity. The primary focus on skills, however, apparently leads to several commonly observed negative outcomes. First, the tendency of many physical education instructors has been to evaluate skill development on an absolute basis, where a premium is placed on correct performance of the skill rather than on effort or relative improvement. Thus the less talented students never do as well as the naturally more talented, and many students quickly learn from this comparison the futility of their efforts.

Second, the emphasis on the correct way of performing a skill through group instruction and demonstration methods dramatically limits the amount of practice each student obtains. This is a significant deficiency because the number of trials is probably the single most important determinant of motor skills development that can be modified. In HRPE improvement in motor skills is an important objective. However, skill development is relative to each student, and the primary pedagogical means of achieving these improvements are practice and specific, individualized feedback. Further, HRPE maintains that the best way to improve students' motor skills is to limit group instruction to a minimum and maximize the number of trials

each student obtains, while the teacher provides individualized instruction and feedback. The primary focus of HRPE is on increasing the amount of class time children spend in enjoyable activity. Hence, it should be at least as successful as the traditional skills approach for improvement, although no empirical tests of this assumption have been reported.

Intensity

The intensity of activity during PE should range from low to vigorous, with most of the activity time at a moderate-to-vigorous physical activity (MVPA) level. MVPA is activity that requires repeated weight transfer, like in running, jumping, swimming, and dancing. A primary teaching concern is to reduce the intensity demands of activities so that participation in the activity during a single bout can be extended. Hence, a clever teacher learns how to mix less intense activities with more intense activities in order to maximize the duration of the bouts and the enjoyment of the participants. Generally, it is reasonable to structure activities to encourage moderately intense activity, allowing individual students to self-regulate their actual intensity level.

Characteristics of Good Teaching

A number of teaching practices are emphasized in HRPE because they increase the efficiency or quality of the class and preserve maximum amounts of activity time (6,25). The administrative actions and teaching methods included in Table 14.1 (page 140) merit special attention because their regular incorporation into teaching practice is essential to fostering maximum participation in enjoyable physical activity.

Relative Advantages of Health-Related Physical Education

Physical education teachers' perceptions of the advantages and disadvantages of HRPE, relative to current practice, dictate the likelihood that HRPE philosophy and practices will be adopted. Some possible advantages of HRPE over current practice are that it

- emphasizes children's fitness knowledge, attitudes, and practices,
- emphasizes children's participation in lifetime PA,

Table 14.1   A Sample of Health-Related Physical Education Objectives, Administrative Actions, and Teaching Methods

A. Student learning objectives: Students will
   1. enjoy participating in MVPA,
   2. develop essential fitness knowledge and attitudes,
   3. develop motor skills,
   4. practice a variety of lifetime physical activities, and
   5. improve lifetime participation in physical activity and physical fitness.
B. Objectives for teachers: Teachers will
   1. maximize enjoyment of physical activity,
   2. maximize the amount of class time devoted to MVPA,
   3. maximize the amount and quality of students' participation in MVPA, and
   4. maximize students' opportunities for practice and feedback.
C. Administration: Teachers will
   1. create a year-long HRPE curriculum plan,
   2. organize the curriculum into activity units (e.g., soccer, basketball, jump rope, fitness stations, dance, etc.),
   3. include running, calisthenics, and a variety of unit-specific activities in each lesson,
   4. establish routines, groups or formations, and a consistent class structure (e.g., warm-up, fitness development, lesson focus, game),
   5. have equipment and facilities ready before class starts, and
   6. minimize unacceptable and off-task behavior by attending to it early, consistently applying established, fair punishment, and reinforcing on-task behavior.
D. Teaching methods: The teacher will
   1. provide brief group instructions,
   2. provide copious individual feedback and instruction,
   3. call students by their names,
   4. provide frequent reinforcement,
   5. make rapid transitions from one activity to another, and
   6. serve as a role model by enjoying regular participation in MVPA during class and remaining physically fit.

- increases enjoyment of PE and participation in MVPA,
- promotes children's physical fitness,
- emphasizes participation in MVPA as the main outcome,
- emphasizes individual and group involvement over absolute performance standards,
- improves motor skills,

- reduces off-task behavior,
- requires effective teaching practices, and
- increases teacher enjoyment of the profession.

The possible perceived disadvantages relative to other approaches may be that HRPE requires advanced planning and efficient class administration and expands the teacher's responsibility beyond PE to after school and later life.

Stages of Adoption

Adopting an innovation, teachers or administrators are likely to pass through the following stages:

- awareness
- trial
- implementation
- maintenance (20)

Although HRPE possesses natural advantages that encourage its adoption, increasing the influence of HRPE requires effort on the part of change agents willing to work for it. Table 14.2 includes selected intervention strategies appropriate for each stage of adoption. Providing information about the nature and relative advantages of the innovation is most important at the awareness and trial stages, as well as knowing about and observing model teachers. Teacher training, reinforcement and feedback, policy statements, and accountability also are important at implementation and maintenance stages. Although examples of HRPE can be found at the elementary school level in most large school districts, apparently only a small minority of innovative teachers and administrators have adopted HRPE (33). As HRPE becomes better known and its relative advantages become apparent more people will adopt the innovation. Indeed, some university professional-preparation programs recently have shifted away from a strict emphasis on skills toward an emphasis on HRPE.

Implementing Health-Related Physical Education

Isolated examples of HRPE can be found in most regions of the country. An ongoing study that assesses the quality of physical education in the several school districts within a large metropolitan area found only one district that reported having district-level policies in support of HRPE (34). Fur-

Table 14.2   Intervention Strategies Employed to Address Each Stage of Adoption of Health-Related Physical Education

Stage of adoption	Strategies
Awareness	Information
Trial	Modeling
	Teacher involvement in curriculum
	Policy statement
Implementation	Training and in-service
	Weekly consultation
	Observation and feedback
	Incentives
	Reinforcement
Maintenance	Feedback
	Reinforcement
	Individualized fitness development

ther, few HRPE programs have been evaluated and reported in the literature.

Several small-scale efficacy studies have been conducted to examine the extent to which and the conditions under which HRPE can be established successfully and the extent to which implementation can affect the desired outcomes (5,7-9,32). Most of these studies share a common focus on increasing the percent of physical education class time devoted to MVPA. The Go For Health study serves as one example.

Description of the Go For Health Efficacy Study

The purpose of the Go For Health project was to increase health, diet, and physical activity behavior at school for elementary school children. The following intervention components were developed and implemented: the Go For Health diet and physical activity curriculum, the New School Lunch, and Children's Active Physical Education (CAPE) (15,30,32). Two elementary schools in a Texas school district were assigned to intervention and the other two to the control condition.

The target population of third and fourth graders had PE daily for 35 to 60 min and were taught by one of the two experienced physical education specialists at each school. Of the four physical education teachers in the two intervention schools, three were certified specialists and one

was a classroom teacher who had switched mid-career to physical education. Facilities at each school included a modern gymnasium and large outdoor playground area. Classes ranged from 50 to 100 students. Sometimes each teacher would have 25 to 50 children; at other times the two teachers at the school would teach the same lesson to as many as 100 children.

CAPE represents only one of many possible approaches to health-related physical education, but the effort to implement it provides a useful context within which to discuss implementation. CAPE is an example of external change agents promoting adoption of HRPE by PE teachers (16). The project had the advantage of a full-time physical education specialist employed exclusively to foster effective adoption of HRPE. It had the disadvantage of being applied in a school district without enthusiasm for HRPE, where administrative support for HRPE was minimal and where the teachers and administrators started at the preawareness stage. There was no budget for equipment or materials. The district director of physical education, typically, was also the athletic director and the high school football coach. Although not impeding the project, he paid little attention to elementary physical education and was content to let each principal provide whatever training and supervision might be necessary. Indeed, the year before the study began, the physical education teachers (who were required by the state to receive in-service instruction the week before school started) attended the in-service training for elementary school math instruction because none was available for physical education.

Periodically physical education teachers were subjected by the school district to mandatory evaluations based on criteria developed exclusively for classroom instruction. These evaluations rewarded didactic, teacher-centered lessons where the entire class did the same thing at the same time—very unlike the highly active, student-centered, multiple-stations approach favored by CAPE.

In order to implement CAPE as part of the Go For Health project, we applied a variety of curriculum development, training, and motivational strategies.

Curriculum Development

The purpose of CAPE was to promote during PE classes the maximum amount of enjoyable MVPA without unduly sacrificing other important objectives. At baseline no curriculum existed, either at the district or school level. Each physical education teacher was personally committed to a few favorite activities (gymnastics, football, or softball) but yearly plans were not available or required. No fitness units were taught, although the AAHPERD fitness testing (not the modern health-related fitness testing) was conducted annually. We involved the intervention school physical education teachers in a 2-year process of selecting activities and creating units for CAPE.

Ultimately, CAPE consisted of five 6-week units that the intervention PE teachers were encouraged to employ exclusively. The curriculum included lessons for each day of the year. Each unit included two or three cardiovascular fitness development physical activities such as dancing, running, aerobic games, jumping rope, and obstacle courses. Each class session consisted of introduction (warm-up), fitness development, game activities, and cool-down. As children's skill and fitness improved over the course of a unit, the duration of the fitness development activity segment increased from about 6 min to as much as 15 min.

Change Agent or Master Teacher

An experienced physical education teacher and fitness specialist served as a change agent, working extensively and exclusively with the four physical education teachers for the duration of the project to foster quality implementation. This master teacher provided training, consultation, curriculum development, and fitness prescriptions individualized for each PE teacher. Gradually, over the 2-year period, trust developed between the master teacher (initially distrusted as an outsider) and the school physical education specialists.

Training for Improved Teaching Skills

The teachers received 16 hr of training each of two summers, plus extensive consultation from the staff master teacher. Training was very practical, increasing the teachers' familiarity with the curriculum and involving them in teaching situations in which they could practice and improve teaching skills with feedback from the master teacher.

Teachers were trained to minimize administrative time by having equipment ready when the students entered the gymnasium or playing field. Students became involved in warm-up activities immediately upon their arrival for class rather than waiting until everyone had arrived, put down their books, adjusted their clothing, and talked with their friends. The teachers were encouraged to serve as models by regularly performing physical activity with the class, although not necessarily throughout each of their six daily classes. Other features emphasized individualized instruction, positive feedback, using children's names, making rapid transitions from one activity to another, moving from one part of the activity area to another throughout the lesson, attending to behavioral problems in their early stages, and establishing and practicing fair penalties for continued unacceptable or off-task behavior. On-task behavior and other evidence of desirable participation were rewarded verbally.

Motivation

To increase interest and motivation in fitness, the staff physical education specialist supervised each physical education teacher during the summer in individualized, personal exercise programs. Teachers were awarded a month's membership in the local fitness center of their choice. To encourage implementation, the teachers at each school were able to earn up to $200 for additional equipment for their PE program.

Results

Using a standard instrument and protocol (14), the amount and type of physical activity were assessed annually by observation of randomly selected children during about 30 classes in each school on randomly sampled days. At baseline the median percent of class time children were observed in MVPA was less than 10% in each of the four classes. At posttest 2 years later, the median percent of class time, which had not changed in the control schools, had increased in the intervention schools to 40% or greater in each school for both third and fourth grades, an increase from baseline of over 400%. Hence, during daily PE at least 50% of the students in the intervention schools obtained 15 min or more of MVPA, compared with less than 5 min for the students in the control schools (32). Informal interviews with teachers 1 year after the end of the program indicated that the teachers in one school had discontinued most of the CAPE principles and activities; in the other school, CAPE was basically still in place, although modified somewhat by the teachers.

Discussion

The results of the Go For Health project demonstrate the efficacy of implementing HRPE in elementary school. Go For Health was a small study conducted to learn about the feasibility of implementation and the conditions under which the target outcomes could be achieved. The researchers were surprised by the lack of structure, purpose, and pedagogy associated with the current elementary school physical education program, and we were not prepared for the strength of the teachers' early resistance to the CAPE innovation. A great deal more time than originally planned was spent with the teachers on curriculum revision, training, consultation, counseling, and attention.

After 1 year the intervention had managed to change PE only modestly in one intervention school and not at all in the other. Only in the second year—with additional training, countless counseling and consulting sessions, and increased participation in personal fitness programs by three of the teachers—were significant increases observed in the average amount of MVPA during class. Apparently, it took a year's tentative experience with the curriculum before the relative advantages of CAPE were appreciated. Also, it may have taken the students a year to adapt to the demand for increased activity during PE. Subsequently, in the absence of continuing education and support after Go For Health was discontinued and without institutional supports and requirements, some teachers, but not all, dropped the program.

Effectiveness and Diffusion

It is clear from the results of the Go For Health program and other small studies that effective implementation of HRPE is possible in elementary schools if sufficient effort by external agents is provided. Also, on the basis of empirical investigation and many conversations with physical education leaders, it appears that HRPE, although rare, has been institutionalized in some innovative school districts without the aid of external agents. It remains for us to learn the extent to which a program of HRPE can be implemented effectively under experimentally controlled conditions so that the results can be generalized to other settings. Further, it is important to assess the efficacy of implementing HRPE in secondary schools.

Effectiveness of a program of HRPE is being tested in a randomized study entitled Children and Adolescent Trial for Cardiovascular Health (CATCH) involving 96 elementary schools in four states (18) randomized to usual or intervention conditions. As part of the CATCH interventions, the effects of health-related physical education on children's physical activity, body composition, and cardiorespiratory fitness will be assessed.

Ultimately, it is desirable to diffuse HRPE broadly among U.S. schools. The tenets of diffusion theory suggest that the spread of HRPE into practice may require a variety of institutional changes such as those included in Table 14.3. The importance of recruiting good people into physical education teaching, improving professional preparation programs, and establishing professional practice standards cannot be underestimated. Professional organizations, such as the American Alliance of Health, Physical Education, Recreation and Dance, and state education departments should establish policy in support of establishing a national K-12 HRPE curriculum. The establishment of a model HRPE curriculum and the development of model HRPE programs and training centers are needed. The profession is in dire need also of evaluation systems that reward teachers for maximizing enjoyable participation during PE.

Table 14.3 Implementation and Diffusion of HRPE

Considerations for implementing HRPE in your school district:
1. Promote the relative advantages and innovative features of HRPE.
2. Identify and train change agents or master teachers.
3. Train teachers already in the field.
4. Provide teacher attention, recognition, and reinforcement.
5. Establish model HRPE programs in schools.
6. Make teachers accountable for children's moderate-to-vigorous physical activity.
7. Hire new teachers from university programs that emphasize HRPE.
8. Make personal fitness an objective for every PE teacher.

Considerations in the diffusion of HRPE:
1. Hire only excellent teachers.
2. Make HRPE the focus of teacher-preparation programs.
3. Establish HRPE practice standards for teachers.
4. Develop model HRPE programs.
5. Create training centers.
6. Establish national guidelines for fair and effective evaluation of HRPE teaching.
7. Establish a national HRPE curriculum.
8. Obtain policy support of HRPE from state departments of education and national professional organizations.

Summary

Health-related physical education (HRPE) emphasizes lifetime participation in moderate-to-vigorous activity (MVPA) as a means of promoting fitness and health. HRPE usually offers classes that devote most of each period to enjoyable MVPA in which nearly all the students participate. HRPE teachers stress effective class management, keep group instruction and demonstration to a minimum, maximize the number of practice trials, and provide frequent individual feedback, instruction, and encouragement. Although HRPE still is uncommon in practice, model programs are available, and some university teacher-preparation curricula now emphasize it. The program's advantages include increased student and teacher enjoyment of PE, improved motor skills, increased participation in MVPA, and improved physical fitness and health. Small-scale studies have demonstrated effective implementation of HRPE in elementary schools in which substantial program attention was devoted to teacher training. Broader diffusion of HRPE is likely, due to its relative advantages over usual practice; innovating the program rapidly, however, will depend on alterations in teacher-training programs and policy support from state and national organizations.

References

1. Blair, S.N.; Kohl, H.W., III; Paffenbarger, R.S.; Clark, D.G.; Cooper, K.H.; Gibbons, L.W. Physical fitness and all-cause mortality: a prospective study of healthy men and women. J. Am. Med. Assoc. 262:2395-2401; 1989.
2. Blair, S.N.; Pate, R.R.; McClenaghan, B. Current approaches to physical fitness education. In: Kratochwill, T.R., ed. Advances in school psychology. Vol. 2. Hillsdale, NJ: Erlbaum; 1982:p. 315-361.
3. Clark, D.G.; Blair, S.N. Physical activity and prevention of obesity in childhood. In: Krasnegor N.A.; Grave G.D.; Dretchmer, N., eds. Childhood obesity: a biobehavioral perspective. Caldwell, NJ: Telford Press; 1988:p. 121-142.
4. Corbin, C.B.; Lindsey, R. Fitness for life. 3rd ed. Glenview, IL: Scott, Foresman; 1990.
5. Coates, T.J.; Jeffery, R.W.; Slinkard, L.A. Heart healthy eating and exercise: introducing and maintaining changes in health behaviors. Am. J. Public Health 71(1):15-23; 1981.
6. Dauer, V.P.; Pangrazi, R.P. Dynamic physical education for elementary school children. 9th ed. New York: Macmillan; 1989.
7. Duncan, B.; Boyce, T.; Itami, R.; Paffenbarger, N. A controlled trial of physical fitness program for fifth grade students. J. Sch. Health 53:467-471; 1983.
8. Dwyer, T.; Coohan, W.; Leitch, O.; Hetzel, B.S.; Baghurst, R.A. An investigation of the effect of daily physical activity on the health of primary school students in South Australia. Int. J. Epidemiol. 12:308-313; 1983.
9. Gafner, L.; Heinrich, J.; Knappe, J.; Holtz, H. Atherosclerosis precursors in school children—results of a two-year intervention study. Cor Vasa 29(6):421-427; 1989.
10. Lohman, T.G.; Boileau, R.A.; Slaughter, M.H. Body composition in children and youth. In: Boileau, R.A., ed. Biological issues. (Advances in pediatric sport sciences. Vol. 1.) Champaign, IL: Human Kinetics; 1984:p. 29-57.
11. Malina, R.M. Human growth, maturation, and regular Physical activity. In: Boileau, R.A., ed. Biological issues. (Advances in pediatric sport sciences. Vol. 1.) Champaign, IL: Human Kinetics; 1984:p. 59-83.
12. Morrison, J.A.; Glueck, C.J. Pediatric risk factors for adult coronary heart disease: primary atherosclerosis prevention. Cardiovasc. Rev. Reports 1981(2):1269-1281.
13. National Association for Sport and Physical Education. NASPE 1988: a year in review. NASPE News 24:1; 1989.
14. O'Hara, N.; Baranowski, T.; Simons-Morton, B.G.; Wilson, B.; Parcel, G.S. Validity of the observation of children's physical activity. Res. Q. Exerc. Sport 60(1):42-47; 1989.
15. Parcel, G.S.; Simons-Morton, B.G.; O'Hara, N.M.; Kolbe, L.J.; Baranowski, T.; Bee, D.E. School health promotion and cardiovascular health: an integration of institutional change and social learning theory intervention. J. Sch. Health 57(4):150-156; 1987.
16. Parcel, G.S.; Simons-Morton, B.G.; Kolbe, L.J. School health promotion: integrating organizational change and student learning strategies. Health Educ. Q. 15(4):435-450; 1988.
17. Pate, R.R.; Corbin, C.; Simons-Morton, B.G.; Ross, J.G. Physical education and the school health program. J. Sch. Health 57(10):445-450; 1987.
18. Perry, C.L.; Stone, E.J.; Parcel, G.S.; Ellison, R.C.; Nader, P.R.; Webber, L.S.; Luepker, R.V.

School-based cardiovascular health promotion: the child and adolescent trial for cardiovascular health (CATCH). J. Sch. Health 60(8):406-412; 1990.

19. Powell, K.E.; Thompson, P.D.; Caspersen, C.J.; Kendrick, J.S. Physical activity and incidence of coronary heart disease. Ann. Rev. Public Health 8:253-287; 1987.

20. Rogers, E.M. Diffusion of innovations. 3rd ed. New York: Free Press; 1983.

21. Ross, J.G.; Pate, R.R. The national children and youth fitness study II: a summary of findings. JOPERD 58:51-56; 1987.

22. Sallis, J.F.; McKenzie, T.L. Physical education's role in public health. Res. Q. Exerc. Sport 62(2):124-137; 1991.

23. Seefeldt, V., ed. Physical activity and well-being. Reston, VA: AAHPERD; 1986.

24. Shephard, R.J. Physical activity and "wellness" of the child. In: Boileau, R.A., ed. Biological issues. (Advances in pediatric sport sciences. Vol. 1.) Champaign, IL: Human Kinetics; 1984:p. 1-27.

25. Siedentop, D. Physical education: introductory analysis. 3rd ed. Dubuque, IA: Little, Brown; 1980.

26. Simons-Morton, B.G. Health-related physical education. In: Wallace, H.M.; Parcel, G.P.; Igoe, J.; Patrick, K., eds. School health. (Principles and practices for school health. Vol. 2) Oakland, CA: Third Party Publishing; 1992:p. 443-452.

27. Simons-Morton, B.G.; Baranowski, T.; O'Hara, N.M.; Parcel, G.S.; Huang, I.W.; Wilson, B. Children's participation in moderate to vigorous physical activities. Res. Q. Exerc. Sport 61(4):307-314; 1991.

28. Simons-Morton, B.G.; O'Hara, N.M.; Simons-Morton, D.G. Promoting healthful diet and exercise behaviors in communities, schools, and families. Fam. Community Health 9(3):1-13; 1986.

29. Simons-Morton, B.G.; O'Hara, N.M.; Simons-Morton, D.G.; Parcel, G.S. Children and fitness: a public health perspective. Res. Q. Exerc. Sport 58(4):295-304; 1987.

30. Simons-Morton, B.G.; Parcel, G.S.; O'Hara, N.M. Implementing organizational changes to promote healthful diet and physical activity at school. Health Educ. Q. 15(1):115-130; 1988.

31. Simons-Morton, B.G.; Parcel, G.S.; O'Hara, N.M.; Blair, S.; Pate, R.R. Childhood health-related physical fitness: status and recommendations. Annu. Rev. Public Health 9:403-425; 1988.

32. Simons-Morton, B.G.; Parcel, G.S.; Baranowski, T.; Forthofer, R.; O'Hara, N.M. Promoting physical activity and a healthful diet among children: results of a school-based intervention study. Am. J. Public Health 81(8):986-991; 1991.

33. Simons-Morton, B.G.; Taylor, W.C.; Snider, S.A.; Huang, I.W. The physical activity of fifth-grade students during physical education classes. Am. J. Public Health 83:262-264; 1993.

34. Taylor, C.B.; Sallis, J.F.; Needle, R. The relation of physical activity and exercise to mental health. Public Health Rep. 100(2):195-201; 1985.

35. U.S. Department of Health and Human Services Public Health Service. Healthy people 2000: national health promotion and disease prevention objectives. 1991. Available from: U.S. Government Printing Office. Washington, DC: (DHHS Pub. No. [PHS] 91-50213).

Chapter 15

Teaching Fitness in the Elementary School: A Comprehensive Approach

Thomas A. Ratliffe
Florida State University & University Laboratory School

Fitness and motor skill development are essential components of the elementary school physical education curriculum and they should complement and contribute to one another. The PE curriculum should help children acquire a mature pattern in the common fundamental motor skills; help develop competence in games, gymnastics, and dance activities; and help them begin to understand and value physical fitness. Numerous articles and curricular packages provide ideas and strategies for teaching specific fitness lessons. Drawing from these resources, this chapter will outline the key elements that comprise a comprehensive approach to teaching fitness in an elementary school setting.

A fitness curriculum like the one described here can be accomplished despite constraints of time, space, and financial resources. I have implemented many such programs in conditions that were far from ideal—for example, with children who have PE twice a week using only a small stage or cafeteria for indoor space and a yearly budget of $150 to $300.

The goals of a comprehensive fitness curriculum in the elementary school can help children acquire the skills, knowledge, and attitudes that lead to a lifetime of physical activity (5):

1. Participation in developmentally appropriate fitness activities in physical education class

2. Learning fitness concepts—lower and higher order objectives (1)
3. Developing a positive attitude about physical activity and becoming intrinsically motivated
4. Regular participation in physical activities in addition to PE classes

Competencies

Children should attain specific competencies during the elementary school years. Students should be able to

1. Demonstrate the correct technique and procedure for performing skill- and health-related fitness exercises.
2. Identify the components of skill-related and health-related fitness.
3. Demonstrate activities and behaviors associated with each component of skill-related fitness (agility, balance, coordination, power, and speed) and health-related fitness (cardiovascular endurance, muscular strength and endurance, flexibility, and body composition).
4. Identify the major parts of the body (organs, muscles, and bones).

5. Describe the function of the heart and circulatory system.
6. Give examples to demonstrate the basic principles of exercise including duration, frequency, and intensity.
7. Identify the benefits of regular physical activity.
8. Identify the risk factors of heart disease and give examples of ways to modify the risk factors.
9. Explain the meaning of caloric balance and the implications for daily diet and activity habits.
10. Describe how muscles increase in size and strength (overload principle) and identify activities that will improve specific muscle groups (specificity principle).
11. Participate in a moderate level of physical activity on a daily basis.
12. Evaluate their own levels of activity and fitness.
13. Design and carry out their own exercise programs.

In the primary elementary grades (K-2), children participate in fitness activities that emphasize competencies 1, 4, 5, 7, and 11. Cardiovascular concepts are introduced using a variety of aerobic activities, for example, chasing, fleeing, and dodging, dance, jumping rope, and fitness walking. Flexibility and muscular strength and endurance concepts can be taught through dance and gymnastics activities. In the upper elementary grades (3-6), these competencies are reviewed and reinforced. The remaining competencies that include more cognitive information are presented, although physical experiences are still a major aspect of instruction. It is important to relate to the child's reality, not the adult's. Children are motivated by fun and achieving competence, not their future health and appearance 20 years from now. In all cases, the emphasis is on successful participation and enjoyment of activities, where cognitive information is presented through hands-on participation.

The following example shows how upper elementary children can be introduced to the concepts of *overload, repetitions, sets*, and the benefits of regular exercise. During a lesson, have children do sit-ups for 30 sec and write down their scores on individual file cards. In the next few weeks, take a portion of each class to practice sit-ups and teach the relevant fitness concepts. Introduce the concept of repetitions and have students do an individually prescribed number of repetitions. This number will vary depending on the individual's capabilities—

some children can do 5, some 15, and some will need to do curl-ups until they develop the abdominal strength to do sit-ups. At this point, discuss sets and have students do three sets of their prescribed dose of sit-ups or curl-ups.

In subsequent lessons discuss the principle of overload and have students do three sets with light resistance (e.g., a milk carton filled with sand). To stimulate thinking about the effects of regular exercise, ask students why they are doing sit-ups every class. The strategy of asking a specific question provides an opportunity for the teacher to check students' knowledge and reinforce their understanding of the concepts. Use visual learning aids to introduce the concepts and to help children remember the words. After a series of lessons, have the students take the 30-sec sit-up challenge again and check for individual improvement. The experience is set up for success and the objective is to learn the fitness concepts of overload, repetitions, sets, and the benefits of regular exercise to improve personal fitness.

Teaching Methods and Strategies

The quality of the teaching will determine the effectiveness of the fitness curriculum. In addition to pedagogical skills, the teacher must value fitness and enthusiastically implement fitness lessons. There is also some evidence to indicate that the teachers' appearance of good health affects how information is received and valued by students (4). The key to teaching children fitness is to keep the activities stimulating, motivating, and fun. This is accomplished by providing developmentally appropriate activities with a lot of activity time, by high levels of success, and by efforts that are reinforced and rewarded.

Children learn best through concrete rather than abstract presentations and by forming mental images of concepts. Learning aids such as pictures, posters, videotapes, models, and equipment will help children understand fitness concepts (6).

A combination of instructional strategies seems to be the best way to teach fitness concepts. At times a series of sequential lessons on a fitness topic are necessary and at other times only part of a single lesson is sufficient and effective. For example, a unit on muscular strength and endurance might include information on and participation in a variety of exercises and activities over a period of several weeks. Stations that relate to the components of muscular strength and endurance could be set up—sit-ups, modified pull-ups, horizontal ladder walk, rope climb, push-ups, and milk-jug arm curls are examples. Over several class periods each student would use a scorecard to record his or her best effort on these station activities. Students would then be shown how to set goals and train for improvement using the principles of overload and progression. Whole class periods or segments of classes could be used to practice the activities. Periodically, improvement can be measured when giving a maximum effort and recording the scores. This strategy offers students the opportunity to practice muscular strength and endurance activities and learn principles of training by personally experiencing the process of working for improvement.

Some objectives can be effectively taught by incorporating the fitness concept into another theme lesson. For example, during active movement experiences, children can be taught facts about the heart, such as its location, size, and function. Another example is to teach the meaning of calories and caloric balance. In the "cookie lesson," each student is given a small cookie, which equals approximately 60 calories, to eat at the start of the lesson. Then, after an active 20-min lesson, the students are asked to remember the cookie and are told that those calories were just used up during the activities. Discussions and activities focusing on the caloric value and balance of foods and exercises can follow in future lessons.

Fitness circuits, par courses, and large-group fitness activities are strategies to involve children in challenging and enjoyable exercise (3). A circuit can include a variety of fitness stations that are identified by the skill- or health-related component that most closely relates to the exercise. Exercise stations can also be used to help evaluate students' knowledge. Ask them to choose between several file cards that you place at each exercise station. Each file card has a fitness component written on it. When students are finished performing an activity, they choose the card with the fitness component (balance, muscular endurance, cardiorespiratory endurance, etc.) that best matches the exercise.

Homework activities can supplement the school class instruction. Children might take their parents' heart rates while resting, after eating, or during exercise. Heart diagrams and work sheets can be taken home to label and color. Students can make a contract to perform various exercises and have their parents initial the contract when completed. Encouraging children's efforts at school and at home helps motivate them and sends the clear message that regular activity is important.

Many excellent resources are available to help teachers design meaningful lessons. The American Heart Association in your community and the American Alliance for Health, Physical Education, Recreation and Dance are two organizations that have curriculum materials for your use in school programs. A list of resources on the topic of teaching fitness in school is included at the end of this chapter.

Out-of-Class Fitness Opportunities

A comprehensive fitness curriculum includes out-of-class opportunities for children to learn and participate in fitness activities (2). The limited amount of physical education class time in most American schools prevents teachers from adequately covering the curriculum goals. Physical education teachers, classroom teachers, administrators, parents, and community programs all must participate in a comprehensive fitness plan.

The Running for Fitness Club is a very successful way to encourage regular, voluntary aerobic exercise. The purpose is to provide opportunity and reinforcement for regular walking and jogging. A walking/running course is marked by tires or stakes planted around the perimeter of the school grounds. A half-mile loop is ideal, although shorter distances can work. Prior to starting the club, support should be solicited from the principal, administrators, and classroom teachers. Basic procedures are introduced and established in one PE class, and charts for recording laps are posted in each classroom.

Teachers establish their own rules for when to record completed laps. A limit should be set on the maximum number of laps each person may record in one day, so that consistent, regular activity is encouraged. The benefits of regular aerobic activity should be taught during short segments of physical education classes so that students begin to associate positive health with regular exercise. As students reach goals such as 10, 25, and 50 miles, the classroom teachers submit the names to the physical education teacher who then rewards each child with a certificate. These certificates should carry a message about the benefits of regular exercise and might also depict figures (young, old, male, female, and multiethnic) engaging in fitness activities.

A fitness project can make a lasting impression on students and encourage in-depth study. Writing a report, constructing a photo collage, making a poster, or designing a play can inspire students to discover new knowledge and learn by doing. Having students show and tell about their projects can help emphasize the importance of the assignments and provide additional information to the class.

Parent involvement and support is another crucial element in a comprehensive fitness curriculum for children. A fitness information night can be arranged to present information about physical fitness, and children could demonstrate correct procedures for fitness exercises such as vigorous walking, bent-leg sit-ups, flexibility, push-ups, aerobic dance, and jumping rope. Parents and children can even participate in some activities together.

A fitness booklet can be compiled with activities and challenges to encourage children to participate in physical activities at home with support from their parents. A remedial program is necessary for some children who have serious deficiencies in fitness components. A special time during the day or after school could be arranged for those students to exercise and practice motor skills. An individualized, written contract with specific goals, requirements, and rewards should be a part of the remedial program. Parental support and involvement is essential in conducting this type of program. Parents can provide support by agreeing to walk or play with their child several days a week, regulate exercise and eating habits, and participate in the reward system.

Assessment

Assessing students' progress is important to inform the teacher of the effectiveness of the fitness programs and to provide objective data for parents, classroom teachers, and administrators who can support the teachers' efforts. Individual items on the health-related fitness test can be administered during the year so that students can begin to evaluate their own fitness and learn ways to maintain and improve their fitness. Pre-, post-, or periodic testing should be used to inform students of their progress and to encourage improvement. Each test item (e.g., sit-ups and the mile run) should be used to explain its relationship to positive health. Students should learn what each test measures, where they rank, how they can determine realistic goals for themselves, and what they can do to improve.

To help children understand the relationship of health and fitness, a "healthy" criterion score can be set for each health-related item. The AAHPERD Physical Best program has established health fitness standards and has record systems, student contracts, activity logs, report cards, and rewards to suit a variety of teaching needs. The Physical Best recognition system is set up to reward participation in extracurricular activities, achievement of individual goals, and mastery of the health fitness standards. (Customizing certificates to recognize particular efforts of students may be necessary.) Recognizing improvement in fitness test items and regular participation in activity should be a consistent aspect of the assessment program.

A convenient method of assessment is to keep records of the children who participate in the fitness clubs. If you are awarding certificates, then you know which children are participating. Work sheets and quizzes are ways to assess students' cognitive understanding of the fitness concepts.

The Congaree Curriculum

The Congaree curriculum is an example of how I implemented these ideas in a public elementary school in South Carolina. Congaree Elementary School is a suburban K-6 grade school of about 320 students. Facilities for teaching physical education consist of a large, sandy field with a wooded, hilly section. This outdoor area has a paved rectangular section slightly smaller than a regulation basketball court. The perimeter of the school and playground area is just over 1/2 mile. Indoor space consists of a cafeteria with portable folding tables and a small stage area. Children at Congaree have two 30-min PE classes per week.

The curriculum topics outlined in Table 15.1 illustrate the major fitness and skill topics that were taught to third-grade children. I developed this curriculum over a period of 5 years. The Congaree children were introduced to and gradually gained competence in fitness and motor skill activities by participating in games, gymnastics, dance, and fitness activities.

During the initial weeks of the school year, PE lessons focused on establishing the learning environment, space awareness, throwing and catching, and cooperation with the teacher and with classmates. At regular intervals during the year, fitness activities were planned to teach concepts to children and to provide opportunities and motivation to learn about and participate in fitness activities.

Table 15.1 The Congaree Curriculum (3rd-Grade Sample)

September
- Establish the learning environment
- Cooperation
- Space awareness and locomotor movements
- Game skills: throwing and catching
- Jumping rope

October
- Preparation and practice for fitness tests
- Fitness tests
- Chasing, fleeing, and dodging
- Throwing and catching (continued)
- Introduce the Running Club: pacing, straw walk

November
- Setting goals for fitness improvement
- Kicking and soccer skills
- Parent-Child Fitness Night

December
- Rhythms and dance
- Heart and cardiorespiratory lessons

January
- Rhythms and dance
  Music and physical education combined classes
  Aerobics dance routines

February
- Gymnastics (floor level): balance, rolling, sequencing
- Introduce the Monkey Bar Club

March
- Gymnastics (with apparatus): weight transfer, jumping and landing, sequencing
- Muscle strength contract

April
- Striking with paddles
- Fitness tests

May
- Field Day
- Striking with paddles and bats

June
- Striking with paddles and bats

Jumping rope was introduced in the first few weeks so that children could participate during recess and at home.

In October, emphasis focused on the health-related fitness items. Several class lessons were used to explain, prepare, and conduct the fitness tests and introduce the Running Club. This was a voluntary club to encourage regular, daily walking and running. Students were introduced to the club in one 30-min class meeting and then were encouraged to participate during recess and classroom breaks with their teachers. Laps were recorded for

students on charts in their classrooms, and when children reached specific goals, their names were posted in the cafeteria and they were awarded certificates. Important lessons centered on *pacing* and the principles of *frequency, duration*, and *intensity*. The straw walk (7) was a successful way to help children learn pacing and the principles of aerobic exercise. A course was set up for children to walk around without stopping. For each completed lap they were given a straw and encouraged to keep walking for the designated time.

In November we scheduled a parent-child fitness night to provide some basic information to parents about the fitness tests and to demonstrate some of the activities children learned in PE. I also explained the fitness opportunities that students had during the year. Examples were the Running Club, the Monkey Bar Club, aerobic videotapes, roller skating, bicycle riding, and playground exercises.

By December and January it was time to blend dance activities with information about health and fitness habits. Using materials (films, posters, and work sheets) from the American Heart Association and stethoscopes from the local nursing school, I taught the function of the cardiovascular system and healthy habits to care for it. The stethoscopes proved very effective as children listened to the sound of the heart during rest, exercise, and recovery. Upper elementary students learned to count heart beats accurately and use a conversion chart to determine heart rate.

Students learned about blood flow and the work of the heart from an American Heart Association film and then traveled through a simulated diagram of the circulatory system made up of a hoop for the mouth, boxes for the lungs and heart, and cardboard and rope tunnels for the vessels. After this hands-on experience, the children completed work sheets that depicted the structure and functioning of the heart and circulatory system. Although many lessons were conducted indoors during these winter months, the Running Club continued to operate, and many children earned 25-, 50-, and even 100-mile certificates.

During the gymnastics instruction in February, flexibility and muscular strength and endurance concepts were emphasized. Segments of lessons (5-10 min) explaining flexibility and demonstrating safe exercises and proper procedures to stretch were integrated with gymnastics lessons on rolling and balance. Flexibility exercises were shown on large posters so that students could look and practice appropriate stretches. Because gymnastics requires substantial arm, shoulder, and abdominal strength, other lessons included segments of instruction explaining and practicing a variety of upper-body strength exercises (variations of push-ups and triceps push-ups) and abdominal exercises (curl-ups and sit-ups). After initial instruction on these strength and flexibility concepts, the subsequent lessons included these exercises in a warm-up period, with the majority of the lesson spent on gymnastics themes.

It is helpful to encourage participation in fitness activities in addition to regularly scheduled PE and combine them with some procedure for reinforcing children's efforts. In February, the Monkey Bar Club was introduced to encourage regular arm and shoulder exercise. Occasional days were taken to observe students maneuver themselves across the horizontal ladder. Names were written on charts in the cafeteria for children who successfully navigated one, two, or three times across and back on the ladder.

March's lessons continued to work on gymnastics themes and progressed to the use of apparatus for developing weight transfer and combining the skills of balance and rolling. At Congaree this meant using the existing outside playground equipment and adding balance beams, tables, and boxes. This was a convenient way to emphasize muscular strength and endurance with an individual program of exercises and goal setting. Two class periods were used to demonstrate the exercises (rope climb, push-ups, sit-ups, ladder climb, modified pull-ups, milk-jug curls, and jump-the-stick), try them out, and help children set realistic goals. Following a trial run and after recording their initial scores for all the exercises, they had to set personal goals. Then time during subsequent lessons was used to practice the exercises and work toward achieving these goals.

April was a good time to review aerobics fitness and encourage regular exercise to prepare for the fitness tests. Certificates were awarded to each child who improved on any of the fitness components or maintained a healthy standard score. The certificate had a spot to check for improvement in each component, so children were acknowledged for their individual progress.

Although the major focus for April, May, and June was striking skills related to racket sports and baseball, lessons or parts of lessons were spent on activities related to the annual field day. Many of the skill- and fitness-related activities that children practiced during the year were displayed on Field Day for observation and participation by parents, classroom teachers, and administrators.

When children only have PE twice a week, the variety and coverage of the curriculum is limited. The Congaree curriculum was designed to develop gradually a program that highlighted certain activities and focused on certain objectives for specific grade levels. Over a 6- to 7-year period children received instruction and developed competence in both motor skills and fitness activities.

Summary

Teaching fitness in the elementary school involves more than implementing curriculum ideas. It takes time and persistence to establish an environment in which children feel competent in movement and where they can appropriately participate in movement activities. Before fitness lessons can be effectively taught, an environment must be created where children feel safe and comfortable in participating, thinking, and learning about physical activities.

Therefore, it is important to realize that a comprehensive fitness curriculum is going to be developed in small steps. Some aspects of the fitness curriculum can be implemented right away, whereas other aspects may take years. Tackle one fitness project at a time and be satisfied with small gains. It should be emphasized that fitness is just one of the benefits of regular physical activity; other benefits include enjoyment, socializing with others, and feeling good. Focus on designing successful experiences so that children develop and maintain their intrinsic motivation toward physical activity and become competent and confident.

Long-range planning (e.g., a 5-year plan) can help the teacher decide how and when to integrate fitness into the total elementary physical education curriculum. This long-range plan should include many of the strategies covered in this chapter—such as providing concrete presentations, combining instructional methods, involving students in fun, challenging exercise, and assigning homework activities—which will help children experience, understand, and value fitness as an essential part of their lives.

References

1. Corbin, C.B. Physical fitness in the K-12 curriculum: some defensible solutions to perennial problems. JOPERD 58(7):49-54; 1987.

2. Corbin, C.B. Youth fitness, exercise and health: there is much to be done. Res. Q. Exerc. Sport 58(4):308-314; 1987.

3. Graham, G.; Holt-Hale, S.A.; Parker, M. Children moving: a reflective approach to teaching physical education. 3rd ed. Mountain View, CA: Mayfield; 1993.

4. Melville, D.S.; Maddalozzo, J.G.F. The effects of a physical educator's appearance of body fatness on communicating exercise concepts to high school students. J. Teach. Phys. Educ. 7(4):343-352; 1988.

5. Pate, R.R.; Blair, S.N. Exercise and the prevention of atherosclerosis: pediatric implications. In: Strong, W.B., ed. Atherosclerosis: its pediatric aspects. New York: Grune & Stratton; 1978: p. 251-286.

6. Sander, A.N.; Burton, E.C. Learning aids—enhancing fitness knowledge in elementary physical education. JOPERD 60(1):56-59; 1989.

7. Sweetgall, R.J. Walking wellness. Clayton, MO: Creative Walking; 1987.

Resources for Fitness Lessons

American Alliance for Health, Physical Education, Recreation and Dance, 1900 Association Dr., Reston, VA 22091.

American Cancer Society (call the local chapter in your city).

American Heart Association (call the local chapter in your city).

Corbin, C.; Lindsey, R. Fitness for life. 2nd ed. Glenview, IL: Scott, Foresman; 1983.

Fit to Achieve (instructional exercise videotape, teacher guide, parent guide, student assignments). Division of Curriculum & Instruction, University of North Florida, 4567 St. Johns Bluff Road, Jacksonville, FL 32224.

FitnessGram. Institute for Aerobics Research, 1230 Preston Rd., Dallas, TX 75230.
1-800-635-7050.

Foster, E.R.; Hartinger, K.; Smith, K.A. Fitness fun. Champaign, IL: Human Kinetics; 1992.

Healthy Growing Up. McDonald's Education Resource Center, P.O. Box 8002, St. Charles, IL 60174-8002.
1-800-627-7646.

McSwegin, P.J., ed. Fitting in fitness. JOPERD 60(1):30-45; 1989.

Petray, C.K.; Blazer, S.L. Health-related physical fitness: concepts and activities for elementary schoolchildren. 3rd ed. Edina, MN: Bellwether Press/Burgess; 1991.

Physical Best: A Physical Fitness Education and Assessment Program. 1988. American Alliance for Health, Physical Education, Recreation and Dance, 1900 Association Dr., Reston, VA 22091.

Priest, L. Teach for fitness: a manual for teaching fitness concepts in K-12 physical education. 1981. Available from: ERIC Document Reproduction Service, Washington, DC: SP 017 370.

Sorenson, J. Aerobic Club for Kids (LP or cassette). Kimbo Educational Records, P.O. Box 477, Long Branch, NJ 07740.

Sweetgall, R.J. Creative Walking, Inc., P.O. Box 50296, Clayton, MO 63105.

Virgilio, S.J.; Berenson, G.S. Superfit: a comprehensive fitness intervention model for elementary schools. JOPERD 59(8):19-25; 1988.

Williams, C.; Harageones, E.; Johnson, D.; Smith, C. Personal fitness: looking good, feeling good. Dubuque, IA: Kendall/Hunt; 1986.

Chapter 16

Super Active Kids: A Health-Related Fitness Program

Melissa A. Parker
Thomas B. Steen
James R. Whitehead
University of North Dakota

Cynthia L. Pemberton
University of Missouri-Kansas City

Brian S. Entzion
River Heights Elementary School
East Grand Forks, Minnesota

Super Active Kids (SAK) is a health-related fitness education program for elementary school children that developed as a collaborative project between a university and a public school (at the request of the elementary school). The school established three program goals (2). The first was to meet the state's schedule recommendation for physical education, which the school's 100 min of PE each week did not do. The second purpose was to encourage spontaneous play and responsible playground behavior. The school staff had become concerned that the children there did not know how to "play" and many youngsters were not participating in physical activity. The third purpose was to enhance students' physical fitness and knowledge about activity and health.

Program Components

To address these concerns the SAK program developers designed a multifaceted extension of the physical education program consisting of four components: noon-hour activities, after-school activities, classroom fitness corners, and a set of

classroom and gymnasium learning experiences for fitness knowledge. Each part of the SAK program had its own objectives and characteristics.

Noon-Hour Program

The purpose of the noon-hour program was to provide two kinds of learning experiences for students, structured and unstructured. The structured experiences, identified as "SAK Day," occurred 1 day a week. SAK Day required the participation of every student and was designed, led, and supervised by the physical education teacher. The objective of SAK Day was to offer an aerobic activity providing students with positive experiences and knowledge about improving their cardiovascular activity. Because it was a required activity, students who missed their SAK Day were expected to make it later in the week.

During the pilot testing period, the primary aerobic activity for SAK Day was the mile run or walk for 20 min. Alternative activities for students who chose not to walk or run were occasionally offered, including ice skating, obstacle course running, jumping rope, or aerobics. These activities were also available for students who finished the walk/run in less than 20 min, and they were available if the weather was restrictive. These activities took place on the playground area of the school grounds while other students were also actively playing in the same area. The 20-min time frame was blocked with the students' lunch period.

On days other than SAK Day, students were free to choose other activities during the noon time that were designed by the physical education teacher and were supervised by the teaching aides (paid adults trained by the PE teacher). Offering a variety of activity choices, this aspect of the program was designed to promote student self-responsibility and to encourage active participation by students.

After-School Program

To promote physical activity outside of the school setting, an after-school component was built into the program. The objectives were to develop self-responsibility and decision-making skills about physical activity habits and to involve family members and peers in the students' physical activity habits. Students were asked to record their out-of-school physical activity experiences. A parent's signature was required to verify the accuracy of the record sheet and was also intended to promote parental involvement in the students' activities. This information was turned in weekly to monitor student progress.

Fitness Corners

The purpose of the fitness corners was to integrate fitness into the classroom setting and to encourage student responsibility for their own fitness level and fitness-related behaviors. The fitness corners were created in an area of each fifth- and sixth-grade classroom. Wall charts, personal records, and materials or equipment necessary for students to perform fitness activities and fitness self-testing were included in each fitness corner. The materials or equipment in the corner included an exercise mat, a pull-up bar, a sit-and-reach box, skinfold calipers, and fitness records. Students used the corner for self-testing aspects of their personal fitness, for personal fitness record keeping, and for cognitive self-testing of fitness-related knowledge. Self-testing was a key component to the development of fitness-related knowledge. Students were allowed to use the fitness corner at the discretion of the classroom teacher.

Fitness Knowledge

Although the major focus of the program was fitness activity, the program was also designed to teach students fitness knowledge (e.g., components of physical fitness, effects of exercise, proper nutrition, etc.). Special PE class sessions on the components of fitness and the fitness corners in the classrooms were ways that fitness knowledge was presented to the students.

Record Keeping

A major part of the SAK program was a record-keeping system to help children track progress and encourage participation. The record-keeping details of the SAK program were designed with two principles in mind: the need for accuracy in the recording of physical activity and the need to minimize and simplify paperwork. Specifically, a system was needed to record the children's exercise at school, after school, and on the weekends. Finally, a method of collating the information into monthly records was required. To meet these needs three recording forms were designed.

The Weekly Exercise Record Form

This form was designed for the students to record the kind and amount of activity performed on a daily basis. On this form a list of physical activities was tabulated opposite boxes for checking off day-to-day participation. One column of check-off boxes was specifically reserved for SAK Day activities and four other boxes were available for activities done on other weekdays. Children circled a box to signify at least 20 min of activity, writing a letter (M, T, W, R, or F) inside of the box to identify the day of the week on which the activity was done. The form also included a space opposite the check-off boxes where a record of after-school and weekend activities could be stapled to complete the weekly record.

The After-School/Weekend Record Form

This form was designed to record activity done out of school and to elicit parent involvement. A column of physical activities identical to the Weekly Exercise Record Form was given with two sets of check-off boxes and recording instructions consistent with those of the weekly record. A dotted guideline around each set of check-off boxes facilitated accurate clipping of the form to fit the space allocated for attachment to the weekly record. There was also space for a parent's signature indicating verification of the activities recorded.

The Monthly Exercise Record Chart

This was designed to encourage participation by providing feedback on the amount of activity performed, besides keeping track of student progress. This chart uses a series of horizontal "thermometers" arranged with the bulb to the left and four graduations along the stem to the right. Each chart had enough space to allow every child in a class to have his or her name at the bulb end of an individual thermometer. The four graduations allowed weekly recording to a total of one month (see Figure 16.1, page 158).

Management of the Records

Each student's weekly record was stored in a safe place in the classroom. The children updated their records when they came in at the end of the noon hour. To promote honesty and cooperation, a student squad leader (designated on a rotating basis in PE class) verified the day's activity by initialing the form—except on SAK days when the physical education teacher initialed the forms. Also on SAK days, the children brought their After-School/Weekend Record Forms (verified with a parental signature) to be stapled to the weekly record and turned in during that day's PE class. After a quick check by the physical education teacher, squad leaders were then assigned to transfer the completed records to the Monthly Record Chart.

For those children who had completed three or four activity sessions during the whole week, a section of their thermometer was colored in yellow; five or more sessions earned a red coloring. Thus the participation of each child in a class, as well as the particular activity level, could be followed as the yellow or red exercise "mercury" rose up the thermometer stem each month.

Time Demands of Record Keeping

A concern throughout was that the record keeping should not become another demand or an additional burden on the teacher's time. Fortunately,

only minimal time was needed after teachers received the initial instructions and understood them, and less than a minute was needed to collect the Weekly Exercise Record Forms in physical education class on SAK days. Such tasks as squad leader verification, thermometer recording, and determining grade stars and yearly awards rarely took more than 5 or 10 min.

Fitness Corner Records: Long-Term Personal Record Keeping

The purpose of the record keeping was to monitor the exercise process; however, the promotion and monitoring of the fitness product was also an important part of the overall plan. In practice, the purposes were accomplished through the use of personal fitness record forms. Forms were kept in a confidential, manila envelope in a file box at the fitness corner. The record cards were specific to each grade and gender and allowed plotting height, weight, and progress on each aspect of health-related fitness.

To move away from norms and toward a more personally meaningful, health-related interpretation of fitness scores (1,3,5), the fitness record cards were designed to categorize scores as "too low," "optimal," "high performance," or "too high" for each aspect of fitness.

Members of the project team determined the SAK program standards. They used professional judgment along with the criterion standards of the FitnessGram (3) and Physical Best (1) fitness education and testing packages. Each card contained instructions for self-, partner, and teacher testing and scoring and was designed to enable monitoring over a whole academic school year. Figure 16.2 (page 159) is an example of a fitness record.

Recognition

The purpose of the records was threefold: to record progress, to reinforce active behavior, and to encourage participation. Display of progress on the exercise thermometers of the Monthly Record Chart provided public recognition of achievement. "SAKids" (children who had completed five or more sessions, including a verified home record) signed their names on a large display poster in the gym, further enhancing achievement recognition.

As an immediate and tangible reward, each SAKid was allowed free time in the gym in the

Teacher: _____   Grade: _____   Dates: ___/___/___ to ___/___/___

Monthly Exercise Record

One week (a good start)	Two weeks (on track)	Three weeks (getting there)	Four weeks (great job!!)
One week (a good start)	Two weeks (on track)	Three weeks (getting there)	Four weeks (great job!!)
One week (a good start)	Two weeks (on track)	Three weeks (getting there)	Four weeks (great job!!)
One week (a good start)	Two weeks (on track)	Three weeks (getting there)	Four weeks (great job!!)
One week (a good start)	Two weeks (on track)	Three weeks (getting there)	Four weeks (great job!!)
One week (a good start)	Two weeks (on track)	Three weeks (getting there)	Four weeks (great job!!)
One week (a good start)	Two weeks (on track)	Three weeks (getting there)	Four weeks (great job!!)
One week (a good start)	Two weeks (on track)	Three weeks (getting there)	Four weeks (great job!!)
One week (a good start)	Two weeks (on track)	Three weeks (getting there)	Four weeks (great job!!)
One week (a good start)	Two weeks (on track)	Three weeks (getting there)	Four weeks (great job!!)
One week (a good start)	Two weeks (on track)	Three weeks (getting there)	Four weeks (great job!!)
One week (a good start)	Two weeks (on track)	Three weeks (getting there)	Four weeks (great job!!)
One week (a good start)	Two weeks (on track)	Three weeks (getting there)	Four weeks (great job!!)
One week (a good start)	Two weeks (on track)	Three weeks (getting there)	Four weeks (great job!!)
One week (a good start)	Two weeks (on track)	Three weeks (getting there)	Four weeks (great job!!)
One week (a good start)	Two weeks (on track)	Three weeks (getting there)	Four weeks (great job!!)
One week (a good start)	Two weeks (on track)	Three weeks (getting there)	Four weeks (great job!!)
One week (a good start)	Two weeks (on track)	Three weeks (getting there)	Four weeks (great job!!)
One week (a good start)	Two weeks (on track)	Three weeks (getting there)	Four weeks (great job!!)
One week (a good start)	Two weeks (on track)	Three weeks (getting there)	Four weeks (great job!!)
One week (a good start)	Two weeks (on track)	Three weeks (getting there)	Four weeks (great job!!)
One week (a good start)	Two weeks (on track)	Three weeks (getting there)	Four weeks (great job!!)
One week (a good start)	Two weeks (on track)	Three weeks (getting there)	Four weeks (great job!!)
One week (a good start)	Two weeks (on track)	Three weeks (getting there)	Four weeks (great job!!)
One week (a good start)	Two weeks (on track)	Three weeks (getting there)	Four weeks (great job!!)
One week (a good start)	Two weeks (on track)	Three weeks (getting there)	Four weeks (great job!!)
One week (a good start)	Two weeks (on track)	Three weeks (getting there)	Four weeks (great job!!)
One week (a good start)	Two weeks (on track)	Three weeks (getting there)	Four weeks (great job!!)

Yellow = 3 or 4 sessions per week.   Red = 5 or more sessions per week.

Figure 16.1 Student monthly exercise record chart.

Grade Five Boys

Name: _____

Skinfolds (Body Fatness)

Instructions:

1. If you are measured by a teacher, record the score using an "**X**"

2. If you are measured by a friend, record the score using an "**O**"

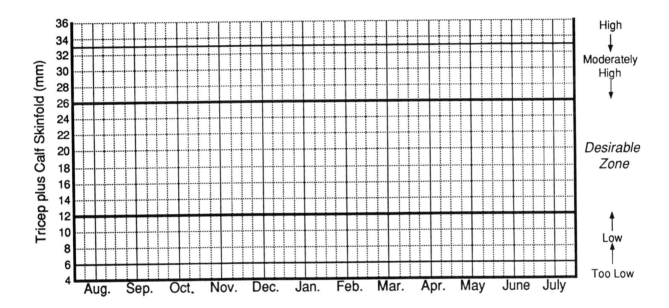

Test Purpose: The purpose of measuring skinfolds is to find out how much body fat you have.

Equipment Needed: A pencil and notepad for recording measurements, and a caliper, ruler, and skin marking crayon for marking and measuring the skinfolds. You should be wearing a short sleeved shirt and shorts so that the measures can be taken easily by a teacher or friend.

Instructions:
1. You should *not* attempt this test yourself unless you and your friend have been taught how to do it accurately by your teacher. If you are not sure, ask your teacher for help.

2. Using the instructions on the wall poster as a reminder, have your friend carefully mark and measure the triceps and calf skinfolds on your right arm and leg. Have each skinfold measured several times until you and your friend are sure that you have the most accurate score.

3. Add the triceps and calf scores together. Carefully record the total of the two scores on this Fitness Record.

Figure 16.2   A sample of a fitness corner long-term record chart.

mornings before school. (It is interesting to note that student feedback indicated that this was the most valued reward of all.) As a more tangible reward, children who achieved SAK status for 80% of a grading period earned a star on their report cards. Those who qualified 90% of the year received special recognition at the awards ceremony at the end of the school year. Finally, to emphasize and personalize the purpose for all SAKids, the following message was written prominently on the SAK instructions: "You can feel good because you are on the way to becoming a fit, healthy kid. Great job!!"

Program Personnel

Numerous individuals committed a substantial amount of time and effort to make the SAK program run smoothly. These included the physical education teacher, the principal, classroom teaching aides, student squad leaders, classroom teachers, and parents. Although each played a different role, each was involved.

The physical education teacher was central to the program: Its success was dependent upon the commitment and ability of this person. The physical education teacher was the coordinator of the program and kept all final records for the students. Beyond the duties already mentioned, responsibilities included preparation of SAK posters and forms; organization of indoor rainy-day and cold-weather activities; giving instructions about record keeping to students, parents, and classroom teachers; and promoting fitness and the program.

The principal was paramount in providing support for the program and gave the physical education teacher advice and encouragement and promoted the program with classroom teachers. In cooperation with the physical education teacher, the principal promoted and explained the program to parents and the community and provided office support and funding for the program.

The classroom teaching aides assisted in the supervision of activity for SAKids, especially in the running activities. They also supervised activity for other children on the playground during their recess time and were responsible for student behavior, including discipline. Their familiarity with the objectives and activities of the program was very important because of their key support role in the program.

The responsibility for supervising other students was given to student squad leaders. The leaders were assigned in PE classes and were rotated on a regular basis (each child was leader at least once during the year). The squad leaders verified the noon-time activity of each student in their squad. Squad leaders were also responsible for transferring their squads' Weekly Exercise Record Forms to the Monthly Exercise Chart.

Classroom teachers played important roles in promoting and supporting the program. Specifically, they allowed the squad leaders to leave class 10 min early for record keeping on SAK Day, and they provided a place in the classroom for students to store their weekly records. They also obtained extra record sheets for students when needed, and they provided time daily for each student to fill out his or her weekly record.

Parents played two roles. First, they had the responsibility to verify the after-school activities of their children. Quite often, the parents themselves became involved in many of the activities. Second, some parents became noon-time volunteers at school whose job was to assist other personnel (e.g., they tied skates and assisted beginning skaters). Because there were many people involved, the burden placed on any one person was not immense.

What Worked

To find out how well the SAK program worked, several different kinds of information were collected. During the planning process, the project team kept journals of activities, thoughts, and opinions, focusing especially on the collaborative work. Once the program was implemented, the team made regular observations of the students in action and kept all the written materials and records of participation. Photographs were taken of such things as the wall charts and playground activities. Toward the end of the first year when the program was tested, a cross-section of students—determined by fitness level, activity level, gender, and grade level—was interviewed for their opinions on the program as it was run during the pilot test period.

An examination of the materials and records obtained revealed that certain aspects of the program had worked well. These can be summarized as follows:

- Playground behavior had improved.
- Many students increased their levels of activity.

- With help, many students had monitored their own progress.
- Many parents became involved.
- The school had successfully used "non-attached time" for educational purposes.

The Students

Soon after the SAK program started it became apparent that playground behavior had improved. The school principal noted a dramatic reduction in the number of conflicts and office referrals for inappropriate behavior. Several members of the staff commented that the children seemed to cooperate better with each other as they organized games, determined sides, and shared equipment.

In addition, many students increased their activity levels. Throughout the program, reminders and the record-keeping system encouraged children to be active. The student records indicated that approximately two thirds of the students participated regularly in some sort of physical activity.

Students also were able to monitor the program mostly by themselves. With daily guidance from the physical education teacher, squad leaders successfully collected the activity records, checked them, and posted the results on the class charts. The teacher checked their work, but it was surprising how quickly the student leaders were able to handle the record keeping. Furthermore, there was little evidence of cheating. Student interviews corroborated that most children reported their activities accurately.

The School and the Community

The involvement of parents was another positive result of the SAK program. Most parents cooperated by verifying student at-home activity, where it was found that many families and parents joined their children in activities (an unintended but pleasant outcome of the program). The school principal reported that several parents jokingly "blamed" him and the program for their participation in SAK activities.

Another benefit of the program was the school's successful use of nonattached time (e.g., the noon hour, time before and after school) for educational purposes. As veteran educators know all too well, it is increasingly more difficult to find curricular time for new programs. Nonattached time has been suggested as one source for additional physical education time (4). However, most schools have

not yet been successful converting nonattached time to a period of teaching and learning. The SAK program using the noon hour helped this school take a part of the school day that was not being used for academic purposes and use it for fitness education.

What Did Not Work So Well

As in most program development projects, there were some aspects of the SAK program that did not work as hoped. The main problems identified during the pilot testing period are described here as cautions for fitness education programming.

Extrinsic Rewards Work for Only Some Children

From observations and formal interviews with students, it was found that the SAK program did not reach all of the children in the same way. In particular, some students found that record keeping became tedious and did not attract them enough to involve them in the program, which thus fell short of its goal to reach all the children. Even with individual encouragement from teachers and squad leaders, some of the children did not record their activity. Although some of these uninvolved children were not actually participating in much physical activity, others, especially highly active children, did not use the SAK report forms because they "didn't need the charts and all that stuff." They said they liked to be physically active and that simply being active was motivation enough for them. They did not want to use records and charts and did not need them as an encouragement to be active.

One Activity Choice Can Be Limiting and Boring

As the program progressed, many students came to view the standard SAK Day activity (the mile run) as a chore—not something they looked forward to and enjoyed. The mile run was initially chosen because it was the easiest activity to supervise and manage, but some variety in the major activities (aerobics, skating, jumping rope, etc.) was necessary to hold the interest of the students.

Fitness Knowledge and Activity Can Be Viewed as Separate Entities

Interviews and observations showed that many children viewed being active and fit separately from knowing about fitness. We had tried to build into the program some learning experiences that helped to develop the cognitive component, for example, classroom fitness corners and lessons in PE. We felt that we had focused most of our energies in this early stage on the noon-hour portions of the program and that we simply had not yet spent enough time developing the cognitive components of the program. However, the disparity between activity and knowledge may be symptomatic of something other than one-sided developmental efforts.

Enthusiasm Can Stall

It was also found that the enthusiasm of the children seemed to stall periodically. There were times of high energy and high enthusiasm (marked by high activity on the playground and regular record keeping), and there were other times when energy, enthusiasm, and program participation waned. Some teachers viewed this as a natural program ebb and flow but saw the need for alternative motivational strategies.

Immediate Program Changes

In light of the first year's experience, the following changes occurred in the second year. The physical education instructor took an additional 5 to 10 min at the end of each day to record student progress. Although this reduced the opportunities for student responsibility and ownership somewhat, it gave the teacher a better understanding of why students chose to participate in or avoid the program. This allowed the physical education teacher to anticipate the inevitable times when student enthusiasm stalled.

A second change was to increase activity choices at noon-time, allowing children to choose from traditional games such as tag, soccer, and jump rope. In the future, to promote spontaneous play, the students will be encouraged to create their own games and activities.

To further encourage spontaneous play and self-responsibility a third modification was implemented. "SAKtivity" leaders were created to promote student management of the SAK Day activities. These student leaders had responsibility for organizing equipment, selecting teams, and mediating conflicts. The physical education teacher maintained responsibility for preparing the equipment for the students, providing alternate methods of team selection, conflict resolution, game adaptation, and meticulous (not meddlesome) supervision of the activities. The early results of these changes indicated that students demonstrated more initiative in the impromptu organization of appropriate play activities.

Future Developments

In the future, the fitness corners in the classrooms will be tied into the health curriculum and will be taught by the classroom instructor. This change should solve the problem for students of perceived unrelatedness between fitness activity and fitness knowledge. The information and concepts from the classroom will then be expanded upon through more frequent lessons in the physical education class. These lessons will be used to strengthen the connection between the classroom and the gym.

As an extension of the "fitness thermometer" idea, another planned addition is the use of "fitness trip maps." Time spent in activity will result in the accumulation of mileage to be applied to the maps.

Summary

With the support of school administrators, physical education teachers, teacher's aides, parents, and students, the Super Active Kids program has achieved positive results. By effectively implementing its four program components, the noon-hour program, the after-school program, fitness corners, and fitness knowledge, the program has begun to achieve its goals of meeting the state's time recommendation for physical education, increasing spontaneous play and good playground behavior, and enhancing children's knowledge about their own health and physical activity.

However, the program is still developing and changes in it will continue as more is learned about the program and the children's responses. The aim is a program that does not "do" fitness to the students but rather helps them to choose fitness activities that are appropriate and challenging. Throughout the development of this program, there have been constant reminders of the substantial amount of work required to implement and maintain a fitness education program that works. The work also has confirmed the idea about good changes not occurring quickly, yet it has also demonstrated that whenever people are willing to work together, it is possible to develop something good for kids.

Acknowledgments

Although not directly involved in the writing of this chapter, Marva Fairchild, physical education teacher, and Dale Taylor, principal at River Heights Elementary School, were central in this project. Without their unending dedication to children and the improvement of education there would be no SAK program. This project was supported in part by a grant from the Collaborative Research Project sponsored by the University of North Dakota Center for Teaching and Learning. Those funds are gratefully acknowledged.

References

1. American Alliance for Health, Physical Education, Recreation and Dance. Physical Best. Reston, VA: AAHPERD; 1988.

2. Entzion, B.; Fairchild, M.; Parker, M.; Pemberton, C.; Steen, T.; Taylor, D.; Whitehead, J. SAK program manual. Grand Forks: University of North Dakota; [1990].

3. Institute for Aerobics Research. FitnessGram. Dallas, TX: Institute for Aerobics Research; 1987.

4. Siedentop, D. Developing teaching skills in physical education. 3rd ed. Mountain View, CA: Mayfield; 1991.

5. Whitehead, J.R. Fitness assessment results—some concepts and analogies. JOPERD 60(6): 39-43; 1989.

Chapter 17

A Health Fitness Course in Secondary Physical Education: The Florida Experience

Dewayne J. Johnson
Emmanouel G. Harageones
Florida State University

The development and implementation of the Personal Fitness course, Florida's physical education high-school graduation requirement, was a result of recent educational reforms. In 1983 the Florida legislature enacted, for the first time in Florida's history, statewide minimum high-school graduation requirements. Beginning with the 1986-87 school year, graduation required the successful completion of a minimum of 24 credits in Grades 9 through 12. Fifteen of the 24 credits are specified by law, including one-half credit in physical education focusing on the assessment, improvement, and maintenance of personal fitness.

In addition to these statewide minimum high-school graduation requirements, district school boards are authorized and encouraged to establish requirements for high-school graduation in excess of the minimum. School district PE requirements for high-school graduation vary—from one-half credit up to two credits. About two thirds of the school districts have requirements beyond the state minimum of one-half credit.

The Personal Fitness Course

The Personal Fitness course is Florida's statewide physical education high-school graduation requirement. The intent of the Florida legislature was

to provide all high-school students with a basic physical education course that would foster the compelling state and national interest in a physically fit population. The passage of legislation requiring the Personal Fitness course was a direct result of successful lobbying efforts by the Florida Association for Health, Physical Education, Recreation, Dance, and Driver Education (FAHPERD).

The purpose of the Personal Fitness course is to provide students with opportunities to

1. develop an individual, optimal level of physical fitness,
2. acquire knowledge of physical fitness concepts, and
3. understand the significance of lifestyle on one's health and fitness.

The content of the course falls into eight categories:

1. Knowledge of the importance of physical fitness
2. Assessment of the health-related components of physical fitness
3. Knowledge of health problems associated with inadequate fitness levels
4. Knowledge and application of biomechanical and physiological principles to improve

and maintain the health-related components of physical fitness

5. Knowledge of safety practices associated with physical fitness
6. Knowledge of the psychological values of physical fitness, including stress management
7. Knowledge of sound nutritional practices related to physical fitness
8. Knowledge of consumer issues related to physical fitness

The curriculum framework and student performance standards for the Personal Fitness course are included in this chapter's appendix. A curriculum framework is a set of broad guidelines that aid educational personnel in producing specific instructional plans for a given course. Course student-performance standards are statements that reflect expected student achievement.

Department of Education Planning Strategies

In preparing to implement the Personal Fitness course, many expressed concern that there would be a diversity of interpretations regarding both the intent and content of the Personal Fitness course and its curriculum framework and student performance standards. In response to this concern, the Florida DOE (Department of Education) formed a task force to provide assistance to school districts implementing the Personal Fitness course. The task force first reviewed all existing materials and determined that, even though some good materials existed, none totally fit the needs of Florida's Personal Fitness course. A decision was then made to develop a teaching syllabus for the course.

The Personal Fitness Instructional Materials Packet was developed by the task force during the 1983-84 school year. The content was based on the course student-performance standards and a year-long analysis of the literature. The packet contained 12 instructional units, each containing a suggested day-by-day teaching outline, teaching strategies, activity sheets, handouts, lab experiences, lab experience work sheets, study guides, and transparency masters.

Teacher Training Activities

Extensive teacher training activities focusing on this teaching syllabus took place on a statewide level and at the school district level. The first statewide training was conducted in June, 1984, during the annual week-long DOE/FAHPERD Health and Physical Education Summer Workshop at the University of Florida in Gainesville. More than 200 high-school physical education teachers received training in the utilization of the Personal Fitness Instructional Materials Packet. Members of the Department of Education Task Force that developed the teaching syllabus served as workshop leaders.

During the 1984 FAHPERD Annual Conference, all high-school physical education presentations focused on the implementation of the Personal Fitness course. Again during the 1985 DOE/FAHPERD Health and Physical Education Summer Workshop at the University of South Florida in Tampa, high-school physical education teachers received training in the Personal Fitness course. This time, the workshop leaders were all public school teachers who had taught the course during the 1984-85 school year and were identified as outstanding teachers. Many of the school districts paid the expenses of selected teachers to attend the summer workshop, with the expectation that those individuals would return to their districts and conduct in-service sessions for those assigned to teach the Personal Fitness course.

We still use the summer workshop and the annual fall conference to provide the Personal Fitness teachers with in-service training in the area of instructional strategies. However, we no longer use all sessions for Personal Fitness. Additionally, for the past several years, the Florida JOHPERD has been committed to soliciting and publishing teaching ideas, strategies, or teaching tips for Personal Fitness.

Data from the districts indicated that most teachers who teach Personal Fitness have now had in-service training by at least one of the three methods mentioned. Unfortunately, 24% of the teachers have received no in-service training. Thirty-one percent of the Personal Fitness teachers have attended at least one summer workshop, whereas 50% have received in-service training at the district level by either local teachers who have attended the summer workshop, by university personnel, or by Personal Fitness teachers from other districts.

Implementation Strategies

The Personal Fitness course was first implemented statewide during the 1984-85 school year. The Florida DOE recommended implementation strategies in eight areas. We will look at each DOE recommendation and then at how the districts have been able to implement that strategy.

• **Scheduling.** Students should take the Personal Fitness course in either Grade 9 or 10 so that they can apply their knowledge of the course content throughout their high school years. The implementation of this strategy by school districts is an ongoing process. Originally, in the 1984-85 school year nearly all districts offered Personal Fitness in Grade 9. By 1987, 40% of the schools had moved Personal Fitness to Grade 10—a trend seen in the last year or two. This adjustment has arisen not because content is too difficult for 9th graders, but because many professionals believe that students entering the ninth grade have enough problems adjusting to the new and different environment of high school. They should be able to deal better with a cognitive-based physical education course at the 10th-grade level after making the adjustment to high school.

• **Laboratory and classroom instruction.** Weekly PE class should be equivalent to 3 days of laboratory activities and 2 days of classroom instruction. Some days may be 100% classroom instruction or lab activities; others may be 50%/50% or 80%/20%. Personal Fitness teachers have been fairly consistent in following this recommendation. Most Personal Fitness classes spend 2 days a week in the classroom and 3 days a week participating in physical activity. However, some teachers will occasionally spend 3 days a week in the classroom, depending on the particular unit of instruction. Sometimes two Personal Fitness classes share a classroom during the same hour using an alternate-days schedule in which, for example, one class uses the room on Mondays, Wednesdays, and Fridays, and the other is in the classroom on Tuesdays and Thursdays.

• **Classroom space.** In addition to recreational or gymnasium space, classroom space should be provided for the Personal Fitness course because of the nature of the class. This was and is one of the recommendations that schools had the most trouble implementing. The enrollments in most Florida schools are increasing, and schools do not have empty classrooms that Personal Fitness teachers can use—despite principals' strong support for needed classrooms. The degree to which this recommendation has been implemented varies (probably due to the different interpretations of "classroom"). Only two thirds of the principals indicated that all Personal Fitness classes at their schools have a classroom; 17% said that none of

the sections of Personal Fitness had a classroom. Data from Personal Fitness teachers (see Table 17.1) help clarify strategies used to provide classroom space for Personal Fitness. Locations for the 40% under "others" category in Table 17.1 include the use of storerooms, gymnasium lobbies, and other such areas where chairs or desks and a portable chalkboard could be arranged.

• **Class size.** Class size for the Personal Fitness course should be consistent with those of other academic courses. Some schools have limited enrollment in Personal Fitness compared to the size of other academic classroom courses. The average class size of Personal Fitness is approximately 33 students, with a range from 16 to more than 58 students. We are having an impact on the attitude of principals, and there is a trend across the state toward placing a cap on the enrollment in Personal Fitness that would be consistent with other subjects.

• **Fitness assessment.** Pre- and postassessment of the health-related components of physical fitness should be conducted. Students should be assisted in selecting planned exercise programs based on their individual assessment results, and they should be encouraged to continue participation throughout the course. Initially, many Personal Fitness teachers were reluctant to switch from the fitness tests they were using, and many

Table 17.1 Data From the Personal Fitness Course Related to Classroom Space and Class Size

Information	Response
From teachers:	
Average class size for the Personal Fitness course	34.92
Range in class size for the Personal Fitness course	16–58
Is the class size for the Personal Fitness course equivalent to other classroom courses?	35.2% yes
Where is the classroom portion of Personal Fitness taught?	
Regular classroom	30.2%
Floating classroom	17.2%
Locker room	6.2%
Bleachers	5.6%
Others	40.1%
From principals:	
Do you think there is a need for a classroom for Personal Fitness?	96.2% yes

did not assess all of the health-related fitness components. Today, however, most are assessing health-related fitness. The real shortcoming at this time is the use of assessment results. Few teachers are sharing results with parents, and only about one half of the schools are using the results in a diagnostic or prescriptive manner. Because Personal Fitness should focus on developing an individual fitness program based on a student's personal level of fitness, we can see that a great deal of work remains to be done to achieve course objectives. Approximately one third of the schools provide remedial programs for extremely low-fit students.

• **Homework.** Assigning both cognitive and psychomotor homework should be viewed as essential elements of the Personal Fitness course. Students should keep notebooks to facilitate tracking of activities from instructional materials, homework, in- and out-of-class assignments, and exercise logs. This recommendation has been implemented fairly well. Most teachers require notebooks and assign written homework. Physical homework is assigned by 38% of the teachers and should be assigned as part of the remedial program just mentioned for students who have a low fitness level in one or more of the health-related components.

• **Student evaluation.** The purpose of evaluation should extend beyond the collection of data for assignment of grades. Evaluation should be viewed as a diagnostic tool to help both the student and the teacher. An effective evaluation system correlates with the course student-performance standards. Student evaluation should include the cognitive, affective, and psychomotor domains. Most schools have implemented this recommendation. We know that, although less common nowadays, a few teachers still grade a student based on fitness test scores. The evaluation method in the affective and psychomotor domains continues to be subjective, or based on participation and dressing out. The quality of the notebook, personal fitness program, homework assignments, and written tests usually make up about one half of the grade.

• **Instructional materials.** Students should have their own individual copies of instructional materials for the Personal Fitness course to enhance acquisition of course content. Some districts or individual schools have gone to great efforts to implement this recommendation. Initially, some teachers took all of the work sheets and lab experiences that were included in the Personal Fitness

Instructional Materials Packet and duplicated them so that each student had a workbook. Other teachers duplicated a few copies for student use or duplicated materials on a day-to-day basis.

During the past several years the state of Florida has adopted textbooks for use in Personal Fitness. Nearly all schools are now using a textbook, but only 37% are using a lab book to supplement the textbook. Schools have used different strategies, generally based on economics, when purchasing textbooks, the ideal being a textbook and a lab book for each student. When this was not possible, the preferred alternative was a classroom set of textbooks and a lab book for each student. Some schools have been able only to purchase classroom sets of each, whereas others have had to choose between the textbook and the lab book. An encouraging trend for schools that have had to settle for classroom sets is that they now may purchase an additional classroom set each year as money is available and will soon have one book for each student. As shown in Table 17.2 principals overwhelmingly support the purchase of textbooks for Personal Fitness and two thirds support the need for a lab book. They are split between a classroom set and student sets, but

Table 17.2   Attitudes About the Relationship of Instructional Materials and the Personal Fitness Course

Questions	Percent answering yes
For principals:	
Do you support the purchase of textbooks for Personal Fitness?	86.1
Do you support the need for a textbook for each student in Personal Fitness?	26.6
Do you support the purchase of lab books for Personal Fitness?	61.4
Do you support the need for a lab book for each student in Personal Fitness?	20.3
For teachers:	
Are you currently using a textbook for Personal Fitness?	84.6
Do you currently have a textbook for each student in Personal Fitness?	35.2
Are you currently using a lab book for Personal Fitness?	37.0
Do you currently have a lab book for each student in Personal Fitness?	20.4

again, this is probably based on economic considerations.

Implementation Problems

The Personal Fitness course was not implemented without the typical problems associated with any major curriculum change, especially a mandated one. Some of the problems have included

• **Initial attitudes of students.** Two questions many students asked Personal Fitness teachers were "Why can't we go to the gym and play?" and "Why do we have to take notes and study in PE?" The initial failure rate created an additional problem. Students did not believe they had to study and pass tests. Teachers indicated that approximately 10% of the students failed Personal Fitness at least one time. However, 20% of the students indicated that they failed Personal Fitness. Failure rates reached as high as 50% during that first year. Today, the failure rate in Personal Fitness is similar to other high school courses.

• **Initial attitudes of some teachers.** Some teachers began the Personal Fitness course by telling the students that they didn't want to teach the course any more than the students wanted to take it, but the state was "making them." Can you imagine how students reacted to Personal Fitness in those classes?

• **Initial lack of administrative support.** Many believe this to be a reflection of the administration's attitude toward physical education in general. This lack of support initially was reflected in a lack of classroom space, large class sizes, and reluctance to acquire additional instructional materials. Administrative support for the Personal Fitness course has increased tremendously in the time since then.

• **Lack of preparedness of individuals to teach the course.** It had been a long time since many teachers had studied the course content, and most physical educators had never received training in teaching methods for a classroom setting. Also, there were few resources for enjoyable, or motivational, lab activities to reinforce the cognitive concepts presented in the classroom. Many of these problems have now been overcome by the state's extensive in-service program. Additionally, to help overcome these deficiencies in teacher preparation for this course, some teacher preparation programs are devoting a portion of their teaching methods

course to Personal Fitness strategies, and two universities have instituted a course focusing on the teaching of the Personal Fitness course.

• **Staffing of the Personal Fitness course.** Initially, school districts took one of two approaches to staffing Personal Fitness: Everyone taught at least one class of Personal Fitness, or only the teachers who volunteered were assigned to Personal Fitness. As time passes, many schools are now assigning Personal Fitness only to the teachers who want to teach it, who have demonstrated competency in teaching the course, or who have received in-service training.

When teachers were asked specifically what problems were encountered when implementing the course, we see that student attitude, class size, and available classroom space were and still are the major obstacles. The other problem areas—lack of textbooks, attitude of physical education staff, and the lack of equipment—are slowly but surely being seen less frequently.

Impact of Personal Fitness

Despite all the problems, the implementation of the Personal Fitness course has resulted in renewed administrative, parental, and student support for Florida's high-school physical education programs. Three separate but related surveys were conducted during the 1987-88 school year by Johnson et al. (3) at Florida State University to determine the impact of Florida's Personal Fitness course. The surveys collected data from high school principals, high-school physical education teachers, and high school seniors. Questions were asked about implementation strategies and problems and about the impact of the course on different individuals' attitudes and lifestyles. We have already discussed some of the data on implementation strategies and problems that were encountered. The exciting thing about the Personal Fitness course, which we want to share, is its impact on attitudes and lifestyles.

Principals' Survey

The first survey obtained information about how the schools implemented Personal Fitness and the perceptions of high school principals about the

Personal Fitness course (see Table 17.3). A questionnaire was mailed to the principals of all 291 public high schools. Responses were received from 158 principals (54.3%). Results of this survey indicated that 90% to 96% of the principals supported the Personal Fitness course, depending on the specific question asked. Over 90% of the principals indicated that Personal Fitness was a valuable addition to the high school curriculum. Most of the 8.2% who indicated that it was not a valuable addition explained that Personal Fitness was a duplication of other courses. This suggests that they were not familiar with or did not understand the purpose and content, the curriculum framework, or the course student-performance standards of Personal Fitness. We may conclude that the physical education staff had not done a very good job of orienting their principal.

We also see that nearly one half of the principals indicated that their attitude about PE in general had improved because of the Personal Fitness course. We would hope that at least one half of the 47% whose attitude did not change already had a positive attitude about physical education. Principals generally held the opinion that the physical education staff were doing a good or great job teaching Personal Fitness, that parents rated Personal Fitness at moderate to high value, and that school board members also would give it this

Table 17.3 The Effects of Personal Fitness on Attitudes of Teachers and Principals

Questions	Percent answering yes
For principals:	
Was Personal Fitness a valuable addition to the high school curriculum?	90.5
Do parents feel that Personal Fitness is a valuable course?	80.3
For teachers:	
Do you agree with the emphasis on fitness in the physical education curriculum?	93.8
Has the implementation of Personal Fitness course improved the attitudes toward physical education of	
School administrators	66.0
High school faculty	58.0
Physical education faculty	67.3
Students	57.4
Parents	51.9

rating. It is disappointing, however, that 18% of the school board members do not know anything about the course. Physical education professionals need to become involved in promoting and marketing the Personal Fitness course, because once people become aware of the nature and purpose of Personal Fitness, they become more positive and supportive of physical education in general.

Teachers' Survey

The second survey asked one physical education teacher in each of the 291 public high schools to answer questions about how their school implemented the Personal Fitness course and their perceptions about the impact of the course. Responses were received from 162 schools (55.6%).

Nearly all of the teachers (93.8%) agreed with the emphasis that Florida has placed on fitness in the physical education program (see Table 17.3). This is a drastic change from 5 years before when little support at the high school level could be found for Personal Fitness, a cognitive-based, classroom course. Additionally, 66% of the teachers felt that the Personal Fitness course had improved administrative support and attitude toward physical education in general. Also, 58% of the teachers who responded to the questionnaire indicated that Personal Fitness had improved the attitude of nonphysical education faculty toward PE. We also see that 67% felt that over the last 4 years the Personal Fitness course had improved the attitude of the physical education faculty. Additionally, physical education teachers generally felt that student and parental attitudes toward physical education in general had improved because of the Personal Fitness course.

Students' Survey

The third survey attempted to determine the impact of the Personal Fitness course on the lifestyles of students. To accomplish this, each principal of the 291 public high schools was asked to administer a questionnaire to one class of seniors. The seniors of 1987-88 were the first students required to pass Personal Fitness to graduate from high school. For many schools, those seniors were the first group of freshmen who were taught the course. Also, many of those schools experienced major problems implementing Personal Fitness that first year—large classes, lack of classroom space, unprepared teachers or teachers with no previous experience teaching in a classroom, and negative attitudes of students, teachers, and administrators. At many schools those problems have now been overcome, and additionally, most schools now have textbooks for the students. Despite these initial problems facing the 1987-88 seniors, the student survey indicated that Personal Fitness had a significant, lasting impact on the lifestyles of the seniors. Responses were received from 201 of the 291 public high schools (69.1%) and represented opinions of 6,118 high school seniors.

Sixty-eight percent of the students are currently involved in a fitness program, most being involved with cardiovascular, muscular strength and endurance, and flexibility components (see Table 17.4). Thirty-six percent of all seniors, or 53% of those who are currently involved in an exercise or wellness program, are involved as a direct result of taking the Personal Fitness course. The attitudes about wellness and fitness of 48.7% of the students were improved by the course. We have to assume that at least half of the 45.5% of the students whose attitudes remained the same already had a positive attitude, because many of them were already involved in a fitness program.

Diets of 43.2% of all students were positively changed, and 46.8% became more concerned about

stress management as a direct result of taking the Personal Fitness course. Amazingly, as a direct result of taking the Personal Fitness course, 37.4% of the students reduced the amount of time they watched television. This probably relates closely to the 36% who became involved in a fitness program. We can see that this may well be a way to reverse the trend of the "couch potato." Students also thought that the information contained in the Personal Fitness course should be taught to high school students (77.5%) and that Personal Fitness should be required (59%). Also, 16% of the students indicated that taking the Personal Fitness course had a positive effect on at least one other member of their family.

These are exciting results about changes in attitudes and lifestyles of high school seniors. What other course can claim this type of impact on lifestyles of students 3 to 4 years later? The true measure of the value of the Personal Fitness course is the lasting impact that the course has on the students who take it. The seniors who were surveyed had taken the course during the 1984-85 school year and appear to have incorporated the concepts they learned into their daily life. If we had this degree of impact that first year, with all our problems, we look forward to the impact we're having today, because we know we're doing a much better job of teaching Personal Fitness.

Table 17.4 Students' Attitude and Lifestyle Changes

Questions	Percent answering yes
Are you currently involved in a fitness program?	67.9
Is your involvement in a fitness program the result of Personal Fitness?	52.9
As a result of taking Personal Fitness, have you made an attempt to positively change your diet?	43.2
As a result of taking Personal Fitness, have you become more concerned with managing your stress?	46.8
As a result of taking Personal Fitness, have you reduced the amount of time you watch television?	37.4
Did your participation in Personal Fitness positively influence other members of your family in the area of fitness?	16.3
Should high school students be exposed to the information contained in Personal Fitness?	77.5

Enrollment Data

Additionally, the enrollment in elective PE over the last several years is at an all-time high in Florida and still on the increase. Those of us who have worked with it would like to credit the Personal Fitness course for this renewed interest in physical education and physical activity.

Recommendations

Three surveys clearly identified some problems related to the implementation of Florida's Personal Fitness course. Ironically, these problems stem from the success teachers are having in Personal Fitness and the positive impact the course has on the lifestyles of students and their families. A number of solutions can be recommended using survey data and the Department of Education's implementation strategies.

Schools should revise implementation in the following areas: class size, classroom space, fitness assessment, homework or notebook requirements, and available copies of instructional materials. Physical educators must continue to work at promoting the Personal Fitness course to parents, administrators, and students. Only through their strong marketing strategy will educational decision makers address the problems. It has become apparent that when administrators know and understand the purpose and nature of Personal Fitness, they become much more supportive of recommendations for the course.

Summary

The education reforms in Florida provided us an opportunity to do what the literature and research indicated ought to happen. By working with the Department of Education, we were able to conduct teacher training activities and work through eight distinct implementation strategies. We also discovered and resolved implementation problems, and finally had a positive impact on principals, teachers, and—most importantly—the students.

Physical education professionals in Florida take pride in the fact that they seized the opportunity and took bold steps to be the first state in the nation to require a cognitive-based fitness concepts course for high school graduation. However, we are equally excited about the national fitness education trend that is growing at the high school level. We hope the impact that the Personal Fitness course has had on the lifestyles of our students and the attitudes of students, parents, and administrators will allow the Florida experience to serve as a model for other states, which thereby will gain support for fitness education as a specific course or one that is integrated into the regular physical education program.

Impact

The implementation of the Personal Fitness course has resulted in renewed administrative, parental, and student support for Florida's high-school physical education programs. Physical education professionals in Florida take pride in having seized the opportunity and taken bold steps to make education reform work for them.

Appendix

Personal Fitness Curriculum Framework and Student Performance Standards

The purpose of this course is to provide a student with opportunities to develop an individual optimal level of physical fitness, to acquire an understanding of physical fitness concepts, and to realize the significance of lifestyle on one's health and fitness.

The content should include but not be limited to knowledge of the importance of physical fitness, assessment of the health-related components of physical fitness, knowledge of health problems associated with inadequate fitness levels, knowledge and application of biomechanical and physiological principles to improve and maintain the health-related components of physical fitness, knowledge of safety practices associated with physical fitness, knowledge of psychological values of physical fitness including stress management, knowledge of sound nutritional practices related to physical fitness, and knowledge of consumer issues related to physical fitness.

After successfully completing this course, the student will be able to

1. Understand the components of physical fitness. The student will
   1.01 define physical fitness,
   1.02 identify and describe each of the health-related components of physical fitness,
   1.03 identify and describe each of the skill-related components of physical fitness, and
   1.04 compare and differentiate between health-related fitness and skill-related fitness.

2. Assess individual fitness levels. The student will
   2.01 identify methods of determining level of flexibility,
   2.02 identify methods of determining level of cardiovascular fitness,
   2.03 identify methods of determining level of muscular strength and muscular endurance,
   2.04 identify methods of determining estimated percent body fat,
   2.05 define ideal body weight,
   2.06 describe at least one method of determining level of flexibility,
   2.07 describe at least one method of determining level of cardiovascular fitness,
   2.08 describe at least one method of determining level of muscular strength and muscular endurance,
   2.09 describe at least one method of determining estimated percent body fat, and
   2.10 describe at least one method of determining ideal body fat.

3. Understand the relationship between physical fitness activities and stress. The student will
   3.01 define stress,
   3.02 identify the different types of stress,
   3.03 identify the positive and negative effects of stress,
   3.04 identify specific health problems that may be caused or affected by negative stress,
   3.05 identify stressful events in his or her daily life,
   3.06 identify positive coping strategies,
   3.07 identify negative coping strategies,
   3.08 identify techniques of progressive relaxation, and
   3.09 describe the benefits of vigorous and nonvigorous physical activities to stress diversion.

4. Understand sound nutritional practices related to physical fitness. The student will

    4.01 identify the basic food groups,

    4.02 explain the FDA's "food pyramid" system of maintaining a nutritionally sound diet,

    4.03 identify the number of calories in 1 lb of fat,

    4.04 identify myths associated with nutritional practices related to physical activity,

    4.05 explain the use of exercise as a method of weight control,

    4.06 explain the use of diet as a method of weight control, and

    4.07 explain the combined use of exercise and diet as a method of weight control.

5. Understand health problems associated with inadequate fitness levels. The student will

    5.01 identify health-related problems associated with inadequate flexibility,

    5.02 identify health-related problems associated with inadequate cardiovascular fitness,

    5.03 identify strength and muscular endurance, and

    5.04 identify health-related problems associated with an abnormal percentage of body fat.

6. Understand consumer issues related to physical fitness. The student will

    6.01 differentiate between fact and fad, quackery and myths related to fitness,

    6.02 determine the validity of marketing claims promoting fitness products and services, and

    6.03 identify consumer issues related to selection, purchase, care, and maintenance of personal fitness equipment.

7. Evaluate physical activities in terms of their fitness value. The student will

    7.01 identify the contributions of physical activities to the development of the health-related components of physical fitness, and

    7.02 identify the contributions of physical activities to stress diversion.

8. Select from a variety of dynamic activities those that will help them to improve physical fitness levels. The student will

    8.01 identify a variety of static and dynamic stretching exercises that promote flexibility,

    8.02 identify a variety of aerobic activities that promote cardiovascular fitness,

    8.03 identify a variety of activities that promote muscular strength and muscular endurance,

    8.04 identify a variety of activities that promote ideal body weight, and

    8.05 identify a variety of activities that promote stress diversion.

9. Design a fitness program that meets individual needs and interest. The student will

    9.01 design a personal fitness program that will lead to or maintain an optimal level of the health-related components of fitness based upon an understanding of training principles, individual skill level, and availability of resources.

10. Understand and apply correct biomechanical and physiological principles related to exercise and training. The student will

    10.01 identify factors one should consider before engaging in a physical fitness program,

    10.02 describe the importance of a warm-up and cool-down period when participating in physical activity,

    10.03 describe the training principles of overload, progression, and specificity (also frequency, intensity, and duration),

    10.04 describe how flexibility is improved through application of the training principles,

    10.05 identify the biomechanical principles related to flexibility activities,

    10.06 describe how cardiovascular fitness is improved through application of the training principles,

    10.07 identify the biomechanical principles related to cardiovascular activities,

    10.08 describe how muscular strength and muscular endurance are improved through application of the training principles,

    10.09 identify the biomechanical principles related to muscular strength and muscular endurance activities, and

    10.10 determine his or her target heart rate zone.

11. Understand and apply safety practices associated with physical fitness. The student will

11.01 describe safety procedures that should be followed when engaging in flexibility, cardiovascular, and muscular strength and muscular endurance activities,

11.02 explain methods of maintaining proper fluid balance during physical activity,

11.03 identify signs of heat illnesses caused by fluid loss, and

11.04 identify precautions to be taken when exercising in extreme weather and/or other environmental conditions.

12. Exhibit an improved state of physical fitness. The student will

12.01 demonstrate improvement in the health-related components of physical fitness as measured by the AAHPERD Health-Related Physical Fitness Test.

13. Assess individual lifestyles as related to quality living. The student will

13.01 identify the primary risk factors associated with disease, disability, and premature death,

13.02 differentiate between changeable and chronic risk factors,

13.03 identify risk factors he or she needs to change or modify to pursue a healthy lifestyle, and

13.04 describe the relationship between one's health and fitness and one's lifestyle.

14. Exhibit a positive attitude toward physical selves and lifelong physical activity. The student will

14.01 identify attitudes that people have toward exercise and physical activities,

14.02 identify reasons why fitness should be a compelling state and national concern,

14.03 describe the benefits of participating in a regular personal fitness program,

14.04 describe the benefits of achieving optimal fitness, and

14.05 demonstrate a positive attitude toward his or her physical self and lifelong physical activity.

References

1. Florida Department of Education. Personal fitness curriculum framework/student performance standards. Tallahassee, FL: Department of Education; 1984.

2. Harageones, M.; Tremor, M. Legislative impact on health and physical education. Florida JOHPERD 21(3):4-5; 1983.

3. Johnson, D.J.; Harageones, M. Impact of Florida's "Personal Fitness" course on attitudes and lifestyles of students, teachers, and administrators. Paper presented at the AAHPERD National Conference. Boston, MA; April 19, 1989.

Chapter 18

Moving to Success: A Comprehensive Approach to Physical Education

Jenifer J. Steller
Dan B. Young
Woodland Heights Elementary School
Spartanburg, South Carolina

Physical education at Woodland Heights Elementary School in Spartanburg, South Carolina, provides for the development of both skillfulness and health-related fitness. The program's goal is to teach and encourage children to be active for a lifetime. Physical education extends beyond PE class time to include daily activities conducted by teachers and volunteers throughout the school year. The physical education program, therefore, is comprehensive in order to provide a variety of motor skill and fitness activities for all students. In this chapter we describe how the program began and the components that make the program comprehensive in nature.

Introducing Moving to Success

Woodland Heights Elementary School calls its comprehensive physical education program "Moving to Success," reflecting the philosophy that in education there is no standing still. Physical education is learning through movement; accordingly, at Woodland Heights, physical education is one means of helping the school's students move toward success.

Moving to Success has evolved over the past 5 years to include many physical activities. The program was conceived in 1987 by the physical education teacher, who was looking for a means to blend fitness activities with the skill-based program. One of the school parents, trained as a youth fitness instructor, volunteered her time to help implement a motor skill and fitness activity.

Woodland Heights Elementary School began Moving to Success with Physical Exercise Revives Kids (PERK) (2). This 5-min early morning activity now is available daily to every classroom, K-5. While selected music is broadcast over the school's public address system, pairs of fifth-grade students, trained as PERK leaders, are responsible for leading each classroom in choreographed routines. Each PERK set includes a variety of motor skills, fitness concepts, and musical experiences. Basically, this activity involves every child and teacher in a warm-up segment, vigorous movements, and a cool-down segment.

PERK became the catalyst that has helped Woodland Heights meet the need for children's fitness activities. The school demonstrated that it recognized the necessity for making time for fitness. With PERK the classroom teachers began to value physical activity as a meaningful part of a student's education, and the students saw PERK as an enjoyable and active beginning to each school day. Very importantly, parents began to support physical activity for their children.

Physical Exercise Revives Kids, therefore, brought together parents, teachers, and students. The parent-volunteer choreographs routines and trains fifth-grade leaders during a scheduled PERK practice. The physical education teacher and the fifth-grade teachers manage the leaders and supervise the daily PERK activity. Student leaders take responsible roles for learning routines, being prompt to school, and showing leadership characteristics in the classrooms.

PERK activity established a framework for the physical activities that were to follow, and every year it added new music and movements. There never was a plan, however, for combining motor skill and fitness activities beyond PERK. The skill and fitness approach developed through support and enthusiasm from the entire school. Moving to Success unfolded one activity at a time, furthered by staff consensus that PERK was to be an evolving program.

An important note is that the time to plan and conduct the many program activities has been dependent upon teachers willing to take on extra responsibilities and on parent-volunteer support to help plan and implement various physical activities. With Moving to Success, teachers and students feel better about physical activity, and the physical education teacher enjoys the support and contributions of other teachers to physical activities at the school. Further, the involvement of the home and community strengthens Moving to Success and sends a message to children that physical education goes beyond the gymnasium and playing field.

Moving to Success provides safe and effective children's activities based on grade-level competencies in the psychomotor, cognitive, affective, and fitness areas as presented in *The South Carolina Physical Education Curriculum Guidelines, Volume One* (8). The program enhances the various motor skill and fitness activities with children's music, fun movements, sports equipment, and a variety of themes and events.

Program Components

Moving to Success activities with motor skill and health-related fitness elements include these resources:

- Physical education classes (K-5) featuring PERK Too and motor skill development
- Physical Exercise Revives Kids (PERK)
- Discover and Understand Communities, Kids, by Walking (DUCK Walking)
- Morning activities for students
- PE Club (running and sport performance troupes)
- Family and community events (see Figure 18.1)

Physical Education Classes

Moving to Success at Woodland Heights Elementary School begins with the twice weekly 40- to 45-min physical education classes. Individual classes arrive at the gymnasium or playing field and immediately begin PERK Too, a 15- to 18-min teacher-directed fitness activity that is choreographed to support the fundamental motor skills being taught in a particular unit. Following PERK Too is the 15- to 18-min motor skill lesson, which incorporates as much aerobic activity as instruction allows. A 3- to 5-min muscle-strengthening segment (Grades 3–5) and a 3- to 5-min cool-down segment (all grades) conclude the class.

PERK Too and the motor skill lesson could each stand on their own; what makes them unique is their interrelationship. For each unit the two share specific motor skills and as much continuous movement as possible. Cognitive emphasis is made through the teacher's instruction when students are asked to say and do (e.g., walk-walk-walk, step-step-step-kick [11]) and by the use of song lyrics in PERK Too (e.g., "The Mighty Pump—The Heart" [10] and "Sports Dance" [7]). There is affective emphasis through teacher encouragement, student feedback, and song lyrics in PERK Too (e.g., "Keep on Trying" [3] and "A Good Friend" [5]). As a result, psychomotor, cognitive, and affective learning alternate between PERK Too and motor skill development throughout the lesson.

PERK Too

The first 15- to 18-min of each PE class provide both a motor skill and health-related fitness emphasis called "PERK Too," because this activity is PERK in an expanded form. Using the basic skills from the unit being studied, PERK Too provides opportunities to practice and refine these skills in an aerobic activity such as choreographing motor skills into aerobic routines. For example, the music

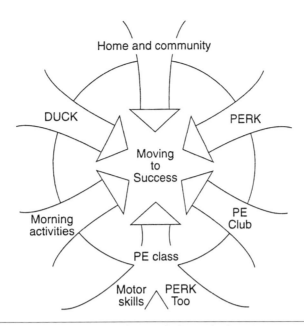

Figure 18.1 Diagram depicting a comprehensive scheme of physical education.

selection and choreography may allow practice of the step-step-step-kick move when the children are studying soccer.

A PERK Too unit is especially designed for the content to implement both psychomotor and cognitive objectives. There are units for locomotor, dance, gymnastic, and individual game skills, singly and in combinations. PERK Too units are designed separately for the kindergarten, first and second grades, and third through fifth grades. After skills and movement sequences are introduced and practiced, music is added. Music selection for PERK Too, along with all other Moving to Success activities requiring music, is made on the basis of established guidelines that have proven to be successful at the school.

Music is chosen appropriate for students' levels of movement experience. To introduce movement sequences, instrumental music may be selected, which allows children to concentrate on the movement rather than on the lyrics. For more experienced movers, however, music selected for its lyrics can be effective in order to utilize the fitness concepts or skills for particular content areas. For example, "Safety Break" (6) provides not only music appropriate for isolating individual muscles during a warm-up but also a good lesson in safety and self-esteem. A fun element is that the song is a rap by children for children. PERK Too music selection gives children a variety of movement and musical experiences using the many choices available in children's music along with rock, country, classical, jazz, and others. In addition, selection of

music with appropriate beats per minute facilitates stretching and aerobic training.

Choices for movements can range from such basics as stretches, bends, curls, twists, walking, running, hopping, jumping, skipping, and sliding to more dancelike movements. Directional patterns can vary greatly: side-to-side, front and back, in-place, squares, diagonals, front-right-front-left, and everywhere. Based on information about children's choreographed fitness workouts, movements and directional patterns are carefully selected to be physiologically safe and appropriate for children (4).

To help the learner feel successful, movement sequences are simple. These sequences begin with the transfer of weight from foot to foot with each beat and use repetitious patterns moving in a forward to backward direction (11). Before second grade, PERK Too provides a great deal of active learning by exploring a variety of sensory and perceptual motor skills. By second grade and beyond, PERK Too elements can work to develop visual correctness (i.e., matching the leader), verbal correctness (i.e., responding with specific right and left), and inhibited movement (e.g., consciously holding one side of the body still while moving the other side). Also, children can move to the song's rhythm if allowed to rehearse to the beat first (11).

PERK Too movements are planned with the specific motor skill unit being taught. For example, during a basketball unit, movement in the PERK Too segment may include the pivot move and a variety of dribbling sequences and defensive moves. Balls, bands, jump ropes, hula hoops, scarves, and streamers can add fun and challenge. Specific choreography provides individualized time for aerobic practice of movements, sequences, and manipulative skills.

The Motor Skill Lesson

Following PERK Too is a 15- to 18-min motor skill lesson. This segment of the class focuses on learning new skills or applying acquired skills. The motor skill lessons follow South Carolina Physical Education Curriculum Guidelines (8). Group sizes are kept small to provide students maximum opportunity to learn, practice, and use the skills. For example, in a third-grade soccer unit, students usually practice individually or in groups of two or three in a noncompetitive or simple competitive game. By fifth grade most students are involved in three-on-three play.

Specific cognitive, affective, and fitness competencies taught in both PERK Too and the motor skill segments are also developed from these curriculum guidelines. Examples shared by both segments follow:

- *Affective*: Accept responsibility for choosing an appropriate piece of equipment for one's own ability.
- *Fitness*: Identify one way aerobic fitness is developed.
- *Cognitive*: Explain how to stop with control.

To present such ideas, the teacher utilizes four wall charts displayed for at least 1 week (see Figure 18.2). Representative of psychomotor, cognitive, affective, and fitness competencies, each chart displays key words and phrases to which the teacher refers before, during, or after the motor skill lesson or PERK Too. Teaching is not limited to ideas displayed; there are many "teachable moments" that can occur. The wall charts, however, provide a specific focus for the teacher and students and send a message to the students that certain ideas are important.

Over the last several years, the amount of time spent in vigorous activity during the motor skill segment has steadily increased. Two reasons may contribute to the increase: First, as students become more skillful and achieve grade-level motor skill competencies, they begin to maintain control and to practice the motor skill longer. The teacher spends less time teaching new fundamental skills (in the upper grades) and more time teaching complex movement patterns. The second reason is that

classes are organized to minimize waiting for instruction or for turns to participate. An example follows:

> In a fourth-grade basketball lesson, the objective may call for one-on-one offensive and defensive play. The students form 12 groups of two students each. They play in six courts that are 15 ft by 45 ft with two groups to a court. The teacher explains and demonstrates the initial task, and then students begin practice. The teacher refines the task for students on an individual basis, stopping the class only when necessary for class feedback or to change the task complexity or difficulty.

Simple checks have shown that student heart rates can be at an aerobic intensity level during the motor skill lesson. Not all motor skill lessons, however, can provide for this intensity level. An example is throwing and catching with stationary partners. Yet every attempt is made to provide aerobic activity during the motor skill segment. A way to maintain continuous movement has developed with the students themselves. Walking in place has been the response to the teacher's "get moving" phrase between PERK Too's music selections. Many students also walk in place during the motor skill segment while listening to the teacher or waiting for their turns to participate.

Class Closure

The last few minutes of PE are spent in muscle-strengthening exercises for Grades 3 through 5 (i.e., upper torso and abdominal muscles) and with a cool-down for all grades (flexibility). Cool-down segments are designed to be appropriate to the sport, dance, or gymnastic activity (1) utilized in PERK Too and the motor skill lesson. During this time the teacher brings closure to the class by reviewing critical ideas from PERK Too and the motor skill lesson.

Positive Results

The combination of motor skill and PERK Too is the most recent addition to Moving to Success. There is much experimentation here and much to learn; however, the motor skill and PERK Too approach have demonstrated positive results. In the 1990-91 school year, the third-grade class average on the mile walk/run pretest was 15:40 min. After a year of various activities provided by Moving to Success, the posttest average was 11:32 min. Adults

I feel I can...	I know how to...
get along with others.	move my body.

I am fit because....	I know soccer skills...
I am active.	Trap Dribble Pass

Figure 18.2   Example of wall charts.

involved in this testing observed a change in attitude from the 1990 pretest to the 1991 posttest. The students seemed to demonstrate a more positive attitude toward running the mile during the posttest than they did during the pretest. The students also appeared to demonstrate real confidence in what their bodies could do, and motor skill acquisition has steadily improved. Using the South Carolina Physical Education Curriculum Guidelines (8) as a major resource, the physical education teacher has observed that the students continue to demonstrate improved skillfulness based on the grade level competencies presented in the guide.

Student testing of both motor skills and health-related fitness has not been given the validity that is needed to demonstrate student success clearly. During the 1991–92 school year, a research project will be conducted to measure all aspects of the physical education program.

Physical Exercise Revives Kids (PERK)

The forerunner of all activities in Moving to Success is PERK, the school's early morning warm-up. Movements are choreographed to allow students to practice a variety of locomotor sequences.

PERK also attempts to accomplish a cognitive awareness of fitness concepts by concentrating on the following: frequency (all classes participate at least 3 days weekly— usually 5 days weekly), intensity (vigorous activity elevates heart and respiratory rates for intensity awareness), and safety (warm-up and cool-down segments are always included). In the affective area, PERK provides an opportunity to develop leadership skills among the fifth-grade students designated as PERK leaders.

Discover and Understand Communities, Kids, by Walking (DUCK Walking)

DUCK Walking, another Moving to Success activity, involves students, teachers, families, parents, and community volunteers. For 2 years DUCK Walking has had 100% participation among students and teachers. It was created by a parent-volunteer and is a 30-week aerobic walking activity. At least 20 min during one school day each week are devoted to aerobic walking. During the 1990–91 school year, 400 students, 21 staff members, and various parent volunteers walked 11,400 aerobic miles.

Individual classes accumulate mileage. Classes may then relate the miles walked to an imaginary tour of South Carolina divided into three regions—the Upcountry, the Midlands, and the Coastal Region. During the 1990–91 school year, each class walked enough miles to equal an imaginary walk through the South Carolina Upcountry area. Teachers enhance the activity by volunteering to use "Extra Mile" Activities as shown in Table 18.1. DUCK Walking becomes an integrated approach to physical education, health, social studies, mathematics, language arts, science, and the fine arts. Teachers, students, and families have found that walking allows doing, sensing, exploring, and discovering, as well as providing healthful benefits (9).

Morning Activities for Students

"Morning Activities for Students" is a before-school component of Moving to Success. For third,

fourth, and fifth graders there are high-energy, self-directed games of tetherball, one-on-one and two-on-two possession basketball, one-wall racquetball, jump rope, two-square, four-square, and six-square.

PE Club

The PE Club is an after-school activity for third, fourth, and fifth graders. The club meets once weekly for 60 min and consists of three interest groups (running, jumping rope, and sport performance) that work independently of each other yet come together for fun and performance.

Family and Community Events

Yearly events involve voluntary school participation with the support of teachers and parent volunteers. Examples of annual Moving to Success activities are the American Heart Association's Jump Rope for Heart event, Sports Night, and the celebration of Physical Education and Sports Week.

Table 18.1 Extra Mile Activities

Health	Social studies	Mathematics	Language arts
Aerobic walking	Communities	Mileage chart	Personal journal
Walking technique	Transportation	Walking time line	Class journal
Warm-up/cool-down	Workplaces	Paces per minute	Family journal
Stretching	Piedmont careers	Distances walked	Letter for information
Pulse rate	Community stories	Temperature chart	Piedmont Pen Pals
Exertion	Local games	Target heart rate	Storytelling
Aerobic benefits	Local folktales	Resting pulse	Class newsletter
Nutritious snacks	Piedmont industries	Calories burned	School newsletter
Food sources	Scenic highways	Counting objects	Trail signs
Healthy recipes	Local festivals	Aerobic time	Walking quotes

Science	Physical education	Fine arts	Family activities
Dressing for weather	Fitness walking	Architecture	Recreation
Observing weather	Active vs. inactive	Walking banners	Family fitness
Nature trail	Strong heart	Composing a cadence	Family nutrition
School terrain	Strong lungs	Local crafts	Sharing "Fit Tips"
Piedmont terrain	Strong muscles	Walking video	Neighborhood walks
Color hike	Strong bones	Community montage	Sharing interests
Litter pick-up	Cardiovascular health	Photography	Sharing talents
Nature sounds	Strength	Walking scrapbooks	"Walkee Talkee"
Signs of seasons	Endurance	Local art museums	Family DUCKs
Insect homes	Healthy body fat	Bulletin board	Piedmont hikes

Family and Community Involvement

Obviously, the support and the involvement of the school staff, parents, and the community are keys to the accomplishments of Moving to Success. For Woodland Heights Elementary School's families there have been DUCK Walking events, newsletters, fitness reports, and parent seminars. Contributions to the *The Scene at Six*, the school district newsletter, announce events and invite other schools to running events, walking events, Sports Night, and sport performances. Articles and pictures of special PE events have appeared on television and in the local newspapers.

Moving to Success has a child-centered emphasis, and the program promotes individual success. As a result each student is active and can also have fun with experiences that demonstrate why and how to get fit. The following are several reasons for sustained interest in the program:

- The individual child can develop motor skills needed to participate effectively. Moving to Success allows every individual to practice and refine motor skills in a variety of aerobic activities.
- Moving to Success has helped to develop the participants' understanding of self-discipline and has promoted leadership roles for students. Activities are designed to encourage everyone's participation.
- Children work with adult role models who enjoy the activities.
- Several activities employ music that relates to children's thoughts and experiences.
- The use of equipment (balls, jump ropes, streamers, etc.) enhances many activities.

Conclusion

The physical education program at Woodland Heights Elementary School effectively combines motor skill and health-related fitness into a comprehensive program called Moving to Success. The school values and supports physical activity as part of the total educational process. Moving to Success successfully blends the school staff, parents, and community, all of whom add assistance and support. The physical education teacher coordinates the program and directly involves the classroom teachers in PERK and DUCK Walking.

Physical education classes blend fitness and learning through PERK Too and motor skill development built into every lesson.

Every attempt is made to implement a student-centered program. Students work on acquiring skills that will help them make intelligent decisions about being physically active young people and adults. A major consideration is planning activities that are positive, fun, innovative, and developmentally appropriate for elementary children. Also, the increased time students spend in the many physical education activities does not have a negative effect on students' academic test scores—which continue to improve at an appropriate rate.

Moving to Success, therefore, focuses on the learner. The process is not merely a string of activities to keep everyone busy. Moving to Success is a foundation for building skillfulness while providing fitness experiences. It is an example of how a school has been able to move beyond the gymnasium to involve the entire school; nevertheless, the program continues to evolve to provide students with learning experiences that will educate the whole child through movement. Most important, all children are active daily and have an opportunity to see that regular physical activity is a means to a lifetime of good health.

References

1. Anderson, B. Stretching. Bolinas, CA: Shelter; 1980: p. 111-149.
2. Guy, M. PERK-ing along: a unique program to improve physical fitness in children. J. SC Assoc. Health Phys. Educ. Rec. Dance 17(1): 20; 1985.
3. Keep on trying. Mousercise. Burbank, CA: Disneyland/Vista Records; 1982.
4. Missett, J.S. Kids get fit school program. Programs for children by Jazzercise, Inc. Carlsbad, CA: Jazzercise; 1991.
5. Rosen, G.; Shontz, B. A good friend. It's the truth. Brattleboro, VT: Rosenshontz Records; 1984.
6. Scelsa, G. Safety break. Kidding around with Greg and Steve. Los Angeles: Youngheart Records; 1985.
7. Scelsa, G. Sports dance. On the move with Greg and Steve. Los Angeles: Youngheart Records; 1983.
8. South Carolina physical education curriculum guidelines. Vol. 1. Columbia, SC: Department of Education; 1990.

9. Sweetgall, R.; Neeves, R. Walking for little children. Clayton, MO: Creative Walking; 1987.

10. The mighty pump—the heart. Slim Goodbody's musical guide to what's inside. Long Branch, NJ: Kimbo Educational; 1986.

11. Weikart, P.S. Teaching movement and dance: a sequential approach. Ypsilanti, MI: High/Scope Press; 1985.

Part III
Fitness in Practice:
Programs to Add to the
Physical Education Curriculum

Each chapter in Part III describes a specific component of successful, health-related physical education. These chapters provide tangible ways for teachers to use the many recommendations advanced in earlier portions of this book.

Chapter 19

In "The Springdale Running Program" Cindy R. Wilkerson and Peter H. Werner report that running programs are inexpensive and can be implemented in most physical education settings. Running programs can be particularly successful when tied into other classes across the curriculum and when they encourage students to run with parents and other family members. Whereas the main goal at Springdale Elementary is to develop children physically, the physical education staff is dedicated to teaching health and fitness as a lifelong commitment to a quality lifestyle.

Chapter 20

Jenifer J. Steller's "The Physical Education Performance Troupe: A Skill and Fitness Approach" explains that designing a program, choosing movements and patterns, and combining skills with a fitness workout are the three components of performance activities and of training a performance troupe. The troupe may help students of all ages meet fitness goals while they refine physical education skills in an aerobic conditioning program.

Chapter 21

Dan B. Young shows how Woodland Heights Elementary School interfaced health, math, science, language arts, and the visual arts with physical education. The fifth-grade students used PE time to administer fitness tests to the school. They tabulated results in the math class, studied health-related fitness in health class, kept journals about their year-long fitness project, and wrote the text for their "Family Fitness Guide" in language arts class.

Chapter 22

Sandra Weigle describes the walking program at Northside Elementary School in Rock Hill, SC, as a model that can easily be copied. By providing organization, walking courses, and incentives, schools can help students reduce stress, improve alertness, talk about health and nature, and enhance communication and activity at home.

Chapter 23

In this chapter Barbara A. Krok describes the process of funding and producing *Citrus County Fitness Break*—a series of fitness and health videos for classroom (not PE) use developed by Krok and

Dianna Bandhauer and starring children from Citrus County schools. This chapter gives teachers advice on how to become producers and includes an appendix with two skits.

Chapter 24

"Fitness—The Ravenel Way," by Adelaide V. Carpenter, describes three program components that have promoted fitness at Ravenel Elementary School in Seneca, SC. The first is the physical education classes, including Fitness Fridays, a class devoted to aspects of physical fitness. The second is the Morning Exercise Program, in which fifth graders lead all the homeroom classes as they perform exercise routines to music broadcast daily over the school's PA system from 7:55 to 8:05 a.m. The third is the Ravenel Ropesters, a trick jump-rope squad that performs in schools, at festivals, and even at college sport events.

Chapter 19

The Springdale Running Program

Cindy R. Wilkerson
Springdale Elementary School
West Columbia, South Carolina

Peter H. Werner
University of South Carolina, Columbia

In her chapter, "Fitting Fitness Into the School Curriculum," Judith Rink offered several approaches for incorporating health-related fitness goals into physical education programs in public school settings. These included programs differentiated for grade level, using school time other than physical education instruction time, approaching fitness as health maintenance, integrating fitness within a motor skill program, designing instruction to facilitate vigorous activity, and integrating fitness within the health curriculum.

The physical education program at Springdale Elementary School offers PE to children in Grades 1 through 5 twice weekly for 30 min each period. Based on sound pedagogical principles and effective instructional practice, children receive a program that focuses on a combination of health-related physical fitness concepts and motor skills acquisition. Because of the limited class time available, choices have been made that reflect several of those Rink proposed for developing fitness in public school settings.

This chapter describes the running program at Springdale Elementary School as it relates directly to cardiorespiratory endurance and to a combination of several of Rink's choices. Other health-related fitness concepts are developed as well during the elementary years but will not be described here.

How the Running Program Works

The running program is generated out of initial experiences during physical education class time each year. Early in each school year, all children Grades 1 through 5 learn about concepts such as running pace, target heart rate, the FIT (frequency, intensity, and time) principle, and so on. In the past decade, four 1-mile runs have been built into the yearly curriculum. Each is centered around a special season or time of year to provide some motivation for students. The Pumpkin Run is held at Halloween, the Reindeer Run is held just before Christmas, the Bunny Run is held in conjunction with Easter, and the Beach Bum Run is held the week before school lets out in May. Family members are always invited to participate in each of the four 1-mile runs.

Each of the four runs is held during class time. Each child's time is recorded annually and kept by the physical education teacher. In addition, each child's time is recorded on a computer-generated certificate or award and sent home to parents. Students may walk or run the course, or a combination of both, and are encouraged to do their best; participation is the key. It is hoped that the children's times will improve in the four runs from October through May. In 1990, 92% of the students improved their times over the year. Although it is

188 Health and Fitness Through Physical Education

not stressed a great deal, the times of the top four boys and four girls in each class are also posted and are published in the school bulletin. At the conclusion of each class on each of the four run days, personal effort, the benefits of a regular exercise program, feeling good about one's self, and accomplishments are highlighted.

Cardiorespiratory fitness cannot be developed during class time in a format of 2 days a week, 30 min a lesson. So at Springdale Elementary School children from Grades 1 through 5 are encouraged to walk and run at times during the day other than in PE, such as before school, during recess, after lunch, and after school. A kilometer track is marked off around the school playground where children are encouraged to walk fast, jog, or run. Classroom teachers keep a chart for children to mark their laps. In Grades 1 and 2 children have a buddy system. Someone must watch them run or run with them in order to get credit for the laps. Third, fourth, and fifth graders work on an honor system. Upon completion of 20, 50, 100, and 200 km students receive individual certificates as awards. It is very exciting to watch children become involved in a running program. Once they become committed, it is amazing how hard they will work to achieve a goal and earn a small award such as a certificate.

Fitness Across the Curriculum

Integrating fitness into other areas of the school curriculum is another program goal. In a 1991 Walk Across America campaign children and their family members symbolically walked/ran across America in 6 weeks. As part of the geography and social science unit, children studied about the states they ran through. Everyone started in California. When classes got to Nebraska, the Cornhusker state, they had a popcorn party. When they entered Wisconsin, the Dairy state, they had cheese snacks. When they arrived at the beach in South Carolina, a day was declared for wearing sun glasses.

A large map of the United States was displayed in the school hall. Each class charted its progress and calculated the mileage of individuals, family members, and the total distance of the class as a whole. The South Carolina Department of Health and Environmental Control provided mileage cards. The local recreation commission provided mile markers for housing developments in the

local community so families could exercise together during the evenings or on weekends. Four local businesses contributed money during the Walk Across America campaign, which was in turn donated to World Hunger.

Other Running Events

Several other events during the school year further emphasize the exercise program at Springdale Elementary School. In January a 100-lap run campaign is held. At the beginning of the school year children are urged to walk/run one lap per day until the 100th day of school. As the day draws near, children often do extra laps to make up for days missed. On the 100th day of school an assembly is held and 100-lap ribbons are given to everyone who reaches the goal.

Toward the end of the school year a Family Fun and Fitness Day is held on a Saturday. 1990 was special because it honored a deceased teacher within the district as well as fathers who were engaged in the Persian Gulf War. Over 300 people participated and entry fees were charged for the run, with proceeds donated to the Epileptic Foundation. Following the run, the school playground was set up for children to show parents the skills they had learned in physical education during the year. Face painting, patriotic songs, and a dance performed by a local clogging group were also featured. The day ended with a hot dog picnic.

As a result of the focus on exercise at Springdale Elementary School, many students have participated in local running events as monitors or runners. Events have included the Turkey Trot, Peach Festival Run, Governor's Cup, Cooper River Bridge Run, and Carolina Marathon.

Motivating All Children to Participate

Elementary school children need very little motivation to run. Certificates and ribbons to all participants who complete goals were the forms of extrinsic motivation that we awarded. We also presented a gold medal to one boy and one girl from each class who completed the most laps during the school year, awarded the last day of the school year at an assembly. Primary motivation is more intrinsic in nature. Lap completions give children a sense of success, be it large or small. Running encourages children to have positive feelings about themselves.

Every child can be successful. Overweight children can complete laps by walking and feel good about it. Children who are handicapped can also participate. The lap tracks can be shortened for disabled children. In the Springdale program children in wheelchairs push themselves around the outdoor basketball court to complete laps.

Summary

Running programs are not expensive and can be implemented in almost every physical education setting. The running program can be particularly successful when it is tied into other classes across the curriculum and when it encourages students to run with parents and other family members. Although the main goal at Springdale Elementary School is to physically develop children, we are also trying to teach health fitness as a lifelong commitment to a quality lifestyle.

Chapter 20

The Physical Education Performance Troupe: A Skill and Fitness Approach

Jenifer J. Steller
Woodland Heights Elementary School
Spartanburg, South Carolina

Children enjoy a variety of aerobic fitness activities—running, walking, swimming, cycling, jumping rope, dancing, and participating in classes, clubs, and favorite sports. Good leaders in these fun activities can educate children to the importance of planning and implementing personal fitness programs. Through these activities elementary students can achieve health benefits, refine their skills, and perceive their accomplishments. Helping children to establish and meet fitness goals, therefore, may motivate them to remain active.

The *performance troupe* is one means that can help teachers and students have fun while achieving health benefits. With the specific goal of public performances, the physical education performance troupe is a group that demonstrates choreographed dance and movement techniques and specific drills that may integrate locomotion, body management, and game and sport skills. An example is a group of boys and girls who perform a 10-min choreographed routine that includes creative movement, ball handling, and rope jumping. To emphasize the fitness approach, practices consist of warm-up routines, movement across the floor, specific movement and skill choreography, and a cool-down with overall body stretches. This fitness approach of warm-up, peak work (aerobic or strength training), and cool-down may also be incorporated into the performance program.

The performance troupe works well for students of all ages because it improves and maintains fitness levels while utilizing locomotion, body management, dance, and game and sport skills. Furthermore, this activity may improve coordination, agility, balance, flexibility, and posture, as well as cardiorespiratory, muscular, and metabolic fitness. Public performances not only promote skill and fitness awareness to the school, family, and community, but also may help troupe members gain self-assurance and poise through positive public response. Most important, fitness with skills helps participants demonstrate both their knowledge of specific motor skills and their efforts to improve individual levels of physical fitness.

There are three components in developing a performance activity and training a physical education performance troupe: designing the program performance, choosing movements and directional patterns, and combining skills with a fitness workout. The logistics of time, location, and student management will vary with each school and the types of activities chosen.

Designing the Program

The first component, designing a performance program, involves several considerations: ascertaining what is suitable for the particular audience and troupe members, selecting the music, and aiding the troupe's memorization of the program.

Knowing the Audience and the Troupe Members

The type of audience and the troupe membership are primary influences in the design of a program. The audience might be adults, or children, or a mix in school or the community. The troupe can be a regular physical education class or an after-school club. Knowing the troupe members by age, skill ability, fitness levels, and memorization ability will affect the selection of music, skills, movements, and patterns.

Establishing skill goals for individual members becomes the next consideration. These skill areas may incorporate many of the physical education content areas. Establishing fitness goals for individuals follows. Developing cardiorespiratory endurance, flexibility, muscular strength, and muscular endurance should be important. Creativity then blends music and choreography with specific skills and a fitness approach to accommodate both the troupe members and the intended audience.

Selecting Music for a Variety of Ages

The creative blend of music, choreography, and skills largely determines the quality of the program. Music that reflects positive and entertaining messages can create a superior performance. For children age 5 to 11 years, some good music sources are albums by Greg Scelsa and Steve Millang for Youngheart Records (P.O. Box 27784, Los Angeles, California 90027) and albums by Hap Palmer for Educational Activities, Incorporated (P.O. Box 392, Freeport, New York 11520). These albums usually list songs for movement, rhythm, and active play. Students of all ages may choose from all music genres, for example, jazz, swing, thematic (i.e., movies, television, and commercials), reggae, bluegrass, classical, kid rap, rhythm and blues, and seasonal. A varied musical selection may further develop students' rhythm skills and musical experiences.

Aiding the Troupe's Memorization of the Program

To help students learn the program easily there are other musical considerations. Lyrical and musical phrasing can simplify children's memorization of movement changes. For example, key words or a repetition of a chorus could signal a change from skipping in place to skipping forward for four counts and backward for four counts. Consistent tempo can also facilitate learning movements, patterns, and their changes. Tempo, too, determines ease of stretching (i.e., slow and even pace), locomotion (e.g., slow to fast pace), and other movement experiences (e.g., slow to fast pace for handling a ball, jumping a rope, or using a hula hoop).

Choosing Movements and Patterns

The second component in developing a performance program is choosing movements and directional patterns. This area interplays with the first component's considerations of audience, music selection, and the troupe members' ages and grade levels. Music may be the foundation of the program; however, the skill elements can determine the choice of the music: These two enhance each other.

Movements and Patterns With Music

Developing movement patterns in conformance with a piece of music requires that the teacher first count out the beat and then replay the music to identify the verse, chorus, bridge, or instrumental sections. In sections where musical patterns repeat, the movement patterns can repeat. Although music is usually written in four-beat time, choreographers tend to count the music in eights. If the song drops a beat, that is, the artist drops the last four counts of an eight-count phrase, this can present a challenge in the performance. These musical "drops" may be used as a transition from one movement to the next by continuing with the previous movement an additional four counts (1).

The suitability of music, however, is not determined by tempo alone. Even if two pieces of music have the same number of beats per minute, they may differ greatly in levels of intensity and may inspire very different types of movement (1).

Movements, Patterns, and Equipment

Movement choices can range from such basic skills as stretches, bends, curls, twists, walking, running, hopping, jumping, skipping, and sliding to such advanced dance techniques as grapevines, flea hops, and jazz squares. Directional patterns can vary greatly: side-to-side, front and back, in-place, squares, diagonals, front-right-front-left, and everywhere. Whatever the movements and patterns chosen, they should be physiologically safe and appropriate for children.

Using balls, jump ropes, hula hoops, scarves, streamers, and other equipment and props adds fun and challenge. Specific drills can provide individualized time for aerobic practice of movements, patterns, and manipulative skills.

Music, Movements, Patterns, Equipment, and Fun

Table 20.1 contains an excerpt from one performance routine for boys and girls age 8 years and older to be performed for children and adults at school or community events. Emphasis is on a light cardiovascular workout, dance technique, coordination, creative movement, and complex locomotor patterns. Although not included in the example here, sport drills with equipment may be utilized toward the end of the song's 3:42 min. "Ninja Rap" might be included in the performance between a warm-up (opening) song and a cool-down (closing) song.

Combining Skills With a Fitness Workout

The third component in training a performance group requires planning for a fitness approach. Practices may be efficient 30- to 60-min sessions. Skill and choreography instruction may come first. Fitness segments follow to refine the performance skills in a safe and effective workout.

Warm-Up Segment

A practice begins with a 5- to 10-min warm-up segment. During this time, the troupe performs overall body stretches and body isolations. The teacher can take this time to lead and oversee the quality of these stretches, discuss the troupe's previous strengths and weaknesses, and give positive reminders of safety and intensity to be followed during the aerobic segment. Music is light or upbeat. Static or preaerobic stretching is best done to

Table 20.1 Routine Excerpt Performed to "Ninja Rap" by Vanilla Ice (from the original motion picture soundtrack, *Teenage Mutant Ninja Turtles II, The Secret of the Ooze*)

Music cues	Movements and patterns
Introduction	• Hold during whistle for 8 counts. • Walk to the beat in place for 8. • During the next 3 counts of 8 peel off into groups to face front.
"Yo"	• Walk while changing lines (Counts 1-8). • Reverse the walk for a count of 8. • Return walking to original positions for Counts 9 to 16. • Walk right (Counts 17-20). • Walk backwards (Counts 21-24). Turn 180 degrees and walk left (Counts 25-28). • Walk backwards (Counts 29-32). Run in place (Counts 33-40) or do the "Running Man" by starting with "funky walks," adding more energy, and sliding each leg behind the body.
"Ninja"	• Face right with left leg bent and arms crossed for a count of 1. • Hold for Counts 2 to 4. • Face front and do a "karate pose" on Count 5. • Hold for Counts 6 to 8. • Reverse for Counts 1 to 4 and Counts 9 to 12. • Let each student choose an individual "karate pose."

Note. Source: J.S. Missett, Kids Get Fit School Program. Programs for Children by Jazzercise, Inc. Carlsbad, CA: Jazzercise, Inc. 1991. Reprinted by permission.

music of about 100 to 120 beats per minute, whereas more upbeat warm-up music may be 110 to 130 beats per minute (1). Here is a chance to use a variety of movements such as turning, twisting, stretching, curling, balancing, and walking.

Peak Workout (Aerobic and/or Strengthening)

The aerobic segment can be 20 to 40 min in length. Music is varied and has 120 to 180 beats per minute (1). Skill movements can be walking, running, hopping, skipping, sliding, galloping, or jumping. These movements can include all kinds of repetitions and combinations of directional patterns, as well as equipment and props. At this time students can utilize skills in the content areas of body management, dance, sports and games, and locomotion. This cardiovascular workout builds in intensity from light to medium to medium-heavy and decreases in intensity from medium-heavy to medium to light.

Following this intensity plan, the aerobic segment can be divided into two practice sessions—one individualized and one "blocked" or staged as a group. For example, during 8 to 15 min of the aerobic segment, an individualized session of "across the floor" work provides a practice breakdown of skills, movements, patterns, and choreographed combinations. For 12 to 25 min of the aerobic segment, a session of group work allows for staged, choreographed performance practice. During this entire segment, individual movement is important.

Cool-Down Segment

A 5- to 10-min cool-down segment gives much needed overall body stretching. As in the warm-up segment, movements are varied and music can be light or upbeat with 110 to 130 beats per minute when walking, stretching, turning, twisting, curling, and balancing. For static stretching, try 100 to 120 beats per minute. The teacher again can oversee the quality of stretches, discuss the practice session's strengths and weaknesses, give positive assurance of progress, and remind everyone to practice or work out at home.

Fitness Approach Benefits

This third component of the performance workout can fulfill aerobic fitness requirements. The three important variables in aerobic training are frequency, intensity, and time (FIT); that is, to achieve and maintain aerobic fitness one needs to exercise often enough, at an appropriate pace, and at least for a minimum time (2).

Frequency requirements can be met when individuals practice at school or at home at least three times weekly. Intensity for the students can be based on their perceived exertion or individual target heart rates during the aerobic segment. For example, children may reach a 140- to 180-bpm heart rate, or they can comfortably talk, sing, and laugh during the vigorous activity (2). Time or duration is achieved with a 30- to 60-min individual session, where at least 20 min of the session is continuous vigorous activity. For children age 6 to 9 years, this time may be 10 to 20 min of continuous vigorous activity (2).

Summary: A Successful Physical Education Performance Troupe

Designing a program, choosing movements and patterns, and combining skills with a fitness workout are the three components in the development of a performance activity and the training of a performance troupe. The troupe may help students of all ages to establish and meet fitness goals while refining PE skills in an aerobic conditioning program. The use of this skill and fitness approach has evolved with the performance troupe at Woodland Heights Elementary School in Spartanburg, South Carolina. This voluntary club began with the skill approach in 1988, added choreography to skill in 1989, then added the fitness approach to skill and choreography in 1990. For the 1990–91 school year 25 third, fourth, and fifth grade boys and girls at all levels of skill and fitness development followed the three components outlined for developing a program and training a troupe. Their 15-min performance began with a warm-up segment using "Boogie and Beethoven" by the Gatlin Brothers to demonstrate stretches, balance, transfer of weight, complex locomotor patterns, and dance technique. The aerobic segment included "Rockin' Over the Beat" by Technotronic to demonstrate dribbling technique and then to demonstrate individual and group jump-rope skills. The cool-down segment included the use of brightly colored, handmade streamers with a dance routine to "Electric Boogie" by Marcia Griffiths. Their performances were well received by students, families, and the community at school and at local high-school and collegiate athletic events.

The performance troupe has worked well for Woodland Heights Elementary School students. Being an after-school club, they did not scientifically measure their individual skill and fitness levels, so there is no conclusive evidence that skill and fitness levels did improve. However, the results of a subjective survey from each troupe member showed unanimous praise for music selections, choreography of movement and patterns, equipment use, the fitness approach, and the element of fun.

Some members suggested a longer practice time and meeting more than once weekly. Some members also suggested new skills, movements, patterns, music, and equipment use. These suggestions provided a plan for the 1991–92 school year to include continuation of the skill and fitness approach to performance, an extended time for practice, new choreographed routines, more public performances, and self-appraisal of skill and fitness levels.

The success of the Woodland Heights Performance Troupe has been its ability to include motor skills in a health-related fitness workout and performance. The reward has been a fun activity that also helps refine physical education skills in a conditioning program.

References

1. Baum, G. Music. JOPERD 62(5):35-37; 1991.
2. Glover, R.H.; Shepherd, J. The family fitness handbook. New York: Penguin Books; 1989: p. 158-169.
3. Missett, J.S. Kids get fit school program. Programs for children by Jazzercise, Inc. Carlsbad, CA: Jazzercise; 1991.

Chapter 21

Curriculum Interfacing Through Physical Education: Health, Math, Science, Language Arts, and Gifted and Talented

Dan B. Young
Woodland Heights Elementary School
Spartanburg, South Carolina

Interfacing subject areas encourages students to perceive learning experiences as interwoven and useful. The first consideration in planning interfacing activities is the content. Each subject area's activities must be able to stand independently. That is, the learning experiences by themselves are valuable; however, they become more relevant and meaningful when interfaced with other subject areas. The purpose of this chapter is to show how a school physical education program can interface health, math, science, language arts, and visual arts.

The critical consideration for the success of curriculum interfacing is teacher planning. It takes time to plan, organize, and integrate learning experiences with activities occurring in other classes. Regardless of how well teachers plan and communicate, conflicts arise that affect the process. Conflicts can be overcome if the time table allows for flexibility.

It may be useful to describe some of the process we used in a year-long project of curriculum interfacing involving all three fifth-grade classes at Woodland Heights Elementary School in Spartanburg, South Carolina. Before the school term began, the fifth-grade teachers met to develop a general outline of classroom learning activities for the school year. The physical education teacher provided all teachers involved with the project a list of PE objectives and activities. Additional meetings were scheduled with the physical education teacher and individual subject area teachers to plan specific interfacing activities. Formal meetings occurred every 6 weeks to review the previous activities and to plan specific activities for the next 6 weeks.

These are the learning objectives and activities that we used to interface with physical education.

Physical Education

The physical education activities were designed to teach the five health-related fitness components, to practice assessing health-related fitness, and to learn when an appropriate level of health-related fitness exists.

Fifth-grade students were first trained to administer a five-component, health-related fitness test (FitnessGram). This included recording information on the student fitness data form shown in Figure 21.1. Each fitness tester (a fifth grader) was assigned to assess four to six students from Grades 1 through 4. Each tester was responsible for assessing, recording, and maintaining the records from the pretest to the posttest. The data cards were kept on file in the math class.

It was important to match the capabilities of fifth graders to the size and grade level of the students being assessed. The most responsible fifth graders were matched with the largest groups or with lower grade students who needed the most leadership. One class was assessed at a time.

The testing environment was arranged into four stations. Each station had enough assessment equipment to handle two test groups. The four stations were height and weight, sit-ups, sit-and-reach, and pull-ups and flexed arm hang. The mile walk/run was set up in a separate area. To increase the efficiency of test administration, the fitness testers practiced giving the test to each other in the test environment.

The test took two 30-min class periods to administer. The mile walk/run was administered during one class, and the other four components were administered in another class. The key to a successful student-administered assessment was the training of the testers and an efficiently arranged testing environment.

Math

The objective in math was to provide students with practical application experiences, requiring that relevant math activities be designed. Each fitness tester entered the data he or she collected into the computer using the FitnessGram software. The information (analysis) was printed out on regular computer paper for the fitness tester to check for accuracy. If mistakes were found, the corrections were made by the tester. FitnessGram cards were printed out for each student after all corrections were made. The FitnessGram cards were sent home for the child and parent to review.

The math teacher planned additional classroom activities using the collected data. Charts and graphs were developed in class to compare one class to another and to compare school scores to state and national norms. Privacy of the scores was maintained. Student activities included using the computer to generate charts and graphs, as well as using paper and pencil activities to make charts and graphs.

Written problems that required computational skills were developed by the math teacher. Two examples of written problems were "What is the average number of sit-ups for boys in second grade?" and "What percent of the students in the third grade completed the mile in less than 14 minutes?"

Health

In the fifth-grade health classes students studied health-related fitness. The objective was to research and identify appropriate activities for a family fitness guide. The learning activities also provided students an opportunity to apply research skills and expository writing.

A family fitness survey was designed using information gathered on health-related fitness topics. The purpose of the survey was to determine current family fitness practices and to determine favorite activities. The survey was sent home to all fifth-grade parents. The surveys that were returned were tabulated, thus identifying the most popular activities.

Students researched health-related fitness topics to identify ideas that could be considered for the family fitness guide and identified topics that could be included in the guide. Topics were then selected based on the information gathered from the family survey. Additional information was gathered on topics that were to be used in the guide. The students worked in small groups to write up the topics, and one group arranged the topics in an appropriate layout for the guide.

Language Arts

Students maintained a journal expressing their attitudes toward personal fitness. Journal writing was a valuable step in the writing process. It was used to increase self-awareness and to utilize higher level thinking skills. The first journal entry was written before the activities began and after each major activity. At the end of the year, students were asked to determine changes in their attitude toward personal fitness.

Student Fitness Data Form

Identification number _____   School _____

Name   Sex
    First _____   (M or F)

    Middle initial _____   Grade _____

    Last _____   Period _____

Date of birth   Notes:
    Month _____

    Day _____

    Year _____

Test Number	One	Two	Three	Four
Month of test				
Year of test				
Height (Record in inches)				
Weight (Record in pounds)				
1-mile run (Record in minutes and seconds)	:	:	:	:
Situps (Record number in one minute)				
Pullups (Record number)				
Arm Hang (Record seconds)				
Sit and Reach (Record in inches)				
Triceps and Calf (Record in millimeters)	/	/	/	/
Shuttle (Record in seconds)				

Figure 21.1   Student fitness data form.

Visual Arts

The purpose of involving visual arts was to have some of the activities in the guide illustrated by students. This provided students an opportunity to apply the concept of line design by producing figure drawings of people in action. Students were given the option of participating in this activity. The sketches were submitted for review. A group of students was selected to review the sketches and identify the pieces that best illustrated the activities in the guide.

Gifted and Talented

The "gifted and talented" classes took the material developed in health classes and used word processing to prepare the guide. The class proofread and edited the guide for spelling and grammatical errors. The guide was printed by the district print shop. It was put together by the gifted and talented class and then distributed to every family of the school. See Table 21.1 for an outline of the family fitness guide.

Summary

At the end of the year the teachers spent some time reflecting on the year-long project. Many valuable learning experiences occurred throughout the process. Positive experiences were the students working together in groups, students working on a similar project in several different subject areas, and teachers working together on a common project. The relevance of the experience, however, was what the teachers valued the greatest.

The activities started with learning how to administer a test and continued with activities that

Table 21.1 Family Fitness Guide Outline

Why your family should exercise

How to start and plan an exercise program

Safety tips for a fitness program

Family fitness exercises
  Walking
  Jogging
  Jumping rope
  Biking
  Swimming

How to warm up and cool down

Taking care of your feet

Additional fitness ideas
  Weight lifting
  Soccer
  Push-ups and sit-ups

Chart for your fitness program

were pertinent to student experiences. Assessing other students' fitness levels, collecting information from a family survey, conducting research, and then using all that information to solve problems and develop a fitness guide created enjoyable and significant learning experiences that enhanced and combined the coursework for fifth-grade physical education, math, health, science, language arts, and visual arts classes. The fifth-grade students will be able to apply what they have learned in future decisions they make in developing a physically active lifestyle. There are no hard and fast rules to this process; each school has its own situation. The number of academic subjects can vary. The only limitations to curriculum interfacing are the creative abilities of the teachers involved. The use of relevant learning experiences for students is enough to justify the interfacing of physical education with other subjects.

Chapter 22

A Walking Program in Your School? Practical Tips to Make It Work

Sandra M. Weigle
Northside Elementary School
Rock Hill, South Carolina

At Northside Elementary in Rock Hill, South Carolina, 25 teachers and staff participated in a walking wellness program. What made our program unique was that it actually got better as the year went on. Participation picked up rather than fizzling out.

Before going into the specifics of what made the program successful, I'll give some background information. In the summer of 1989 I attended the Brightside Health Conference at Furman University in Greenville, SC, where Robert Sweetgall, a well-known fitness walker, presented a workshop. I left convinced that a walking program at a pace of 3.5 miles an hour for at least 20 min three times a week would make a significant difference in my overall health and well-being. I committed to do this for 6 weeks, and as a result I lost weight, increased my energy, and developed a better overall feeling about myself.

Starting the Program

At the beginning of the school year I presented the idea of a walking program to our faculty and staff of 40. To get their interest and attention I asked the following questions:

1. Who is completely satisfied with their physical health and well-being? (One person said yes; the others said no.)
2. Would anyone like to improve their physical health and well-being? (All answered yes.)

At this point I shared briefly my experience at Brightside and my own walking program and results. The biggest cost, I pointed out, would be time and a good pair of shoes.

We agreed that I would mark off the inside of our building in miles and make a walking course outside, which I did with the help of a tape measure and some donated tires. Walking was also allowed in neighborhoods or at local parks and tracks. I expected 14 participants, but 25 people signed up. By the end of the year, 5 more signed up, bringing our total to 30 out of a staff and faculty of 40.

Incentives

During the first year, I used several simple yet effective incentives to enhance interest and enthusiasm.

1. Each participant had an accountability partner. The partners checked weekly to see if

their commitments were being kept. "Ruthless compassion" was encouraged.

2. I posted a chart near the physical education room where teachers, students, and parents could see our progress. Teachers charted their own mileage in 5-mile blocks. Peer pressure and student interest proved to be good motivators.

3. At certain intervals (25 miles, 50 miles, etc.), teachers were given homemade pins—miniature chalkboards to which I hot-glued a clasp—the total cost was about 50 cents each. Everybody loved the pins, but we found that after the 50-mile pin, people were more interested in the walking than the pins. By that point the prize was the walking!

4. Each Friday a "walking report" was included in the school's morning announcements, detailing each walker's progress and the total miles walked.

Involving the Students

The children were observers to all of this until midyear. Except for walking in their physical education class, the students (those who were interested) only walked during recess on their own. Rob Sweetgall did a walking workshop in our school district, and the entire faculty from Northside School attended. Afterward the teachers who were already committed to walking became fanatics, and those who were not yet committed joined in with enthusiasm.

An outgrowth of their commitment and enthusiasm was that many teachers decided to begin walking during the school day with their classes. A chart similar to the one used by the teachers but marked off in 1-mile increments was put up in each classroom. Teachers made stickers or used stars for rewards. During Friday announcements, student walkers were added to the list. Total mileage for teachers and students was announced. By the end of the school year, well over 3,000 miles had been walked! Our school–business partner, Hoechst Celanese Corp., offered to reward the top three teachers with monetary prizes. These were not necessary to the success of the program but were appreciated by all.

Benefits of the Walking Program

There were many side benefits of the walking program, in addition to the improved physical well-being of the whole school.

1. Less stress in the classroom (especially for those who took a 10-min walking break at 10 o'clock). Teachers and students enjoyed the mental and physical break from the classroom routine.

2. More alert children and teachers due to the newly-discovered physical effects. (Nothing like fresh air to awaken the senses.)

3. Noticeable appreciation for nature. Some classes did writing activities about what they saw, heard, or smelled on their walks.

4. Opportunities to talk about and experience healthful living. Many teachers used the walks to carry over into health lessons about clean air and other environmental concerns like pollution and littering.

5. Improved discipline. No names on the board by 10:00 a.m. meant that the class could walk. Teachers were delighted with the positive effect on overall class morale.

6. Children walking on their own during recess. Keeping their mileage record served as an incentive for many children to walk on their own; and, as one first-grader said, "It's fun!"

7. Improved communication in families. Walking after dinner became standard for many. One family reported that it had become their favorite part of the day.

8. Establishment of a regular habit of exercising. It was a goal of the program to encourage a lifestyle that included regular exercising—which happened for many teachers and students.

Making a Walking Program Work for You

A walking program in your school or workplace can succeed. You need two things:

1. Education—Provide information about why walking is an excellent exercise choice. (It's easy to do, it's not expensive, it has a low incidence of injury, it has lots of benefits, and it's fun!)

2. Motivation—Provide incentives. (Inexpensive pins, charts, public announcements, and surprises go a long way toward keeping the walking fun.)

Summary

Everybody wants to feel and look better. Walking on a regular basis can help accomplish these goals. At Northside there has been an overall increase in health awareness since starting this program. The Wellness Committee, which is made up of one teacher from each grade level, the guidance counselor, and the PE teacher, continually looks for ways to keep the program interesting. The committee meets monthly to share ideas, which is vital to keeping in touch with the needs of the participants.

In conclusion, a walking program at your school can be a success. By providing some organizational skill, creating some walking courses, offering unique incentives, and involving the students, your school can enjoy benefits such as reduced stress, improved alertness, opportunities to talk about health and nature, improved discipline, and improved communication and activity in families. All people want to look and feel better. That desire, coupled with some organization, can provide an opportunity.

Suggested Readings

1. Floyd, P.A.; Parke, J.E. Walk-jog-run-for wellness. Winston-Salem, NC: Hunter Textbooks; 1990.
2. Hawkins, J.D.; Weigle, S.M. Walking for fun and fitness. Englewood, CO: Morton; 1992.
3. Seiger, L.H.; Hesson, J.L. Walking for fitness. Dubuque, IA: Brown; 1990.
4. Sweetgall, R.J.; Neeves, R. The walking wellness teacher's guide. Newark, DE: Creative Walking; 1987.
5. Sweetgall, R.J.; Neeves, R. Walking for little children. Newark, DE: Creative Walking; 1987.

Chapter 23

Citrus County Fitness Break: Funding and Developing Fitness Videotapes[1]

Barbara Bradford-Krok
Floral City Elementary
Floral City, Florida

In Citrus County one of the goals in our *Administrative and Instructional Handbook for Elementary Physical Education* is to "make a contribution to the personal fitness of each child based on the health-related components of fitness." Because most schools in our county schedule the students only twice a week for PE, improving fitness, along with teaching movement concepts and skills and providing practice time for skill improvement, is a virtual impossibility. We have a state demonstration school for physical education in our county that has daily physical education to meet requirements for state recognition, some of it taught by the classroom teacher. Some Citrus County schools have recess and some don't, but the appropriateness of the activity during recess is often suspect.

We know children need daily physical activity and time to learn and understand the components of health-related fitness. We do not want students to leave our classes never having heard such terms as *target heart rate*, *duration*, and *intensity*.

We felt that the only way to offer children daily physical activity was to involve classroom teachers, but we realized that they could help us only if we gave them something they could do quickly and easily. They would not be willing to spend their time planning additional activities, preparing materials, getting their classrooms ready for activity, or moving to another site.

Borrowing an idea from Palm Beach County, we decided to try making a set of videotapes that classroom teachers could use with their classes in their classrooms. That these videotapes were for the classroom teacher is a key point. We hoped they would be used particularly on days when the class did not have PE.

Making the Grant Application

In April of 1988 we applied for a Local Education Improvement Grant. We called the project "Citrus County Fitness Break"—because it was to be a break from the regular classroom routine for some exercise or activity. It was not intended to be another PE class or to replace the regularly scheduled

[1]Dianna Bandhauer (at Lecanto Primary School) and Barbara Bradford-Krok (at Floral City Elementary School) co-wrote a grant to fund the development of a set of fitness videos in Citrus County, Florida. This chapter is based on their experience.

physical education. In June of 1988 we were approved for $1,740, the full amount of our request.

In the grant application we gave three reasons for our project. First, we cited the fitness scores in our county. The results were taken from the Physical Best health-related test from AAHPERD, which we are required to give twice a year. Second, we cited the classroom teachers' general lack of knowledge regarding the health-related components of fitness and their inability to design fitness activities for their students. Even if they knew the concepts from their own participation in fitness activities, they probably would not have the knowledge to design fitness activities that would be appropriate for young children. Finally, we cited the lack of time in our physical education schedules to provide sufficient opportunities for each child to have daily physical activity.

We proposed the development of a series of videotapes to be used by the classroom teacher. Each tape would start with a short skit dealing with either a fitness component or a concept pertinent to our physical education classes. We wanted our skits to be fun for the students to watch as well as informative. We knew we were competing with commercial television and Nintendo, so we needed a quality product. Our skits range from how to take your heart rate to body composition to appropriate dress for safe participation in PE. The students themselves would be the actors.

We would also have an activity session or workout, tied to the concept introduced in the skit when appropriate, although most often aerobic in nature. The exercise routine would be repeated a second time on each tape with a lead-in statement of "one more time." Before each routine we would spend a short time showing the steps or movements that the children would need to know to participate.

Although we were not so naive as to think that this few minutes of activity would dramatically improve fitness levels, we did feel it would get our students up and moving on a daily basis, limited as that might be. And even a small amount of activity is better than none at all! We also felt that it would be an activity they would enjoy, especially because it was students on the tape and often students they knew. It would also be done in a nonthreatening environment. And, finally, we hoped that the fact that the classroom teacher was doing it—not only the physical education teacher—would help the students view activity and fitness as more relevant to themselves and their lives rather than something done only in physical education class. We've all heard about the little boy who was asked, "What is math?" He thought for a bit, and then said, "I guess it's something we do at 10 o'clock in the morning." We don't want activity and fitness to be only "something we do in PE."

One of the criteria in determining the recipients of our Local Education Improvement Grant is how many students are actually involved and how directly they are impacted. We proposed filming the exercise routines at each of the school sites (eight, at that time). One of the schools involved was a self-contained, special education school for the severely and profoundly physically, mentally, and emotionally impaired. At that school the routine was based on flexibility rather than aerobic endurance. By doing the filming at all the elementary schools and by having the students be the "stars," our initial effort involved many students.

Also, knowing that a feeling of ownership plays a key role in the change process and maintenance of that change, we hoped that filming at each school site would give the schools a feeling of ownership and they would be more likely to use the videotapes. Therefore, we felt justified stating in the grant proposal that *all* of our elementary students *could* be directly affected if the tapes were used. We also made a special effort to involve all the elementary physical education teachers in an attempt to foster a higher level of cohesiveness among our group.

Our proposal then was to develop a set of eight minitapes and to provide a complete set of tapes to each elementary school. Our grant monies were spent for substitute teachers at a cost of $1,260, which was a majority of the funds. We also purchased half-hour videotapes for $380, so that each school would have eight separate tapes for eight different teachers to use at the same time (compared to one long tape, which could be used in only one classroom at a time). And we used $100 to print "Fitness Break" T-shirts with our logo for the students to wear during the taping of the exercise routines.

Making the Tapes

In the fall of 1989 we brought all of our teachers together at our District Media Center for 1 day to begin the process of developing the skits and routines. At that first meeting we also selected two of the teachers to be in charge of the actual filming at the individual school sites and to do most of the editing. Although Mrs. Bandhauer and I cowrote the grant, we wanted all of our teachers involved and working together—an objective almost as important as making the tapes. (She and I did not do the actual filming, though we did most of the editing.)

Originally, we intended to do the filming ourselves using school or personal video cameras and doing the editing and copying at our District Media Center. However, Mrs. Bandhauer called our local cable television station to see if its staff members could help (they had previously assisted her in filming a demonstration school videotape), and they agreed to do the filming for us and to assist in the editing process using their equipment. The station is required to donate a certain amount of time to community service projects, and this was an excellent way to do that. So the filming was done on a TV camera by a professional cameraman filming at the individual schools. The editing was done at the TV studio and then transferred from the master tape to the individual VHS tapes, which greatly improved the quality of each tape. The television station did all of the copying for us.

When the exercise routines were ready, we arranged a schedule to film at each school site with the on-site teacher responsible for finding a place to film (usually the library, a classroom, or stage). The teacher also picked 15 students from all grades and had their release forms signed and returned. (We have since decided to decrease the number of students to 8 or 10.) Each of the two teachers filming had 4 days of release time and filmed two schools each day over approximately 2 mo. On-site teachers had one-half day of release time while the filming was being done at their schools, so they could assist as needed. The two teachers arrived at the school site, taught the routines to the students, and led them from off-camera during the taping. The music and cues were done with the taping, although we had the capability to dub later as needed.

As the skits were written (a really major job!), they were filmed at Lecanto Primary School. All the skits were filmed there for several reasons: first, its proximity to the television station; second, the size of the student body and the school facilities; third, Mrs. Bandhauer's key role in writing the skits; and finally, the invaluable assistance we received from the teachers of both special education and gifted education at Lecanto Primary School in the preparation, rehearsal, and presentation of the skits. (See the appendix.)

The editing, completed at the TV studio using its equipment, gave us many more options for on-screen visuals, such as fade-ins and -outs and rolling credits. However, juggling schedules—when we could meet, when the studio was available, when the cameraman was available—lengthened the process appreciably. Nevertheless, the improved quality of our finished product was well worth the extra time involved.

Results

On the whole the project went well and we are pleased with our product. The only real problem was time: We simply did not realize how big a job we had taken on and failed to allow enough time (i.e., substitute days) to complete the work. The filming itself was accomplished without difficulty, but writing the skits and routines and editing the tapes took much more time than we could have anticipated. For a second attempt I would probably double the number of days needed for completion.

The tapes are placed in each school's media center for checkout by *classroom* teachers who have received in-service instruction from the physical education teacher as to the tapes' availability and their intended use. I've also had a number of parents borrow the tapes, especially if their child is featured. A log is kept to show how often the tapes are used, and critique sheets are filled out to gauge teacher, student, and parent reaction to the tapes.

Summary

Move over Jane Fonda and Richard Simmons! Here come the youthful, energetic stars of our own fitness videos, the students of Citrus County. We wanted our students to learn that physical fitness is fun and makes you feel good, to learn about fitness, and to learn to enjoy participating in regular exercise and activity. And, finally, we wanted to try to find a way to provide some time every day for our students to move and be active. We feel that our "Citrus County Fitness Break" has accomplished all of these goals.

Although the project was not particularly difficult, it was time-consuming. But it is a project that any teacher, school, or district could do with some planning and work. So turn on the creativity, write your grant proposals, involve your school district's audiovisual department (or solicit help from your local cable TV station), find your own fitness stars, and get those cameras rolling! Soon you'll have your own fitness videos guaranteed to please the users.

Appendix

Two Skits From the "Citrus County Fitness Break" Videotape Series

Skit 3: "Time Warp"

CAST: one "old" lady, several other girls and boys

PROPS: junk food, restroom signs, old-lady outfit, old-man outfits, rocking chair, smoke or something to visually cue a "time warp"

Skit begins with three to four girls stuffing their faces with junk food. Two boys pass by on their way to the restroom (restroom in background). Girl #1 gives her junk food to a friend to hold while she goes to the restroom. By mistake Girl #1 goes into the boys' restroom (despite her friends yelling and telling her it is the *wrong* restroom).

Girl #1 goes into the boys' restroom, the boys yell at her, the lights flash, and Girl #1 is engulfed in smoke. The camera goes back to the restroom door, and Girl #1 and the boys leave the restroom as *old* people.

Scene changes to the old lady talking to the boys and girls as they sit on the floor in front of her rocking chair.

Girl #1/Old lady: "I went into the boys' restroom by mistake and a very strange thing happened to me. I entered a time warp. I was able to see the years of my life unfold in front of my eyes. I have called you all here today to share some things that will make your life better for you.

"I know what I will say is hard to believe, but the things you do right now will affect your health the rest of your life. Recent physical fitness tests show half of America's children are not physically fit. That means their msucles are not in good working condition. A person who is physically fit is able to work and play for many hours without getting tired.

"You have probably thought of being physically fit as an important part of being healthy and feeling well. But you may not have realized that being fit could actually save a person's life. If you are strong enough to run for help, to tread water after a boating accident, or to hold on to a rope while waiting to be rescued from a fire, you might win in a situation in which someone less fit might lose out.

"I didn't take care of my body as a youngster. I did not work very hard in my physical education classes. I ate too much junk food and never ate any vegetables. I liked to watch TV more than I liked to go outside and play. But I *was* smart enough not to take drugs. I did not look overweight, but I was not taking care of myself.

"Now I have high blood pressure and high cholesterol. I take 10 pills a day the way I used to eat a package of Doritos and drink several Cokes a day. I worry every day because I ate too much and did not get enough of the right exercise. In fact, now I can't even tie my shoes without the help of others; I can't walk to the mailbox or play outside with my grandchildren. All I can do is wish I had not been so mean to my body when I was young. The risks I took were controllable by me. I did not make wise choices.

"The reason I am telling you these things is that you are still young enough to change your ways if you don't want to end up unhealthy like me."

The old woman gets up and begins to walk out of the room. She walks out the door, camera focus changes to the outside of the restrooms. Girl #1 walks out of the girls' restroom "normal." She passes the boys who were on their way to the restroom in the first scene. Her girlfriends are standing there and hand back her Coke and bag of chips. She takes them and drops them in a nearby trash can.

Girl #1 (to her friends): "Let's go to the fruit stand. I suddenly have this urge to eat something healthy."

(Other girls respond by dropping their junk food in the trash.)

Girls #2 and #3: "Yeah, it has been a long time since I have eaten an apple."

Skit 6: "Fat Cells"

CAST: 2 actors

PROPS: 1 extra-large sweatsuit, lots of tennis balls

Actor #1: "Fat has a bad name these days. Too much fat in our food makes us gain weight. Too much fat in our body is hard on the heart. Some fat is good. It gives you energy. But fat is bad when you eat too much of it. It will make you gain extra pounds.

"Fat is in many foods. Some foods have more fat than others. Foods with lots of fats are french fries, potato chips, and ice cream. Foods low in fat are fruits, vegetables, pasta, grains, and beans.

"The body keeps the extra fat stored in cells in your body. This tennis ball represents a fat cell. Each time you eat food with a lot of fat, the extra fat is stored in the body like this."

(Actor #1 puts the tennis ball into the other actor's sweatsuit, which is already filled with tennis-ball "fat cells." Continue to put tennis balls into the suit, then fade.)

Actor #1: "Exercise is a good way to keep the fat cells out of your body."

(The person in sweatsuit starts to do jumping jacks.)

Actor #1: "As you can see, the fat cells begin to fall out when a person exercises. To make sure you only have good fat in your body you need to cut down on the foods you eat that are full of fat and get plenty of exercise. To have a healthy body composition with less fat you need to exercise at least three times a week for 20 minutes, but daily exercise is better."

Both actors (rap this song):
"Challenge our muscles everyday
to keep those ugly fat cells away.
Physical fitness can be fun,
if your play is properly done.
Veggies, fruits, and juices too,
can make your body work the whole day through."

Chapter 24

Fitness—The Ravenel Way

Adelaide V. Carpenter
Ravenel Elementary School
Seneca, South Carolina

During the 1989–90 school year at Ravenel Elementary School in Seneca, South Carolina, the physical fitness program was affected by three separate factors: physical fitness training during physical education class, the morning exercise program, and the jump-rope team—the Ravenel Ropesters. The purpose of this chapter is to explain these three areas and how they influenced the physical fitness level of the students at Ravenel. To quote Dauer and Pangrazi,

> All children have the right to become strong, sturdy, quick, agile, and flexible. It is the responsibility of the school to provide opportunities for them to achieve this physical goal—developing and maintaining a level of physical fitness that allows them to live fully and achieve well. (1)

The primary goal of these fitness factors is to help students reach their potential. Students could feel better about themselves and their activity level and thereby reach higher goals in physical fitness. Dauer and Pangrazi further state, "The key thought lies in motivating the child to take responsibility for his or her own fitness" (1).

Ravenel's student population is approximately 400, with the children evenly divided among the school's five grades (1–5). Although most of the students live in single-family neighborhoods, they represent a wide range of socioeconomic levels.

Physical Education at Ravenel

As Ravenel's physical education teacher, I am responsible for implementing physical fitness training. Because I was assigned to Ravenel 4 days a week, my schedule allowed me to meet with my students once a week for 45 min and every third week for two 45-min periods. The extra physical education class always occurred on Fridays and it became known as "Fitness Friday," because this class was always used for physical fitness training and information about fitness. Fitness Friday occurred approximately 12 times in the year for each class. Instead of having PE 36 times, the students met for a total of 48 times, with 12 of these lessons devoted fully to the different aspects of physical fitness. The focus of Fitness Friday was to emphasize the importance of fitness, allow further practice time, evaluate levels of fitness, and present new fitness information. Students adjusted well to the fitness training that took place during the extra class.

On Fitness Friday at the begining of the school year, the younger students were introduced to the physical fitness components. These were sit-ups, pull-ups, sit-and-reach, and the endurance walk-run. Other items such as push-ups, rope jumping, active games, and other activities were included. In all the first-grade classes, I taught one fitness component at a time, such as sit-ups one day and pull-ups another day. In teaching sit-ups, I used two first-grade students as models and showed the position of each and what they were supposed to do. I would let the students see the exercises done correctly and also point out ways they might be done incorrectly. Students loved it when I would do the skill wrong and they could explain why it was wrong. First-graders also had to learn to count sit-ups correctly, and this was a skill we practiced.

After teaching a skill such as sit-ups to first-graders, a vigorous activity was planned. The older students were given practice time to work on fitness skills, and games were played that encouraged fitness development. The older grades were able to practice fitness components with only a brief review of correct and incorrect techniques. Students would rotate in groups to different stations to work on skills such as strength, endurance, agility, flexibility, and others. After station work, a vigorous activity was usually planned. The third-, fourth-, and fifth-graders kept index cards for their fitness goals and for their scores.

Every physical education class started with a 5-min warm-up designed to get students moving at the beginning of class; students did sit-ups with a partner, push-ups, and individual rope jumping. When they became familiar with the warm-up, they could complete the exercise while I was busy with other tasks, such as equipment changes or discussion with a teacher or student. First-graders did not use ropes during warm-up until later in the year. Activities using locomotor skills were used in place of the ropes.

The physical fitness program "Physical Best" was our countywide instrument for testing. This program was discussed from the beginning of the school year, and students were informed of testing dates. Health-related fitness standards were explained and posted on a wall in the physical education room.

The Physical Best testing began in February and concluded in March. Clubs were established called "I'm Fit" and "I'm SuperFit." The "I'm Fit" club used the health fitness standard according to the Physical Best booklet. A higher level of achievement was established for the club called "I'm SuperFit." Students' names were displayed in the hall outside the PE room when the students were able to meet their standard. During the year more and more names were added to the lists as students improved and met their goals. These club lists were displayed in the hall from December until May, which motivated the students and improved self-esteem.

All students who met health fitness standards were recognized as members of the appropriate club. These students received certificates at the awards day ceremony. Top achievers also received a gold-painted, wooden medallion to wear. Students were encouraged and praised for improving fitness scores. A fifth-grader who was an outstanding exercise leader and a Ropester (programs discussed later in this chapter) made tremendous progress on her body composition, reducing her percent body fat by 12%. She and her parents were thrilled with her advancement, which occurred over 12 months.

The school record for each event was posted for all students to see. The records have improved each year. The school record for the 1-mile run (6:50) was 13 sec better than the year before. Sit-ups (96) showed an increase of 38 from the previous year. The sit-and-reach and pull-up school records showed improvement, but the margin of improvement was not as great. The testing results showed that Ravenel students scored well on flexibility and abdominal strength and endurance. The student scores on aerobic endurance and upper-body strength and endurance were much lower. Table 24.1 shows the percentage of students who met the health fitness standard.

The South Carolina Physical Education Curriculum Guidelines were used throughout the year for the development of lesson plans. Many lessons targeted skill development, but fitness components were included as often as possible. One example of this integration of goals was my lesson on soccer punting. Students were arranged in groups of three, with two students staying active by retrieving, running, and passing the soccer ball. During a unit on rope-jumping skills, task cards were utilized. Students worked at their own pace, and partners were used to check progress. Other

Table 24.1   Percentage of Students Who Met the Health Fitness Standard

	Grade level		
	Second	Fourth	Fifth
Flexibility	78	83	78
Aerobic endurance	30	43	31
Body composition	74	55	62
Sit-ups	86	85	88
Pull-ups	41	37	27
Total number of students	74	81	78

topics such as heart rate, target heart rate, intensity, and other terms were included in the unit on rope jumping. For a first-grader, heart rate was shown by placing a hand on his or her chest after jumping hard. Older students were taught how to find their target heart rates.

The Morning Exercise Program

The past school year was the first year for the morning exercise program at Ravenel, which was implemented to increase daily PE time and to improve student physical fitness levels. Another reason for starting this program was to provide our fifth-graders with a challenge and to promote leadership and responsibility. Support from the principal, Cathy Watson, was instrumental in getting this program on its feet. She provided encouragement in the planning stages and much help when small details presented problems. Much of the success of the program was due to her commitment to this project.

The exercise program was scheduled for 7:55 a.m. to 8:05 a.m., with the tardy bell ringing at 8:05 a.m. Two fifth-grade leaders were assigned to a homeroom and arrived early to class. The cassette tape was played over the school intercom system, and all classes began simultaneously. The first step in setting up the exercise program was tryouts for the fifth-grade leaders. All fifth-graders were allowed to try out and they attended the training sessions mornings between 7:50 a.m. and 8:10 a.m. Students were given handouts of the routine, which was also printed on the chalkboard and on signs in the room. After a week of following the routine and becoming familiar with it, students who were having difficulty were asked to try out again at the next training session. The remaining students were selected as leaders and continued to practice the routine until all were very comfortable leading it, which included being able to count out the routine and give directions as needed. One of the pair was in charge and the other assisted. The training and selecting of leaders usually took 2 to 3 weeks.

During the 2 weeks the fifth-graders were training for the program, I assisted by presenting the routine to every homeroom class in the school at their PE time. This gave all students a chance to learn the exercise. At this time I discussed proper technique, reviewed safety precautions, and talked over counting sequences.

Once a session began, each lasted approximately 6 weeks. Total time for a session, including the leadership training, was about 8 or 9 weeks. This worked well with our 9-week grading periods, and we completed four different routines during the year. As the year progressed the fifth-graders became more skilled at leading, and the new routines were easier for them to learn.

Homeroom teachers aided in the morning sessions by exercising along with their students while keeping order in the class. They also assisted by selecting leaders who were doing an outstanding job. After each session ended the leaders selected as outstanding were recognized formally; their names were announced over the intercom system by the principal and displayed in the hall. They also were given outstanding leadership certificates, and other students looked up to these prominent leaders.

The professional quality of the routines made them both fun and challenging, one reason for the program's success. Credit for this goes to a personal friend, an aerobics instructor, who wrote the routines and helped train the leaders. A caution should be added about selecting music. We used current popular hits that the students enjoyed in our routines and we listened very carefully to the lyrics to be sure the songs were appropriate for a school setting.

The Ravenel Ropesters

The third element in our fitness program was the Ravenel Ropesters, a jump-rope demonstration team. This group of 24 students presented over a dozen performances throughout the year—at Ravenel, other schools, festivals, and during half-time at a basketball game. The jump-rope team became the envy of all students because of the trips and special activities in which they participated.

As a result of the Ropesters' popularity, the students did much more rope-jumping at recess, PE, and elsewhere. The Ropesters became teachers to the other students and taught many skills and tricks they had learned at team practice. A favorite memory is seeing the many students who worked hard to learn the trick we called "Leg Over," which is performed with the leg over the arm holding the rope. Almost all students were fascinated with this trick and tried to learn it. Many succeeded. The Ropesters had a huge impact on the student body at Ravenel.

Jump Rope for Heart was held in March and all PE classes participated in jump-rope activities prior to the event. Task cards provided the necessary information for advancing through the different levels of jump-rope skills. Students worked in partners and progressed through the skills at their own pace. The task cards were divided into clubs representing three levels: the Red Club, the White Club, and the Blue Club. Many students advanced much further than they thought possible. The Jump Rope for Heart event was a success, raising almost $2,000. I believe the Ropesters were a great motivation for the students at Ravenel.

Summary

Physical fitness at Ravenel has always been a vital part of the physical education program, a commitment that will continue into the future. This chapter has explained the factors that affected the physical fitness level of the students at Ravenel—without comparisons of past years' fitness scores. Rather than show student scores, I tried to show the elements that influenced the scores. I will end with some remarks the principal gave:

> During the 1989–1990 school year, our physical education program inspired the majority of our students to participate in the varied experiences which would lead them toward

fitness. For example, students were involved in task-oriented jump rope and gymnastic activities. I saw students excited about accomplishing feats they thought they could not achieve. One fifth-grader became frustrated at her inability to master some skills. At this time Mrs. Carpenter developed a personalized program in order to provide a plan at which she could succeed.

The Morning Exercise Program not only provided a leadership role for fifth-graders but instilled pride in these students. The morning fitness time ensured that students had exercise each day rather than once per week.

The Ravenel Ropesters, comprised of students of all ability levels, were instrumental in inspiring the entire student body to develop jumping skills and physical stamina.

The physical education program at Ravenel is geared to encourage and provide the means by which all students can begin to make fitness a regular part of their lifestyle.

Reference

1. Dauer, V.P.; Pangrazi, R.P. Dynamic physical education for elementary school children. Minneapolis: Burgess; 1979.

Summary

Health-Related Physical Education—
A Direction for the 21st Century

Russell R. Pate
Richard C. Hohn
University of South Carolina, Columbia

Each of the preceding chapters was written by an author who presented his or her individual viewpoint on a particular aspect of health-related physical education. Accordingly, the careful reader will have noted that not all the authors' viewpoints are in perfect agreement; not all the procedures recommended would be perfectly compatible in the field setting. However, we believe (and we hope that the reader agrees) that several broad, cross-cutting themes are evident in the material in this book. It is our view that these themes constitute a foundation upon which to build a truly new approach to physical education.

1. *Promotion of lifelong physical activity and fitness should be the primary goal of physical education.* Perhaps the broadest and most fundamental of the themes in this book is the view that physical education should be designed with the student's future health and fitness in mind. As noted by several authors, it is clear that higher levels of physical activity *maintained through adulthood* promote health, prevent disease, and enhance fitness. The challenge to physical education is to provide programs that increase the likelihood that today's students will become physically active adults.

2. *The physical education curriculum should be balanced so as to function effectively in all three educational domains.* Physical education, by virtue of both its

purpose and the environment in which it occurs, is geared toward physical activity. Accordingly, it is appropriate that major emphasis be given to learning in the psychomotor domain. However, a major theme in this book is that physical education programs that focus exclusively on motor skill acquisition are too narrow and shortsighted. The authors in this book recommend repeatedly that the cognitive and affective domains should be given much more time and attention than traditionally given in physical education. So, it is recommended that physical education at once become both broader and narrower. That is, narrower in the sense that programs should focus more on promotion of lifelong activity and fitness, but broader through greater emphasis on knowledge and attitudes.

3. *Youngsters should leave their physical education experience with a heightened sense of "physical activity competence."* A major theme that cuts across this book is that long-term activity behavior can be effectively promoted in PE by enhancing the student's self-efficacy as it applies to activity. Youngsters who feel that they are competent in physical activities and that they are able to control their activity seem likely to exercise lifelong. Conversely, those who have had repeated failures in activity settings and who feel incompetent appear less likely to exercise regularly as adults. Accordingly, it seems important that physical education

experiences be structured to provide youngsters with movement successes, not failures.

4. *Physical education should provide meaningful amounts of physical activity.* Several authors in this book decry the fact that, for a great many youngsters, physical education is a rather sedentary undertaking. Therefore, a clear recommendation is that physical education lessons be designed so as to provide youngsters with moderate to vigorous physical activity in doses that are physiologically meaningful. Although the amount of activity needed for health and fitness in childhood is not known with certainty, it seems reasonable to recommend that a youngster engage in at least 1 hr of moderate to vigorous activity per day. We cannot expect PE to meet this entire requirement, but it should make a major contribution. That it currently does not suggests that physical educators should reconsider the priorities they apply in selecting instructional methods.

5. *Physical fitness testing procedures should be designed to promote attainment of long-term activity and fitness objectives.* Different authors in this book express rather different positions on the proper role of physical fitness testing in physical fitness. However, one common theme concerning fitness testing is discernible. Fitness testing procedures and the reward and recognition systems often used in conjunction with them should be designed first and foremost to promote physical activity behavior. An important secondary objective is to enhance cognitive learning of health-related physical fitness. Accordingly, it is recommended that fitness tests be administered in a manner that maximizes the likelihood of the child (a) experiencing success, (b) avoiding embarrassment and failure, and (c) learning about the health-related physical fitness components. The results of fitness tests should be used in meaningful ways—ideally, by communicating the results to youngsters and their parents in an understandable fashion, and by providing effective remediation to those who are found to be in need of improvement.

6. *Physical education programs should meet the needs of all youngsters, and in particular those who have special needs and/or are low fit.* The predominant philosophy expressed in this book calls for physical education to focus primarily on promoting active lifestyles. The underlying purpose of this orientation is to enhance the public health. Because most of the health benefits of regular exercise accrue to persons who avoid a sedentary lifestyle (i.e., they are at least moderately active), it has been argued that physical education could have its most beneficial effect on public health by attending first to the needs of those youngsters who are most likely to become sedentary adults.

Accordingly, a major theme in this book is that physical educators should strive to deal more effectively with low-fit youngsters. Because low fitness may predispose youngsters to negative exercise experiences, direct, short-term intervention to improve fitness may be appropriate. Beyond that, however, the low-fit and inactive youngster may benefit most from development of positive attitudes toward exercise and from acquisition of behavioral skills that will promote future activity. In short, low-fit kids may need us the most, and at present they probably are not getting our best service.

7. *Professional preparation programs should prepare future teachers of physical education to develop balanced curricula and to deliver instruction that is effective in all three educational domains.* No chapter in this book is dedicated to the specific issue of preparing professionals to deliver health-related physical education. However, a clear implication of the material in this book is that pedagogical programs in physical education must change if health-related physical education is to become widespread in the United States. The traditional focus of teacher training programs in PE has been on delivery of motor skill instruction. Therefore, it is not surprising that a "good physical education program" usually is seen as one in which the teacher effectively promotes mastery of fundamental or sport-specific motor skills.

The authors of this book as a group would agree that physical education teachers should be competent skill instructors. However, they would also agree that this is not enough. In health-related physical education, skill acquisition is an objective, not a goal. The goal is promotion of lifelong activity and fitness, and this requires physical educators to promote relevant learning in the cognitive and affective as well as the psychomotor domains. Most current professional-preparation programs fail to develop these competencies. Health-related physical education will not become a professional norm until this changes.

Goal Clear, Strategy Uncertain

This book has been dedicated to a discussion of why and how one specific component of the American educational system, physical education, could be refocused on the goal of promoting adoption of one particular health behavior—regular participation in exercise.

Neither the process of education nor the process of promoting health behavior change are pursuits that can be reduced to rigid guidelines and computer programs. This is so in part because both effective education and health promotion are somewhat intuitive, individualized processes. We do not expect this to change. However, at present a lack of knowledge limits our ability to generate guidelines for delivery of health-related physical education. We fully anticipate that this *will* change. The pages of this book are filled with suggestions and recommendations that appear to be appropriate and useful. Few of these have been tested by research, but we hope that this, too, will change—sooner rather than later. Until such research is conducted we will remain uncertain about the most effective ways to promote lifelong physical activity through school physical education.

Although the relevant educational strategies are not yet fully developed, we submit that there is no uncertainty about the appropriateness of the major goal espoused in this book. We believe there is compelling evidence that physical education should focus its attention first and foremost on promotion of lifelong physical activity, and we think that the rationale for this position is powerfully logical. It can be summarized by the following points:

1. Lack of physical activity during adulthood is a major health problem.
2. A great many adults are physically inactive.
3. Adult physical activity behavior is determined in part by experiences during childhood.
4. School-based physical education has the capacity to provide the population of American children with experiences that can promote adoption of physically active lifestyles.

So, although we readily admit to uncertainties about optimal educational strategies, we fervently endorse the goal: The institution of physical education should, perhaps must, focus its massive energy on promotion of lifelong exercise behavior.

The Challenge of Change

Changing physical education so that it places primary emphasis on promotion of lifelong exercise will probably be, at one level, slow and difficult. Current practice in physical education has evolved from deeply entrenched school policies and regulations, the perceptions of numerous education power brokers, and an array of professional beliefs and expectations that have developed over time. The physical education program envisioned by the authors of this book is in fundamental ways very different from today's typical PE program. Changing the norm will require major modifications in school policies, state regulations, and professional preparation curricula. The expectations of school administrators, parents, and public agencies will have to change. Furthermore, the day-to-day practices of tens of thousands of physical educators will have to change. Clearly, the enormity of the task of markedly changing an institution as large and tradition-bound as physical education could be intimidating, akin to a supertanker making a 180° turn. We must expect that this is going to take some time.

On the other hand, at the grassroots level, change in educational practice can occur with lightning speed. In contrast with subjects such as math, science, and English, physical education curricula and teaching techniques are relatively unregulated in most school districts. Professional preparation programs in physical education must meet established accreditation standards; however, these standards tend to be rather flexible. In most colleges and universities the principle of academic freedom gives individual professors the latitude to design course content and choose what types of research they will conduct.

Because the most important activity in physical education is that which *directly* impacts the students in our schools, it is possible to make changes at the most critical level on an immediate basis. If you are a teacher of physical education, you could make a change in your curriculum or teaching methodology *today*. If you are a professor in a physical education professional-preparation program, you could make a change in your course content *today*. If you are a researcher, you could begin designing a study to identify effective health-related physical education practices *today*. So, although we may be striving to turn a profession that has the inertia of a supertanker, as individuals each of us is a speed boat that can turn on a dime. The authors of this book invite you to turn . . . *today*.

Index

Goals, of programs. *See* Fitness goals and objectives,
　　program; Objectives, of programs
Go For Health study, 141-143
Goodbodies program, 108, 109
Gortmaker, S.L., 107
Gottlieb, N.H., 32
Gould, D., 84
Grading
　　in Corbin's five-step curriculum model, 62, 63
　　motivation and, 78, 87
Greendorfer, S.L., 35

H
Haddock, C.K., 37
Hanson, C.L., 37
Harvard Alumni Study, 11-12
Health belief model, 32, 33-34, 35
Health curricula, 72-73, 198
Health-exercise relationship, 11-19, 22, 137
Health-related physical education (HRPE). *See also*
　　Fitness programming
　　description and implementation of, 137-144
　　future directions for, 215-217
Health-related physical fitness. *See also* Fitness
　　programming
　　definition of, 99, 101
　　in Ratliffe's comprehensive approach, 151
　　Super Active Kids program, 155-163
Health-Related Physical Fitness Test Manual
　　(AAHPERD), 27
*Healthy People 2000, National Health Promotion and
　　Disease Prevention Objectives,* 6, 17, 29, 92
HELP philosophy (Corbin), 60, 63
High school curricula. *See* Secondary school (high
　　school) curricula
Holt, K., 83
Homework
　　for cognitive learning, 95, 149
　　for Florida Personal Fitness course, 168
　　motivation and, 78, 95
　　for obese students, 108
HRPE. *See* Health-related physical education (HRPE)
Hypoactivity, 99, 100

I
Impaired students, 99-107, 189, 216
Incentives. *See* Awards/rewards; Motivation;
　　Recognition
Independence (self-direction), 62, 73
Information processing theory, 45, 48-50, 52
Instructional methods. *See also* Planning instruction
　　cognitive principles for, 48-50
　　in Corbin's five-step curriculum model, 62-65
　　for elementary fitness lessons in general, 78, 80
　　for facilitating vigorous activity, 72
　　for fitness testing, 124-127, 134
　　for Florida Personal Fitness course, 167-169
　　for health-related physical education, 139, 141
　　for motivation, 77-78
　　in Petray's Physical Best . . . Plan, 94-96
　　for positive attitude development, 76-77, 78, 107
　　problems with, 73
　　in Ratliffe's comprehensive approach, 148-150
　　in Ravenel Elementary School program, 211-212
　　in Woodland Heights's Moving to Success program,
　　　178-180, 181, 183

Integration, of fitness into school day
　　Citrus County Fitness Break for, 205-209
　　for cognitive learning, 95
　　curriculum interfacing, 197-200
　　in elementary school in general, 71
　　in Ravenel Elementary School program, 213
　　in Springdale running program, 188
　　Super Active Kids program for, 155-163
　　in Woodland Heights's Moving to Success program,
　　　177-178
Integration, of impaired students into regular classes,
　　106
Intellectual skills in cognitive learning, 46, 47-48, 50,
　　53
Intensity of activities/exercise
　　in health-related physical education in general, 139,
　　　216
　　for impaired students, 105
　　influence on physical activity behavior in general,
　　　33, 40
　　learning correct, 75
　　for low-fit students, 116-117
　　for obese students, 108
　　in positive attitude development, 76
Intentions, in reasoned action theory, 32, 34
Interpretation zones, 87, 88
Intrinsic motivation
　　practical application of, 84-85, 86-89, 126
　　theory on, 82-84

J
Jump-rope demonstration teams, 213-214

K
Kern, K.A., 94
Klesges, L.M., 37
Klesges, R.C., 37
Knowledge. *See* Fitness knowledge
"Know Your Body" curriculum, 83
Koestner, R., 83
Kopperud, K., 95
Koslow, R.E., 17
Kreisel, P.S.J., 83-84

L
Language arts curricula, interfacing with, 198
Learning oriented goals (mastery goals), 50-51, 52-53
Learning theory, 45-53. *See also* Cognitive learning
Leeds, Margaret, 94
Leon, A.S., 12
Lesson planning. *See* Planning instruction
Lifetime fitness programming
　　Corbin's five-step model for, 60-66
　　current status of, 22
　　determinants of behavior and, 40-41
　　and exercise-health relationship, 16-18
　　goal orientation and, 51
　　in health-related physical education in general, 137,
　　　138, 139, 215
　　NCYFS study on, 24, 29
　　rationale for, summarized, 217
Lindsey, R., 95
Lipid Research Clinics Study, 14
Location. *See* Facilities
Locker rooms. *See* Showers
Long-term memory, 49
Looney, M.A., 132, 133
Los Angeles Public Safety Workers, study on, 13-14

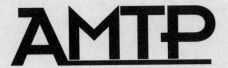
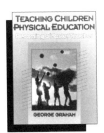
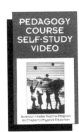
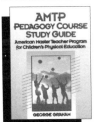
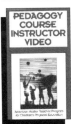
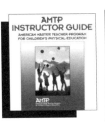
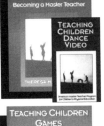
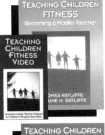
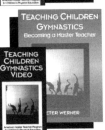
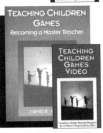
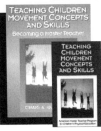